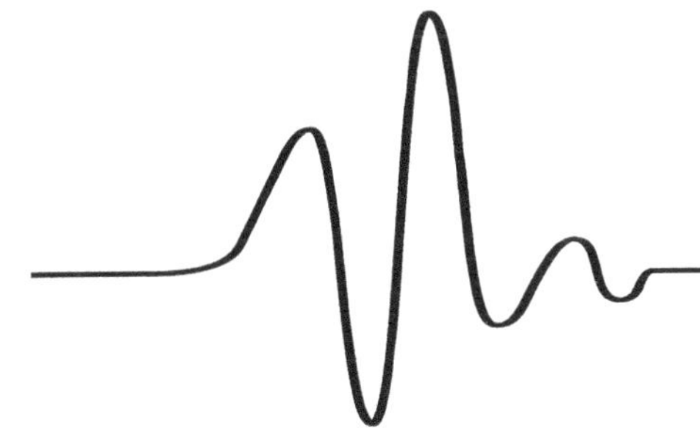

An Acupuncturist's Guide to

Medical Red Flags & Referrals

David Anzaldua, MD

Published by:
BLUE POPPY PRESS
A Division of Blue Poppy Enterprises, Inc.
1990 North 57th Court, Unit A
Boulder, CO 80301
www.bluepoppy.com

First Printing, November 2010
Second Printing, February 2012
Second Edition, January 2013
Fourth Printing, April 2013
Fifth Printing, August 2013
Sixth Printing, July 2014
Seventh Printing, January 2015

ISBN 1-891845-54-3
ISBN 978-1-891845-54-3
LCCN #2010940482

Page layout: Honora Wolfe
Cover design: Eric Brearton
Illustrations, David Anzaldua, MD and Eric Brearton

COMP Designation: Original work

10 9 8 7

Printed at Frederic Printing, Denver, CO

This book is dedicated to my teachers and students: past, present, and future.

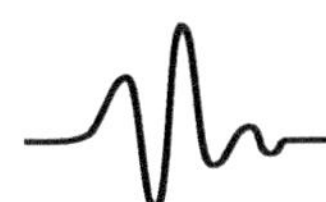

ACKNOWLEDGMENTS

After many years as a clinician and educator in modern scientific medicine, I discovered the treasure of Traditional Chinese Medicine and added that perspective to my clinical approach. I had many excellent teachers in both arenas along the way. I am more deeply appreciative of these individuals than I can express in mere words. This book arises directly out of my desire to give to others a small portion of the knowledge that I have been so generously given.

I also want to acknowledge a few of my former Chinese medicine students who have inspired me by their diligence, open-mindedness and eagerness to learn and who have matured into stellar practitioners themselves. Several reviewed early versions of this work and offered useful suggestions. These included Dadali Ziai, MTCM, L.Ac and Richard Esquivel, OMD, L.Ac. I am especially indebted to Anthony Von der Muhll, MTCH, L.Ac, for his valuable insights regarding this material.

My most valuable ally in my quest to make this material useful and readable, however, was my wife, Danielle Dufayet. Not every author is lucky enough to marry an English major and writer. Beyond her proofreading efforts, which were prodigious, Danielle helped me to realize and continue to remind me of the necessity and usefulness of this book during my busy medical practice and teaching schedule. She inspired and unselfishly supported me throughout this effort and I thank her for it.

Several esteemed medical doctors also looked at early versions of this work. I want to thank David Clark, MD, for doing so from the cardio-pulmonary point of view. His comments were valuable and helped guide me along the way. Finally, Bruce Robinson, MD, a prominent and well-respected medical emissary to the TCM community, did me the dual favor of looking over parts of this manuscript and also introducing me to my publisher, Blue Poppy Press.

Finally, I want to thank the entire Blue Poppy team, from the reception staff through the managers and editors, for their far-ranging vision and excellent support throughout this project. I can't imagine having had a finer group of people to work with on this venture.

David A. Anzaldua, MD, ABFP, ABAARM

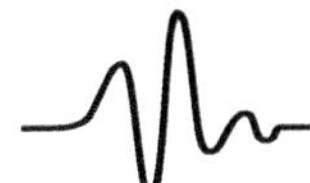

FOREWORD

Here are a few brief comments about some of the terminology in this book.

I have streamlined some terms for ease of reading. For example, I often say "acupuncture" as shorthand for the collective practices of indigenously-derived East Asian styles of medicine like Traditional Chinese Medicine (TCM) while being aware that acupuncture is only one modality in TCM. Sometimes I say "Chinese medicine" as shorthand for TCM while also being aware that Chinese medicine may combine modern scientific medicine with TCM. Similarly, I sometimes say "Western medicine" to mean the kind of scientific medicine now being practiced around the world, including in China and East Asia.

I use two key words when describing the frequency of certain conditions and disorder in the U.S. population that are essential to understand; incidence and prevalence. Incidence is the frequency at which a certain condition arises in a specific population during a given unit of time, often over one year. 1000 cases of X condition in the U.S. population per year, for example. Prevalence, on the other hand, is the number of cases that can be found in a certain population at a given moment in time, let's say 1000 cases of condition Z are found to be present on July 30, 2010.

A condition like the common cold would have a much higher incidence than prevalence because, while many people get a cold each year, it doesn't last long enough to be nearly as prevalent at any given moment in time as it is incident. In contrast, back pain has both a high incidence and prevalence. Many people get it yearly and it can last long enough so that the likelihood of finding people with back pain at any given time is also rather high.

It's important for all modern health care practitioners to understand as much medical terminology as possible in order to communicate with other modern practitioners and because an exploration of medical terminology often rewards the practitioner with insights about disease processes. For this reason, I include a lot of medical terminology in this book. When I do, however, I often present the technical language in parentheses after a more user-friendly description of the condition is given.

David A. Anzaldua, MD, ABFP, ABAARM
October, 2010

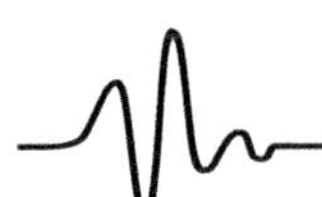

INTRODUCTION

An Acupuncturist's Guide to Medical Red Flags and Referrals

While I was packing books into my briefcase one spring evening after a long day of teaching, a student from acupuncture rounds came rushing into the break room, eyes wide with excitement. It seems there was a male patient with a "possible broken arm" in one of the treatment rooms. The students and their Traditional Chinese Medicine (TCM) faculty member were concerned about this patient and wondered if I might take a look at him.

The patient was a 20-year-old man who had been riding a skateboard to his acupuncture appointment. He had fallen off while trying to jump a curb and broke his fall by catching himself on his outstretched right hand and felt immediate pain in his wrist and elbow. The pain had grown worse in the time it took him to be checked in and led to a treatment room where he now sat in obvious discomfort.

The patient's face was pale. There were beads of sweat above his lip. He was holding his right elbow with his opposite hand. It was obviously swollen. As concerned students looked on, I carefully palpated the patient's right wrist and forearm to check for tenderness, leaving the area I knew would be most tender for last. The patient winced when I finally touched his elbow. There was enough tenderness there to make me think he had a fracture, but something else concerned me even more.

When I checked his radial pulse on the right and compared it to the left, I found it to be weaker, barely palpable. I recognized the combination of a **swollen, painful elbow with a diminished radial pulse in the affected extremity** as a red flag for a *supracondylar fracture of the elbow*. The patient was sent immediately to the emergency department (ED) of a nearby hospital because pressure from swelling and/or bone fragments in the antecubital fossa of the elbow pose a grave risk of neurovascular damage to the distal hand.

This is the way red flags pop up in clinical practice, suddenly and often without warning. It's fortunate for our patients that serious conditions marked by red flags are relatively less common than nonurgent problems. We can't let their relative rarity lull us into a false sense of security, however. We must be ready to promptly and accurately recognize them when they appear, whether they are rare or common and refer them when necessary.

The purpose of this book is to give acupuncturists the ability to promptly, accurately, and consistently recognize red flag signs and symptoms that indicate the possibility of serious conditions and confidently seek consultation for these conditions in a way that protects the patient's health and builds collegial consultative relationships. These consultations, incidentally, don't necessarily have to be with medical doctors, although that may well be what you choose with many of the conditions in this book. You might even have the special skill set needed for some of these. The important thing is to be able to recognize red flags and consult about or refer them when necessary.

About the red flags in this book

The red flags in this book are derived from the author's greater than 30 years of primary care clinical experience as the head of integrative medicine clinics working side-by-side with acupuncturists and other physicians, as well as cases derived during the supervision of acupuncture students for many years. They are meant to cover the problems most often seen by acupuncturists in the U.S., listed below in rough order of most to least frequent ("The Practice of Acupuncture, Who Are the Providers and What Do They Do?" *Annals of Family Medicine*, March, 2005, Vol. 3, number 2).

- Musculoskeletal
- Psychological and mental
- Neurological
- Digestive and gastrointestinal
- Respiratory
- Genitourinary
- Gynecologic

- Cardiovascular
- Infectious diseases, skin complaints and cancer

Standardized presentation of red flags

The red flags in this book could have been organized in an organ system format similar to the above list, but I have chosen not to do so here. Rather, they are organized by symptoms using patient's terminology whenever possible. The main reason for choosing a symptom (problem-oriented) format for red flags is because that's the way patients present them to us. They complain of "bloody urine," rather than "hematuria", for example. This is also the favored approach in modern clinical medical education.

We are particularly concerned with several types of conditions in this book.

- Conditions most likely to present in acupuncture practices in the U.S. because they have a high incidence and prevalence in the general population and might present to acupuncturists even more frequently than to other types of practitioners.
- Conditions with the greatest risks of not having been previously or adequately assessed by other medical professionals because they can be tricky to identify by patients and practitioners alike.
- Conditions that are extremely dangerous and, if caught early, can make a huge difference in a patient's life.

The best way to use this book

Each red flag is written to stand by itself and has sufficient background material included with it to make it understandable without reference to other reference texts. They can therefore be read in any order, depending on your interest or needs in your education and/or clinical practice. You may want to look them up as you see patients, for example. They do build upon one another in many cases, however, so readers who want to read this material from "front to back" will pick up valuable self-reinforcing information by doing so.

What is the likelihood of encountering rare red flags in acupuncture practice?

It may seem unlikely that you'll see some of the rarer red flags in this book. A word of caution is appropriate in this regard, however. If the average busy acupuncturist sees 30 patients a week for 48 weeks a year (1,440 patients a year or 43,200 patients in 30 years) he or she will encounter multiple red flags for conditions with even low incidence. Pneumothorax due to acupuncture, for example, occurs in 1/5000 patients (see incidence section in "Pain, chest"). Using these statistics, it will be encountered 8.64 times during this average lifetime practice.

While it is true that many patients with severe conditions will self-refer to medical doctors rather than seeing an acupuncturist, many will not. Patients may also seek care while they are in early or subacute phases of serious conditions. It's therefore important to realize that there's really nobody "out there" to do the job of red flag detection for you. It's a responsibility all health care practitioners share.

Understanding that red flags mark end points in disease evolution

Patients can present in many different stages of their serious condition, from mildly to severely ill. This fact directly influenced my decision about the red flags selected for this text. Deliberately omitted are some red flags that mark the end stages of specific diseases. For example, because it is unlikely (though not impossible) that acupuncturists will see patients with massive myocardial infarctions (MI) the red flag for MI is not included in this book. The red flag for angina is, however, because angina is an earlier evolutionary point in the progression of coronary artery disease (CAD) more likely to be seen by acupuncturists.

All red flags, however, are signs and symptoms of advanced enough stages of their underlying conditions so they are easily recognizable by sufficiently educated clinicians. Master clinicians will recognize even earlier signs and symptoms than those listed in this text, however, and it would be remiss of me not to mention that one of my goals in writing this book is to help clinicians recognize ever more subtle signs and symptoms of underlying illness so that earlier intervention can occur.

This can be accomplished by something I call "mentally running the red flag backward" to determine what earlier signs and symptoms might be. For example, long before patients with low blood oxygen (hypoxemia) become blue around the lips (cyanotic), their complexion is sallow and pale. Similarly, long before a patient with multiple sclerosis (MS) loses bladder control or a patient with a nerve root compression of the lumbosacral region loses the ability to move the big toe upward (dorsiflexion), there is tingling (paresthesia) in affected regions.

Examples like these abound and are the most enjoyable and exciting part of red flag education for me. I hope the prospect for early recognition of illness and prevention of illness will be as exciting and rewarding for you as well, and will add to the well-being of all our patients.

Areas specifically not covered in this book

There are a few areas deliberately left uncovered in this text because they are not the focus of this work, would require a voluminous text, or are well covered in other standard texts.

- It is not the purpose of this book to explore treatment options for red flag conditions, although some treatments are included if they make the red flag more interesting, easier to remember, or strengthen an understanding of the underlying condition.
- As a corollary of the above, this book does not explore the relative efficacy of TCM treatments versus modern scientific medicine (MSM) treatment. The ability to deal with red flags is essential regardless of the efficacies of different healing styles.
- Although the subject of differential diagnosis (a list of all possible diagnoses) inevitably comes up in the course of considering red flags and is briefly discussed in some situations, this book does not attempt to list all possible diagnoses for each red flag.

The final result

It's impossible to include every possible red flag in a book of this length. I expect some honest disagreement among experts about some of the red flags chosen and the criteria used to select them. Regardless of this, this material is deep, rich and accurate enough to be useful to acupuncture students and practitioners as a solid beginning exploration of red flags. They have already proven enjoyable and useful in red flag seminars and classes for acupuncture students and acupuncturists.

I invite your thoughtful comments and questions so that future editions of this book will best fit the needs of acupuncture students, practitioners and especially our patients.

David Anzaldua, MD
June, 2010

TABLE OF CONTENTS

Chapter 1: Medical Red Flags

What are red flags? How do we notice them and how do we miss them in the clinical setting? What are the main differences in types of red flags? How significant does a sign or symptom need to be to compel us to refer for further screening?

Red flags are signs and symptoms that indicate the possible or probable presence of serious medical conditions that can cause irreversible disability or untimely death unless managed properly. The purpose of this book is to give acupuncturists the ability to spot red flags easily and consistently in the normal course of practice and to consult with other practitioners of their choosing so suspected "red flag conditions" can be ruled in or out and treated. Chapter 2 goes into detail concerning the consultation process. In this opening chapter we consider:

1. The dangers of missing red flags and benefits of picking them up and referring them.
2. The difference between highly diagnostic and less diagnostic red flags.
3. The distinction between "general red flags" versus "specific red flags."
4. Cautions about "sleeper" presentations of red flags.

Possible dangers of missing and not referring red flag conditions

The short scenarios listed below illustrate some ways in which an acupuncturist might miss red flags and some possible consequences of doing so.

- Wrongly accepting the patient's self-diagnosis as definitive: A patient presents with a chronic cough says it is "my allergies." The acupuncturist identifies and treats a defensive qi vacuity pattern without recognizing that the persistent cough also indicates the possibility of lung cancer. The cancer metastasizes, leading to an untimely death.
- Wrongly assuming that a prior physician workup and referral for acupuncture ensures that the patient's condition carries no risk of disability or death: A patient is referred for treatment of persistent wrist pain following a fall on an outstretched hand. The acupuncturist treats qi and blood stagnation for weeks without reporting back to the physician that the wrist pain has not improved. The physician assumes all is well because she has not heard from patient or acupuncturist. An occult fracture not identified on original x-ray becomes necrotic, leading to permanent disability.
- Mistakenly treating symptoms without understanding they reflect a serious underlying medical condition: A patient complaining of chronic fatigue and daytime sleepiness is treated by the acupuncturist for qi and yang vacuity without recognizing red flags for severe sleep apnea. The patient subsequently falls asleep at the wheel and suffers a fatal motor vehicle accident that kills several other people also.
- Mistaken assumptions about abnormal reactions to medical care and failure to understand the normal course of recovery: A patient referred for postsurgical acupuncture suffers from increasing pain, swelling, stiffness and sensory abnormalities in a limb is mistakenly assumed to have normal postsurgical pain while a permanently painful and disabling complex regional pain syndrome (CPRS) develops.
- Failure to note or understand a painless red flag sign: An elderly male patient tells his acupuncturist during routine history that he painlessly passed bright red blood in his urine the day before. Because there was no pain, the patient and acupuncturist minimize the event. The patient dies of avoidable metastatic bladder cancer one year later that could have been easily treated after the first bleed.

The bottom line is this: No medical practitioner can automatically assume that red flags have already been picked up by other health care providers. Even the most skilled practitioners miss them. Furthermore, stable conditions may become unstable, nonthreatening conditions may become threatening, and new conditions may arise. Acupuncturists are in a position to avert catastrophe by prompt and accurate red flag recognition and timely consultation. Patients, acupuncturists, and the public all benefit from this patient-centered approach.

Benefits of consultations and referrals

Western medicine (WM) assessments can help, rather than hinder, the acupuncturist in providing safe and effective Chinese medicine (CM) treatment in a number of ways.

- Acupuncturists can use WM assessments to refine their impressions about severity of conditions as well as the course the illness is likely to take.
- WM assessment can shed additional light on the pathological mechanisms at work in an illness, which can aid in the selection of CM modalities and techniques.
- Understanding WM pathological mechanisms can sometimes aid in identifying important cautions and contraindications to acupuncture, herbal medicine, tui na, gua sha, and other CM modalities.
- WM assessment can provide quantitative and qualitative baselines against which to measure outcomes of CM treatment.
- Evidence for many conditions in this book is accumulating that simultaneous multidisciplinary care works best in improving outcome.

Proper consultation and/or referral as outlined in this book rarely, if ever, results in the patient quitting acupuncture. On the contrary, proper referral typically results in increased respect for the acupuncturist for recognizing the serious illness. Referred patients typically continue acupuncture care with greater confidence that serious diagnoses have been ruled out by a multidisciplinary approach.

Highly diagnostic versus less diagnostic red flags

It will be evident as we proceed through this material that not all red flags have equal diagnostic power. Some are highly diagnostic (*i.e.*, highly indicative) that a particular serious condition is present. Others are far less diagnostic, but still make it likely enough that a serious condition is present so we must assume it is present until proven otherwise.

An example of a highly diagnostic red flag is neck pain followed by numbness in one arm and hand. By far the most likely explanation for neck pain with arm numbness is a compression of one or more spinal nerves in the neck, a serious condition that can lead to lasting pain and disability. Other conditions that might cause neck pain with associated arm numbness are rare, making this red flag highly diagnostic.

An example of a less diagnostic red flag is one-sided ankle swelling, which can be caused by several relatively common conditions, like skin infections. Even though other causes may be likely, one-sided ankle swelling can also be caused by a calf vein deep venous thrombosis (DVT), a serious condition that can turn rapidly fatal if a clot breaks loose and travels to the lung in the form of a pulmonary embolism (PE)—see red flag for PE below.

The above example brings us to a secondary guiding principle about red flags. The more dangerous the possible underlying condition is, the more we need to rule it out, even if the red flag could be explained by less serious causes. The seriousness of calf vein DVT requires that we assume its presence unless proven otherwise, even if we think it more likely that the patient is simply suffering from poor circulation, lymphatic swelling or a localized infection.

The additional presence of chest pain and shortness of breath following unilateral ankle swelling is a red flag for the dreaded consequence of PE mentioned above. We shouldn't wait for this PE to develop, however, before referring the patient with the red flag for a DVT to an urgent care facility where a venous ultrasound can easily rule DVT in or out. Recognizing and acting on red flags signs and symptoms as soon as possible is far better than waiting until the condition has progressed to serious consequences.

General red flags versus specific red flags

This book lists and examines both general and specific red flags under various symptom categories.

1. General red flags are signs and/or symptoms that signal dangerous conditions with multiple possible explanations or that can manifest in many different anatomical areas. An example is headache with a neurological deficit, which is a general red flag for some type of intracranial lesion, tumor, or bleeding, for example.
2. Specific red flags signal specific illnesses or are present in specific anatomical regions. An example is persistent double vision after a blow to an eye, which is a specific red flag for a "blow-out fracture" of the orbital bones of the eye socket with entrapment of an extraocular muscle in the fracture.

General red flags are important, not for their specificity, but for their wide reach. No single text can cover all the red flags for every serious injury or illness. By knowing general red flags like unexplained weight loss, however, the astute clinician can recognize when serious illness is likely to be present even if the exact illness is unknown. The ability to recognize general red flags is at least as important as being able to recognize specific red flags and that is why we also emphasize them in this book.

"Sleeper" presentations of red flags

Chest pain and shortness of breath following unilateral ankle swelling is a dramatic presentation of a PE. We must also be on the lookout for sleeper presentations, red flags that present with far less drama. Sleeper presentations generally include common symptoms and/or signs like constipation or low back pain that often have non-serious causes and may therefore lull the practitioner into a false sense of security. Even common and mild signs and symptoms can indicate serious illness, however, when combined with other specific signs and symptoms.

Constipation, for example, accounts for more than 2.5 million visits in primary care offices every year. It is not a red flag by itself, but when we combine constipation with unexplained weight loss, for example, the combination is a red flag for possible colon cancer. We could make the red flag even more diagnostic by adding clinical context like patient age $>$ 50 years old, but we don't need to do so because constipation with unexplained weight loss alone makes it likely enough that colon cancer is present that we are obliged to rule it out.

Another example of a sleeper presentation of a red flag is one episode of painless bloody urination in a man $>$ 50 years old, a red flag for carcinoma of the urinary tract. A single instance of painless hematuria is easily ignored by patients and clinicians. Yet, its presence in a man over 50 years old makes it likely enough (and the consequences of missing it are dire enough) that we must assume the patient has cancer until proven otherwise. Carcinoma of the bladder can be easily removed through a scope at this early bleeding stage, but is often lethal if we wait.

Back pain can also present in certain contexts as a sleeper presentation. Back pain is ubiquitous. More than 80% of adults will have back pain at some time in their life. It is the most common complaint of patients under 45 of people who see primary care providers, and accounts for a great deal of the traffic in any primary care provider's office. As with constipation, the presence of a few additional common symptoms and signs together with back pain can make us suspect a serious cause for it.

Such was the case with a seemingly healthy 23-year-old man who walked into my office complaining of low back pain. The only clues that this young man's back pain was not a garden-variety, non-serious back pain was the steadily progressive nature of the pain (steadily progressive pain is discussed as a general red flag in the chapter dealing with "pain in general") and a 10-pound weight loss over a month that was not attributable to dieting or increasing aerobic exercise.

In fact, this young man was trying to gain weight by increasing calories and drinking protein shakes along with weight-lifting. This young patient with unexplained weight loss and progressive back pain had cancer of the spine and underwent urgent surgery to excise the tumor just in time to save his life. Unexplained weight loss is, by itself, so indicative of the possibility of some type of serious illness that it can be considered a general red flag on its own and is treated as such later in this book.

Summary

All red flags, whether highly diagnostic or not, general or specific, presenting with drama or as sleepers, warn us of the possibility of disabling and life-threatening disorders. It's important to remember that they only need to be sufficiently suggestive to compel us to rule out a serious condition to be a red flag, not absolutely diagnostic. Our goal is to help practitioners identify the red flags in this book and guide them with the referral process, the latter being the subject of the next chapter.

Chapter 2: CONSULTATION AND REFERRALS

Knowing how to consult other healthcare professionals regarding red flag conditions is a crucial skill for acupuncturists. This chapter shows you how to do it to get optimal benefits for your patients and your practice.

The ability to identify red flags is a crucial skill. So is the ability to effectively and efficiently consult other health care providers about them. The consultant you choose is up to you. It doesn't necessarily have to be a medical doctor, but it does need to be someone who can competently determine if the condition you are concerned about is present or not. The material in this chapter applies regardless of who you consult.

Often enough, however, due to the conditions we cover herein and because we are talking about consultations in the U.S., the consultation will be to a medical doctor. Unfortunately, consultation skills are generally poorly covered in acupuncture and medical schools. Students and practitioners are often left to learn this skill on their own, leaving a lot of room for mistakes. This chapter is designed to give you the preparedness you need to effectively and even enjoyably consult other practitioners. You may want to read through it quickly and refer back to it at the time of actual consultation later.

This chapter will cover several levels of consultations and referrals.

1. 911 type referrals.
2. Sending a patient to a hospital emergency room (ER) or emergency department (ED) of a hospital.
3. Consultations on a semi-urgent basis (within the same day to several days).
4. Consultations in a timely manner (within several days to two weeks).

The first two, though dramatic, will be covered only briefly because, despite the seriousness of the situation, the level of effort and finesse on the part of the acupuncturist is minimal compared with consultations that involve semi-urgent or timely consultations and referrals.

911 situations

Let's say you have an urgent situation that develops in your clinic. A patient is on the table getting acupuncture and begins having severe shortness of breath, for example. In the cases of emergencies that require activation of the medical emergency response system, you call 911.

Below is a streamlined guide for how to handle 911 emergencies, a summary, not a substitute, for guidance provided in standard Basic Life Support/First Aid manuals as published by the American Red Cross.

1. Call for help and dial or have someone in your office dial 911 to activate the emergency services system.
2. Provide CPR, basic life support, and first aid if needed until emergency services personnel arrive.
3. Maintain communication with the 911 operator and ensure that the patient and the office are prepared for emergency services personnel.
4. You will be asked some basic questions about the patient's situation by the medical response team that comes to your office. These concerns will be forwarded to the waiting ED staff.
5. You should meet the patient at the ED if your treatment caused the harm, e.g. pneumothorax.

ED referrals

Sending a patient to an ED *without a 911 call* (with a family member driving the patient, for example) takes a little more finesse. This is because you will ideally call the ED beforehand to give the triage nurse or attending physician a "heads-up" about your patient before he or she arrives.

Neither the 911 situation or the direct ED referral, however, requires the kind of communication skills of timely and semi-urgent consultations, the subject matter for the rest of this chapter.

Timely and semi-urgent consultations

Consultations regarding patients who need to be seen on a timely or semi-urgent basis require more sophisticated skills than referring emergency patients. In these cases, you will be consulting practitioners that you may develop collegial relationships with over the years. The difference between uncomfortable and ineffective versus mutually rewarding and beneficial consultation is often determined by the attitude and degree of preparedness of the referring practitioner. This chapter shows you how to do it well.

Consultation and referrals

First, let's define what we mean by "consulting" and "referring". Basically, consulting a practitioner is the same as referring the patient, but the words "consultation" and "referral" have somewhat different connotations worth exploring. I prefer to say that we are "consulting regarding a patient," rather than "referring the patient" because "consultation" connotes a sense of collegiality and ongoing conversation between equals, whereas "referring" can imply that we are sending a patient to be "taken over" by a consultant because we "can't handle it."

The latter is certainly not the case, which should be obvious by the tone of this chapter. If we remove this negative connotation to the word "referral," however, we can use the words "consultation" and "referral" interchangeably. Whatever we call it, the consultation is a request for specific services you wish to have rendered to your patient. It can be accomplished in a way that is beneficial for you, your patient, and your consultant. The more specific the information is about the patient, and the more specific you are about what you want the consultant to do, the better.

It is your prerogative to set up the parameters of the consultation relationship with your consultant to accomplish your intended goals (see step 2 below on determining what services you want for your patient).

Six steps to successful referral of timely and semi-urgent patients

After you have spotted and thought about the red flag, the six steps you must take for semi-urgent referrals are the following:

Step 1 – *Determine* who you want your consultant to be

Step 2 – *Determine* what service(s) you want your consultant to perform and the role you intend to play in your patient's ongoing and future care (see Appendix A)

Step 3 – *Prepare* yourself with the right "mind-set" for the referral

Step 4 – *Organize* your clinical data logically for presentation

Step 5 – *Contact* your consultant and present your referral in a clear, concise, standardized way

Step 6 – *Document* your referral in the patient chart so you are in a strong medico-legal position in the event that if the patient suffers a poor outcome regardless of your best efforts

Step 1 – DETERMINE who you want your consultant to be

If you want to consult another specialized acupuncturist or alternative practitioner, you can go through the professional listings for these practitioners to find the ones you want if you do not already know them. In the case of medical doctors or institutions, you can choose from a variety of physicians listed in the phone book or online under the specialties if you do not already know your consultant (you should have this information ready ahead of time).

Referring directly to a specialist, however, is probably not the optimal way to refer red flag patients most of the time. Rather, it's best to refer a patient with a timely or semi-urgent condition back to their primary care provider (PCP) first, if one is available, rather than attempting to send the patient directly to a specialist. See break-out box for reasons to consult to a PCP.

By PCPs, we mean doctors of medicine or osteopathy from three specific specialties: family practice, pediatrics and general internal medicine. Such physicians are considered "primary care specialists," or "primary care providers" because that's the function they perform. (We use "PCP" for this group for sake of brevity while fully recognizing and respecting the fact that acupuncturists are also PCPs in some states.)

Step 2 – DETERMINE what service(s) you want your consultant to perform for your patient and the role you intend to play in your patient's ongoing care

Your communication with your consultant should clearly state what service, from those listed below, you would like them to provide for your patient and how you will interact with them and your patient in the future (see sample consultation form and letter, appendix A).

1. You are sending the patient for evaluation and suggestion of treatment options which you will then discuss with the patient to help them make decisions.
2. You are sending the patient for evaluation and co-treatment of the condition.
3. You are sending the patient for evaluation and total treatment of the condition. You will see the patient for other problems and will continue to care of the patient after treatment for the referred condition.

Step 3 – PREPARE yourself with the right "mind-set" for the referral

Communicating with other health care professions doesn't come naturally to everyone. When difficulties in referring patients are encountered, it's also common to feel some anxiety, distress, and frustration. Acupuncturists accustomed to a slow-paced and informal style of communication may feel distressed by contemporary medicine's demands that only the most pertinent information be transmitted in the minimum time necessary.

Common fears that some acupuncturists may feel when referring patients include:

1. Anxiety that their concerns about the patient may be perceived as overblown or their diagnostic impressions inaccurate.
2. Fear that they may be perceived as having misled or mistreated the condition, if found to be more serious than originally believed.
3. Fear they may encounter veiled contempt for, or abrupt dismissal of, their form of medicine.
4. Fear of loss of respect and status in the eyes of patients, peers or physicians if patient's case seems to require further assessment and intervention beyond their own clinical practice.
5. Fear of responsibility for the patient's condition if the patient's health is endangered by unnecessary medical procedures or therapies.

It may offer some small degree of comfort to know that these types of feelings are not unusual. In fact, they are even the rule among a variety of practitioners from many different healing systems, especially when starting out in clinical practice. Acknowledging them and using the antidote for them, as outlined below, will help guide you to effective consultations.

The antidote for fear of consulting—the proper mind-set

The ultimate antidote for emotional turmoil regarding consultation and/or referral is to constantly remind ourselves of why we're referring in the first place – out of concern for the well-being of our patient. All other considerations pale in comparison. If we remind ourselves that we must make our best effort at consultation because of patient needs, it is easier to face challenges we may encounter.

It is also important not to prejudge how the process will go before it happens. Unless consultation has been attempted according to the helpful guidelines in this book, it is difficult to estimate how future consultations will turn out by looking at the results of past attempts. All clinicians, in fact, stand an excellent chance for successful and collegial consultations if the methods in this text are used regardless of healing tradition.

We should also remind ourselves that many patients actually need multiple approaches to health care. Patients may have strong preferences for one type of care or another, but it is the rare patient that will not need different approaches at different times. Our true role is as part of the total health care team.

Step 4 – ORGANIZE your clinical data logically for presentation

If your telephone calls or letters of referral are organized according to the accepted standard framework for referral, you will be pleasantly surprised by the positive response you'll receive. Consultants can forgive a lot of things, including a neophyte status in the referring practitioner, but they don't like a disorganized presentation that rambles and doesn't give them the information they need to make decisions efficiently, any more than you would.

Don't underestimate the importance of a standardized patient presentation when it comes to referrals. Referrals should be organized strictly by **patient ID, history, physical exam, assessment, and plan**. This is not the time to stray from this tried-and-true formula. Never get on the phone or write a letter to a consultant until you've first taken the time (usually minimal) to organize your data. Jotting down a few notes to keep you on track ahead of time will help when you start out.

Step 5 – CONTACT your consultant and present the patient in a clear, concise, standardized way

When referring the patient to their PCP, it's best to contact them directly by phone, fax, or secure e-mail. It's second best to leave a phone message with the receptionist. If you leave a message for the receptionist it will only add a layer to the communication process and the receptionist may not have the training to recognize the semi-urgency of the situation.

It's also advisable to provide the patient with contact information for the physician's office and encourage them to follow up directly with the physician if an appointment cannot be made while you are on the phone with the consultant's office. Providing the patient with physician contact information is not a substitute for your direct communication with the physician's office, however. If you simply hand the patient a business card or a slip of paper with phone numbers and say "give them a call," the patient may decide otherwise.

Remember that if the patient's primary care physician does not respond, that is a problem with their response system, not your referral efforts. The final section of this chapter deals with situations in which the consultation doesn't go as smoothly as you would like.

The presentation, sample dialogue:

Hello. Is this Doctor Jones? Thank you for taking my call. Yes, this is Richard Needles. I'm a local acupuncturist seeing your patient Henrietta Smith, date of birth 01-10-1980. I'd like to give you some important information about her. Do you remember her offhand, or do you want to get her chart before we talk?

This is it in a nutshell, Doctor Jones. **History:** Mrs. Smith came to see me for back pain today, but claimed she's also had a swollen left ankle since returning from a trans-Atlantic flight last week. **Physical:** Her left ankle is indeed swollen and measured 4 cm larger in diameter than her right ankle 5 cm above the medial malleolus.

Assessment or **Impression:** I'm concerned about the possibility of a DVT in her left calf. **Plan:** I wonder if you'd have the opportunity to see her for this today.

The referral can turn in a number of different directions at this point, depending on what the PCP says. Perhaps her PCP is late on his way to catching a flight out of the country. Perhaps he thinks the patient needs to go directly to the ED or wants to see her in his office right away. In any case, you've fulfilled your obligation. You've made your best effort to contact the patient's PCP, which is always the best first step for timely or semi-urgent referrals.

Step 6 – DOCUMENT your referral in the patient's chart so you are in a strong medico-legal position in the event that the patient suffers a poor outcome regardless of your best efforts

Whatever method you have implemented, it's important to document what you've done in the patient's medical record. One time-efficient method is to fax or mail a copy of your written referral (Appendix A) to the physician's office, provide the patient with a photocopy and also file a copy in the patient's medical record. It also is advisable for someone on your staff to call the PCP's office to ensure they have received the referral.

Delays are common in accessing physician care in settings other than same-day urgent care or emergency room facilities, which is another reason it's advisable to initiate the referral the same day the condition is detected, preferably before the patient leaves your office. This is particularly true if you are referring the patient to a PCP who may need time to refer the patient to another series of specialists.

What do you do if, despite your best efforts, a referral "goes bad?"

By "going bad" I mean:

1. The consultant seems poorly responsive to your referral, and you get little or no feedback from them regarding your patient's case.
2. The patient keeps an appointment but has personality or communication issues with the consultant or their office that preclude an effective rapport between them.
3. The apparent seriousness of the medical problem does not seem to be adequately addressed or even recognized by the consultant.

With the exception of out-and-out rudeness, which is always inexcusable, we need to be careful before concluding that a consultation was unsuccessful due to lack of receptivity on the consultant's part. Except in the case of a consultant not taking your call (you can always fax them or write a letter) there may be reasons for what seems like a less than enthusiastic response that has little, if anything, to do with you.

If the patient did not obtain a satisfactory consult, it's possible that the patient presented a different history to the consultant than you obtained, misunderstood the consultant, or was misunderstood by the consultant. The patient's condition may also have changed (hopefully better) between the time they saw you and the consultant.

Consultants should let you know about some of these occurrences by calling you or sending you a note, but it is always possible for you to call the consultant and ask for his or her opinion regarding the referral. Communication is a two-way street. Referring acupuncturists and consultants don't always walk it perfectly, but the effort is important on the patient's behalf. Personality clashes are also possible. If they happen between your consultant and your patient, there is nothing you can do about it.

Let's say, however, that your patient returns to you and, after careful thought, you conclude that their problem was not adequately addressed for whatever reason. There are still options. You must remember the primary principle: we are referring for the benefit of the patient and for no other reason. The patient's needs must come first. What is the patient's need in this situation? It is clear. The patient needs another referral for a more satisfactory consultation.

We have to be creative in this case. Why needlessly offend a consultant who might be needed for future consultation or someone who might have simply botched a particular referral? What we have to do in this case is put the decision making power squarely back in the hands of the patient, where it belongs, but also guide the patient to exercise that choice for another consultant.

Sample dialogue with a patient if you or patient are not satisfied with the consult:

YOU: I understand you didn't feel that Doctor W. understood your problem.

PATIENT: He didn't listen to me at all. He just rushed me in and out.

YOU: I wish there were something we could do the change that, but it's out of our hands. My primary obligation remains to help you. Even though I don't know exactly where the "disconnect" occurred with Dr. W., I'm still concerned about your symptoms.

PATIENT: You and me, both...What do you suggest?

YOU: I can't tell you what to do. Ultimately, who you see is your decision. If I were in your shoes, however, I would seek a second opinion.

PATIENT: Who would you suggest?

YOU: I'll give you a list of consultants. Since your situation is not an emergency, I suggest you check with your insurance to see which of these you might be able to see on your plan. Then give me a call back and I'll send them a note to introduce you and your problem.

7 important reasons to refer the patient to his or her PCP rather than directly to a specialist

1. The PCP might be more accessible and is more likely to have a close relationship with the patient and more ready to "go the extra mile" than a specialist who doesn't know the patient.

2. The PCP probably has additional medical and family history that will be useful to all consultants who may eventually attend the patient.

3. Many PCPs have contacts and knowledge of specialists within the consultant community that make further referrals to the best specialist or institution more likely.

4. Many patients are insured under managed care plans, which will require a referral from a PCP within the patient's managed care network before they can access a specialist.

5. Many specialists will only accept referrals directly from a PCP. Valuable time can be wasted trying to refer the patient to a specialist only to have the patient informed that a referral is required from his or her PCP for insurance or other reasons.

6. When you refer to PCPs you begin to build a rapport with them that may well encourage them to send patients back to you — a practice-builder.

7. Not referring a patient back to his or her PCP could be interpreted by the PCP as a sign that you do not understand the importance of the PCP relationship and/or importance of coordinated care.

For these reasons, our recommended default for nonemergency referrals (semi-urgent or timely referrals) is that they be made to the patient's primary care physician, or to a free-standing medical or urgent care clinic (not in a hospital) if no primary care physician is available.

In this latter case, the physician in a free-standing medical or urgent care clinic temporarily plays the part of the PCP and can refer the patient further. Referral to a walk-in clinic may also be an option if a patient has an unsatisfactory relationship with their PCP or the condition you are concerned about has already been dismissed by the patient's PCP—an unfortunate situation that does arise occasionally.

There are a few circumstances, however, in which referral directly to a specialist may be an appropriate option.

1. A patient's PCP asks you to send the patient directly to a specialist.
2. The patient's current PCP is inaccessible, no free-standing clinic is available, and the case is urgent enough to warrant referral directly to a specialist.
3. You are serving as the patient's PCP (they have no medical PCP), you have an established referral relationship with a specialist whom you consider appropriate, and managed care insurance is no obstacle to a direct referral

Chapter 3: ALTERED MENTAL FUNCTION

There is nothing as basic in assessing a patient's overall well-being as noticing their level of consciousness. Is the patient alert and oriented or lethargic? Acupuncturists need to be aware of situations in which variations from normal indicate trouble.

The ability to maintain mental attention, focus, and orientation while awake is often taken for granted, but like many other processes, mental sharpness is actually the product of a delicately balanced set of conditions that allow for optimal function of brain neurons. Two critical factors that must be present are the plentiful delivery of blood rich in just the right amounts of glucose and oxygen to the brain. Anything that can alter the concentration or delivery of glucose and oxygen can cause a change in consciousness by causing neuronal dysfunction.

Other factors that can cause neuronal dysfunction include toxic substances in the blood, bleeding in the brain, seizure activity, direct pressure from tumors and imbalances in specific hormones and neurotransmitters. Neuronal dysfunction, from any or all of these causes, can result in disorders ranging in severity from minor inattention, dizziness and drowsiness, fainting or loss of consciousness, to deficits in thinking and full-blown dementia, depending on what area of the brain is affected and how acutely or severely it is affected.

One of the symptoms in the above list, dizziness, must be clearly distinguished from vertigo through detailed questioning on the patient interview. Dizziness is the feeling of light-headedness, fainting or weakness. Vertigo is the feeling that you or your surroundings are spinning or moving. This distinction of dizziness from vertigo is necessary because conditions that cause vertigo (under hearing and balance in this book) have more to do with the inner ear than with inadequacy of brain nutrients.

This critical distinction of dizziness from vertigo also tells us who the ultimate consultant will be, often an ears, nose and throat physician (ENT) or neurologist in the case of vertigo, or a cardiologist or pulmonologist, in the case of dizziness.

General red flags:
Progressively decreasing mental function at any age

This is a general red flag for ***degeneration and death of brain neurons*** from a variety of possible causes that can eventually progress to dementia. Dementia is a progressive, degenerative disorder that affects memory, language, attention, emotions, and a patient's problem solving capacity and general intelligence. This is a general red flag because it has many possible causes. It is likely to be missed in early stage and on the average causes death about four-and-one-half years after diagnosis .

Causes of dementia, also called senility, include Alzheimer's disease, tiny strokes (lacunar infarcts), tumors, metabolic problems or toxicity due to drugs or substances and neurodegenerative disorders. According to the year 2000 World Health Organization (WHO), *up to 10% of the U.S. population 65 years and older has dementia, with Alzheimer's disease accounting for two-thirds of cases.* The percentage goes up to 45% in those 85 years and older. These are sobering statistics for all clinicians because of the havoc that dementia causes patients, and often their families.

Declines in mental function and memory are seldom reported by patients, however. Rather, family members, coworkers, friends, or other associates are usually the first to note decreasing cognitive function and memory. Common early warning signs are difficulties managing finances and time, including tasks such as balancing checkbooks, paying bills and making appointments. If there is reason to suspect mental decline, clinicians should administer the Mini-mental Health Status Exam (MMSE), a standard test for measuring and tracking cognitive impairment can be downloaded for use at www.medicine.uiowa.edu/igec/ tools/cognitive/MMSE.pdf .

By the time the MMSE or the red flag listed in this chapter for dementia is recognized, dementia is fairly advanced. There has already been considerable neuronal death and dysfunction. As in all red flags mentioned in this book, we urge the practitioner to "play the red flag backwards" to find the earliest manifestations of the disorder so that interventions, whatever type the practitioner is competent in providing, can occur in the earliest stages possible. This means that the earliest stages of mental decline should be recognized.

Dementia is often preceded by years of lesser dysfunction. There is often a tendency, both among patients and health care professionals, to accept such decreasing function as "normal" in aging. There is even a category for this in some medical texts called "age associated mental decline" (AAMD). Declining function, though common, need not be accepted as a normal consequence of aging, however, because evidence shows that those who aggressively pursue mental and physical challenges can maintain and even expand mental capacity at any age in many cases.

In fact, some types of mental decline can be reversed with early intervention and most types can be slowed. The key to understanding how this could happen is to understand the inherent plasticity (ability to make new brain tissue) inherent in the brain, a concept poorly understood until recently.

For many years the regenerative capacity of the brain was thought to be extremely limited. We knew that, after the age of 20, thousands of brain cells die off every day. We thought that was the end of it. In the late 1990s, however, Elizabeth Gould at Rockefeller University uncovered evidence that a large number of new brain neurons are also born every day, perhaps as many as 5,000–10,000 new neurons that arise as stem cells (pluripotential cells) in the hippocampus, an area of the brain involved with learning, memory and mood.

That gave new hope for brain health, but there's a catch: Animal research shows that the great majority of these new brain cells will shrivel and die if conditions aren't right for them to mature into well-functioning neurons. What appears to make them mature optimally is learning; not any kind of learning, but learning that challenges and pushes us out of our "comfort zone." The need for challenging learning to save brain cells has been well demonstrated in animal studies and evidence points to this being true in humans as well.

An additional factor to consider in the generation and maturation of new neurons, however, is exercise. Exercise causes the release of "brain derived neurotropic factor" (BDNF) in the brain. BDNF is to neurons what Miracle Grow® is to plants. It nourishes brain cells and helps them develop and mature. When a person combines exercise with challenging learning material, the beneficial effects on new brain cells is maximized. This is the ideal recipe for continued mental sharpness at any age.

General red flags:
Chronic or repeated dizziness occurring other than when standing up

This is a general red flag for *cerebral neuronal hypofunction* from a variety of possible causes, all of which can lead to disability or death. It is also a common complaint presenting to acupuncturists that affects 10–40% of people in the U.S. population over the age of 60.

Because occasional dizziness is often easily dismissed, the significance of persistent or recurrent non-orthostatic dizziness may be underestimated by patients and clinicians. History, symptoms, and physical findings of different types of chronic non-orthostatic dizziness depend on the various causes, which are listed and examined below.

1. Decreased perfusion of blood to the brain from arrhythmia or heart weakness

Symptoms: If the dizziness results from an arrhythmia, we would expect a history of sudden dizziness as the heart goes into an abnormal rhythm, which can become recurrent. Dizziness from decreased brain perfusion because of a weak heart muscle would tend to be more constant and could be expected to be worse with exercise. The patient might also have a history of shortness of breath and/or chest pain with dizziness from heart problems.

Signs: With arrhythmias the clinician may be able to palpate abnormal pulses, either the extremes of bradycardia or tachycardia or some type of irregular rhythm. With dizziness from decreased brain perfusion because of a weak heart muscle we might find low blood pressure, a weak pulse and possibly bilateral pedal edema if heart failure was present.

2. **Normal perfusion, but decreased oxygen to the brain.** In some cases dizziness is caused by inadequately oxygenated blood reaching the brain due to decreased oxygen capture by the lung (pulmonary causes) or decreased red blood cells (RBCs) to carry oxygen or decreased hemoglobin in RBCs (hypoxemia due to anemia).

   Symptoms: Patients like these would tend to have more chronic and less episodic dizziness and shortness of breath (SOB).

   Signs: In the case of anemia, we might see pallor of the face, nail beds and palpebral conjunctiva. With dizziness from decrease lung function we could hear abnormal lung sound compatible with chronid obstructive pulmonary disease (COPD), bronchitis or pneumonia and fever with the latter.

3. **Decreased glucose in blood.** Since glucose is the main fuel for brain neurons, anything that decreases the glucose concentration in the bloodstream beyond a certain critical amount (below 50 mg/dl) can cause neuronal dysfunction even in an abundance of perfusion of oxygen rich blood. This happens most commonly when diabetics take too much insulin by mistake or sometimes when people have recurrent low blood sugar ("reactive hypoglycemia") 1-3 hours after eating (which is not as serious).

   Symptoms: Patients like this tend to look and feel "jittery" as well as feeling dizzy because there is a compensatory release of catecholamines (epinephrine and norepinephrine) by the body to try to increase blood sugars from stores in muscle and fat leading to symptoms and signs indistinguishable from the flight or fight reaction.

   Signs: The physical signs accompanying low blood sugar are those of the stress reaction: sweating, fast heart rate, tremors and hypervigilance. This could be expected 1-3 hours after meals (postprandial timing) in the case of reactive hypoglycemia and after insulin administration in diabetics.

4. **Toxins in the blood.** Many medicines and substances can cause drowsiness and dizziness so the patient's intake of these substances should be ascertained to see if there may be an easy explanation for the dizziness.

   Symptoms and Signs: The dizziness associated with toxins and medications tends to be more episodic, though often long-lasting due to the extended half-life of many substances, and continual in patients who maintain a steady state of a substance due to repeated dosing.

5. **Seizures.** Sometimes simple seizures (non-generalized) can cause recurrent dizziness. In these cases, search for a history of seizures, head injuries, etc.

   Symptoms and Signs: Simple seizures (non-generalized) do not always stay simple, but may also be intermixed with generalized seizures, observable as tonic/clonic epileptic episodes. Also, other manifestations of simple seizures like stereotypic movement may be observable.

6. **Intracranial masses**

   Symptoms: In this case, we would expect to find other symptoms like headache, etc.

   Signs: With intracranial masses, we would expect to find neurological signs compatible with location of the lesion.

Despite our desire to isolate vertigo from dizziness because of the differences in etiology we again mention that patients, and sometimes physicians, blur or mix up the two conditions so we must be aware that patients and physicians may mean vertigo when they say "dizziness" and vice versa. We must also remember that the two conditions can coexist.

Specific red flags:
Increasing confusion in an elderly person days, weeks, or months after minor head trauma

Condition assumed present until proven otherwise:
Chronic subdural hematoma (collection of bleeding under the skull between the dura mater and the brain tissue usually from trauma)

Possible consequences of missing the condition:
Mental deterioration, coma and/or death

Stabilization, referral, and management:

1. **Stabilization:** There are no specific stabilizing steps to take.

2. **Consultation and Referral Options, Transportation:** If the neurological presentation (confusion, etc.) is neurologically severe and rapidly progressing, but the patient is stable from a cardiopulmonary point of view (stable blood pressure, pulse and no SOB or chest pain) the patient can be transported directly to the hospital ED by a family member. If there are also cardiopulmonary concerns, a 911 call is warranted (as is always the case with cardiopulmonary problems). Less severe cases can be referred to their primary care provider on a semi-urgent basis.

Relevance to acupuncturists: Because the symptoms of chronic subdural hematomas in the elderly progress slowly, sometimes appearing several weeks or even months after what may seem like an insignificant head trauma, the confusion can be assumed by the patient and family members to be "normal" for an elderly person or a sign of early Alzheimer's and a subdural hematoma can be missed.

ACTUAL CASE

- **History:** A 75-year-old patient was brought to the office by his son because of concerns that his father, a retired lawyer who had always been "sharp minded," was now becoming forgetful and confused for the prior two months. When asked about this, the father said, "I guess it's age catching up with me." Neither the son nor his father could remember anything toxic that the father could have ingested and the father did not drink alcohol. On repeated questioning regarding possible head trauma, the son finally remembered his father hitting his head against an open kitchen cabinet door approximately three months earlier.
- **Physical findings:** The father was oriented to person, place, and time but answered questions slowly and seemed to be almost in a stupor at times.
- **Impression:** Possible subdural hematoma
- **Plan:** The patient was sent to his PCP who then referred him to a neurosurgeon.
- **Follow up:** A CT scan of the head showed a large subdural hematoma. This was evacuated by drilling four surgical burr holes into the skull and draining the blood. The patient made a dramatic recovery over the next few days and returned to his usual cognitive state.

DISCUSSION

History and Symptoms

The actual case sums up much of the usual history obtained in regard to chronic subdural hematomas. It should be stressed, however, that the changes in overall neurological function can run the gamut from mild to profound depending on the size of the hematoma and also, on how rapidly the blood builds up. The symptoms and signs are worse in the case of rapidly forming and large hematomas. The presenting symptoms may be exceedingly subtle at early stages and patients may not give a history of hitting their heads, or may give a history of a seemingly insignificant trauma.

Patients can present with a slow onset of symptoms (and signs) over days, weeks or even months. Confusion is most common, but the family and patient can also note slurred speech and difficulty balancing and walking, headache or lethargy. Many of the symptoms (and signs) of chronic subdural hematoma in the elderly can be missed if the patient already has dementia. A faster than normal decline in mental function is a tip off that a subdural hematoma may also be present.

Physical Exam Findings

The mental status exam part of the physical exam may be profoundly abnormal with a patient being disoriented to person, place and time, or it may be normal as in our actual case study. The Mini-mental health screening exam (MMSE) will also be positive for decreased mental facility. As noted above, new confusion may be masked by antecedent dementia. The neurological exam is often normal. In more advanced cases, we would see stupor and more severe confusion.

Incidence and/or Prevalence

Incidence of chronic subdural hematoma is 1.72/100,000 /year in the average population and increases steeply with advancing age up to 7.35/100,000/year in the 70–79 year age group.

Risk Factors

- Anticoagulant medication (blood thinners including aspirin)
- Long-term abuse of alcohol
- Recurrent falls
- Repeated head injury
- Elderly age

Mechanism Producing the Red Flag

Subdural hematomas occur when tiny veins between the surface of the brain and its outer covering (the dura) stretch so much that they tear and bleed. The blood collects under the dura, putting pressure on the brain thereby impairing neuronal function (see figure 1, meningeal layers). Elderly vessels are particularly fragile because brain shrinkage that normally occurs with aging stretches and weakens veins that bridge the dural space, making them more likely to break with minor head injury. In fact, they can become so weak that a subdural hematoma can rarely occur without trauma. The relative lack of focal neurological findings (unilateral paralysis, etc.) in favor of a more generalized finding like confusion is due to the fact that the entire brain is compressed, rather than a single locus.

Other Important Considerations

- This is a well-known neurological emergency that is fairly frequent in the elderly and completely reversible with appropriate care. The slow bleeding from small, low pressure veins inside the skull is vastly different from the bleeding that results from arterial rupture in the subarachnoid space (reviewed elsewhere).
- Not considered here are acute subdural hematomas that occur in young people as well as the elderly due to trauma.
- A misleading factor ("red herring") may be the patient's acceptance of the idea that "age is catching up with me." Although age does undeniably "catch up" to all of us, this reference should in no way obscure the detection of subdural hematomas.

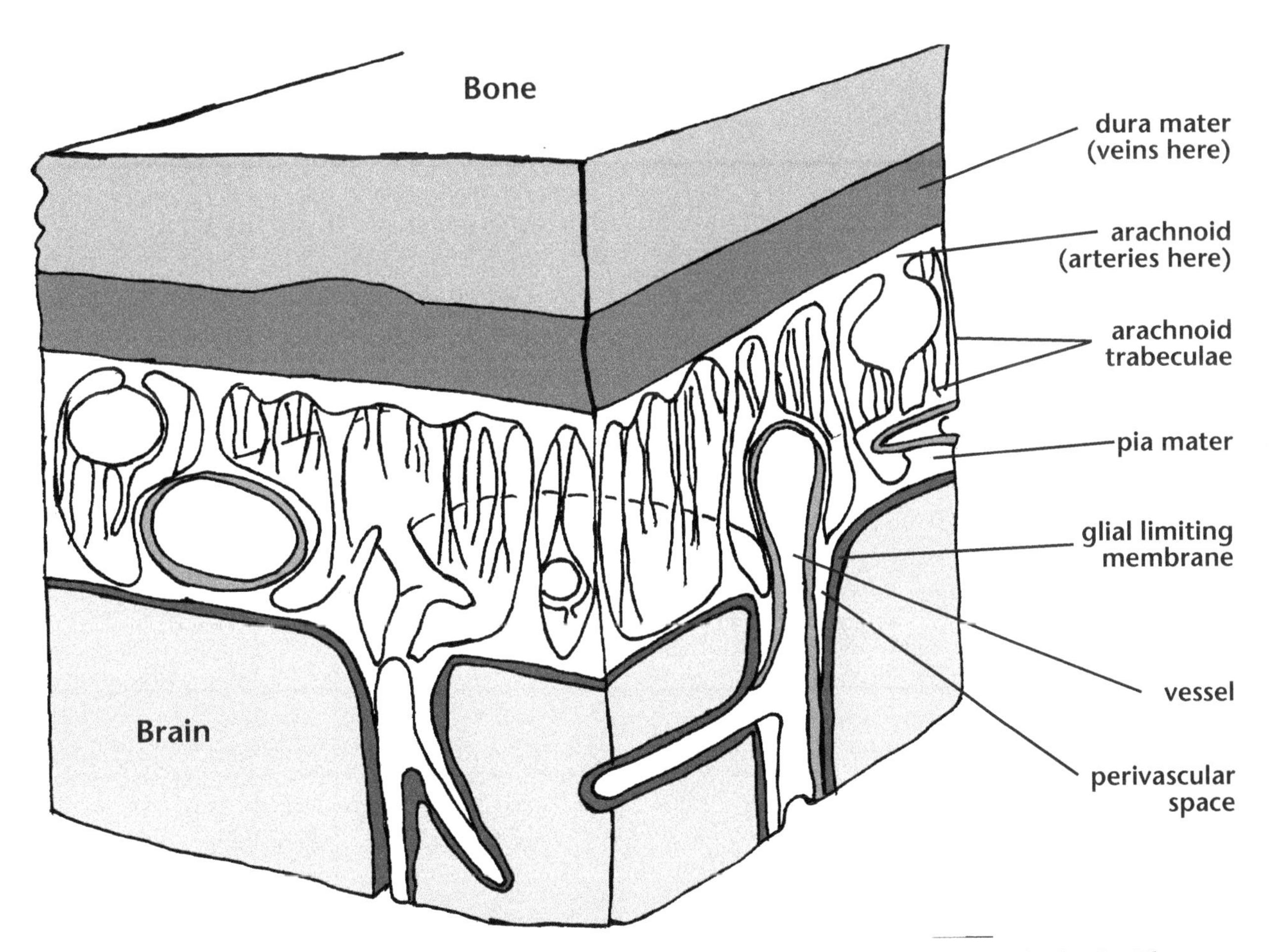

Figure 1. The meninges lie between the brain and the skull. The pia mater is closest to the brain. The highly vascular arachnoid is the next membrane. Just underlying the skull is the dura mater. Veins can rupture between the dura and the skull causing slow bleeding–a subdural hematoma.

Specific red flags:
Severe dizziness immediately after standing up

Condition assumed present until proven otherwise:

Severe orthostatic hypotension (Sudden drop in blood pressure when going from lying or sitting to standing posture–only a red flag if symptoms are severe, *i.e.*, fainting is imminent)

Possible consequences of missing the condition:

Possible syncope and falling, especially in elderly, causing fracture and possible death

Stabilization, referral, and management:

1. **Stabilization:** The only stabilizing step is to remind the patient to rise slowly from sitting or lying to standing position to allow blood pressure equalization.
2. **Consultation and Referral Options, Transportation:** Patient should be referred to their primary care provider for possible adjustment of medications and/or diagnostic workup to determine the cause of orthostatic dizziness.

ACTUAL CASE

- **History:** A 65-year-old Caucasian female presented with the complaint of severe dizziness and almost passing out every time she stood up suddenly. Her only medical problem was high blood pressure that was "under control" with medications.
- **Physical findings:** The patient had a normal physical exam. Her seated blood pressure was 110/70mmHg, but taken immediately after standing her blood pressure dropped to 95/65 mmHg.
- **Impression:** Orthostatic hypotension ("orthostasis"), probably from too much antihypertensive medications
- **Plan:** Patient was sent back to her PCP.
- **Follow up:** The physician caring for this patient's hypertension realized eventually that the patient had "white coat syndrome," which made it appear that her blood pressure was higher than it actually was because her readings were high every time her physician took them. Because of this overestimation of her blood pressure, her physician had continued to increase the dose of her antihypertensive medi- cines leading to overmedication and orthostatic hypotension. The patient is now taking her own blood pressure reading at home and using those readings to titrate her medication dose. She is on lower doses of antihypertensive meds and no longer has orthostatic hypotension. Her usual blood pressure is close to 120/80 mmHg.

DISCUSSION

Typical History and Symptoms

Additional symptoms, beyond the red flag symptom of dizziness vary with the underlying causes of the hypotension. The list of possible causes for orthostatic hypotension includes simple dehydration causing low volume of fluid in the circulation (hypovolemia), overmedication with antihypertensive medication, and more complex dysfunctions of the cardiovascular, neurological, endocrine or renal systems.

Physical Exam Findings

The patient may have an entirely negative exam. Blood pressure cycles up and down many times during the day and may be higher or lower than the patient's average reading at any given reading. Therefore, the best way to determine the patient's true blood pressure is to average many readings. Individual readings that are suspected to be inaccurate should always be repeated in different settings.

Although somewhat arbitrary and variable, the classical confirmatory sign of orthostatic hypotension in the literature is a decrease of 20 mmHg or more in systolic pressure or a decrease of 10 mmHg or more in diastolic pressure with the patient going from the lying to standing or sitting to standing position (or on a tilt table). Some patients get symptoms with lesser decreases in blood pressure drop, however. We must remember that this is a symptomatic condition, so the blood pressure reading alone is not sufficient to make the diagnosis. It is only confirmatory if symptoms exist.

Incidence and/or Prevalence

Orthostatic hypotension is extremely common, but there is much debate about its true prevalence. It has been reported to be between 5–30% in *normal* elderly subjects, many of whom are on medications. This red flag only considers severe orthostasis, however, enough to represent a danger from falling. The incidence of falling (from all causes) in community residents 65 and older is 30% (one fall/year) and 15% for recurrent falling. This latter number represents a huge threat because many of the elderly have osteoporosis and are at high risk for fracture and many never recover from the complications of their fractures. We must assume that orthostatic hypotension contributes significantly to falling, along with other obvious factors like muscle weakness, etc.

Risk Factors

- Age 65 or older (less sensitive baroreceptors, heart not as responsive to demands)
- Medications, including diuretics and other drugs for high blood pressure, beta-blockers, anti-Parkinson's drugs, tricyclic antidepressants, sildenafil (Viagra®), particularly in combination with nitroglycerin, narcotics, and alcohol
- Cardiovascular, neurological, renal, and endocrine problems
- Heat exposure and dehydration
- Bed rest (causes weakness)
- Crossing legs at the knees for prolonged periods (venous pooling)
- Pregnancy (lower blood pressure)
- General debilitation and malnutrition

Mechanism Producing the Red Flag

Orthostatic hypotension is caused by a temporarily inadequate supply of blood to the brain and subsequent neuronal hypofunction.

Another Important Consideration

- Acupuncture treatment of patients with severe orthostatic hypotension should be performed with patient lying down in a stable position, and should be carefully monitored for syncope upon arising after treatment. Acupuncture treatment can reduce blood pressure, generally a benign side effect, but fainting may be a result in those prone to orthostasis.

Specific red flags:
Dizziness and slow heartbeat (< 60 bpm) that does not increase with activity in an elderly person

Condition assumed present until proven otherwise:
Sick sinus syndrome (SSS)

Possible consequences of missing the condition:
Debility, falling and possible death

Stabilization, referral, and management:

1. **Stabilization:** Patients should not physically exert themselves or engage in activities where sudden syncope could have serious consequences (such as driving, equipment operation, etc.) until their condition is addressed through referral.
2. **Consultation and Referral Options, Transportation:** If the patient is not presenting with severe shortness of breath (SOB), they can be referred to their PCP on a timely basis, but should not drive themselves. If presenting with the above, they should be referred on a semi-urgent basis. As always, a 911 call should be placed with patients with syncope, severe SOB at rest (dyspnea at rest), chest pain or falling blood pressure. We would not expect these latter symptoms with SSS unless other heart and lung problems were present.

Relevance to acupuncturists: The mild and nonspecific symptoms of sick sinus syndrome may easily mislead both patient and practitioner from diagnosing a condition which can cause serious injury or even death by falling.

ACTUAL CASE

- **History:** A 60-year-old sedentary African-American female complained of mild shortness of breath and dizziness with mild exertion. She denied chest pain or syncope.
- **Physical findings:** The patient was 5'2" and 160 pounds. She seemed slow to respond to questions and paused several times to take a deep breath. Her resting pulse was 55 bpm and regular after a full minute of timing. Her heart tones were normal and her lungs were clear. There was no ankle edema.
- **Impression:** Possible sick sinus syndrome
- **Plan:** Patient was referred to a cardiologist who saw her the next day in his office.
- **Follow up:** The patient had a full cardiac workup in the hospital after a near syncopal attack at the cardiologist's office. She was found to have moderate coronary artery disease (CAD), and due to continued symptoms from her SSS, a cardiac pacemaker was implanted. The patient is doing well and is asymptomatic one year after the referral.

DISCUSSION

Typical History and Symptoms

Patients with sick sinus syndrome almost invariably complain of fatigue, weakness, and dizziness, especially with exertion. Symptoms indicating instability include shortness of breath, chest pain, and near-syncope or syncope. Falling episodes can result with deleterious results including fractures, head/brain injuries, etc. A history of risk factors for coronary and other types of heart disease (see chest pain section) should always be obtained whenever dizziness, shortness of breath, chest pain, abnormal heartbeats (palpitations) or other symptoms associated with cardiopulmonary disorders are suspected.

Physical Exam Findings

The patient may appear weak or hypo-responsive to normal stimuli, like normal conversation. The finding of a low pulse rate of <60 in an elderly, poorly conditioned person who obviously does not have athletic bradycardia (see mechanism of red flag) is a clear indicator of SSS.

Incidence and/or Prevalence

Best estimates are that 3% of people with slow heartbeats suffer from sick sinus syndrome, but the exact prevalence is unknown.

Risk Factors

The risk factors for sick sinus syndrome are the same as those noted for angina and heart disease under the chest pain red flags in this book and include:

- Coronary artery disease
- High blood pressure
- Heart valve disease
- Advanced age
- Lipid abnormalities
- Diabetes mellitus
- Lifestyle factors such as smoking, obesity, stress, lack of exercise, excessive use of caffeine or alcohol, or a diet high in animal fats and cholesterol also are associated with heart disease.

Mechanism Producing the Red Flag

Normal heart rate (at rest) is between 60-100 (bpm). In SSS, the heart cannot beat faster than approximately 60 bpm because the sinoatrial (SA) node (the heart's natural pacemaker) does not generate enough spontaneous beats. In contrast, the heart rate is slow in athletic bradycardia because the heart is so strong that it doesn't need to beat as often to supply the needed blood to the body because of a greater "stroke volume" with each beat.

SSS can also cause bradycardia-tachycardia syndrome (heart rates that fluctuate between being too slow and too fast) and can give rise to other arrhythmias that can be fatal. Any disorders that affect the coronary arteries or the myocardial muscles like arteriosclerosis can also produce diseases of the specialized tissue of the SA node and decrease its capacity to generate and transmit electrical impulses. The symptoms of sick sinus syndrome result from decreased perfusion of oxygen-sensitive tissues: brain, kidneys, and the myocardium itself.

Another Important Consideration

- This red flag could have easily been placed under the "slow pulse" category, but was placed under dizziness instead because that is usually how patients with this condition present.

▶ Specific red flags:
Adult or child with inattention and/or hyperactivity severely interfering with daily function

Condition assumed present until proven otherwise:
Attention deficit hyperactivity disorder (ADHD)

Possible consequences of missing the condition:
Increased risk of bipolar, conduct disorders, oppositional-defiance disorders, impaired self-esteem and self-confidence, decreased performance at school and/or work, social isolation and dysfunction, depression, possible death from substance abuse, and risk-taking behaviors

Stabilization, referral, and management:

1. **Stabilization:** There are no immediate stabilizing steps to take
2. **Consultation and Referral Options, Transportation:** The referral is certainly not an emergency, but should be on a timely basis. Treatment of ADHD is a hotly debated issue. In fact, its very existence is questioned by some people and health care providers. There is very solid evidence, however, that the disorder is real and can have a powerfully detrimental influence on some patients. An expert, or a group of experts, should be consulted for treatment of severe ADHD. This may include a skilled acupuncturist, family physician, psychologist, psychiatrist, dietician or neurologist. No special transport requirements are needed.

Relevance to acupuncturists: According to many sources, ADHD is common (see incidence below). If so, it will be encountered frequently by acupuncturists. ADHD signs and symptoms are not often self-reported, however, and may be dismissed by clinicians or parents as "normal,". Difficulty of treatment and risk of poor outcomes rises with delayed assessment and intervention of significant ADHD.

ACTUAL CASE

- **History:** The patient was a 25-year-old engineer recently promoted to supervision of all electrical systems of a large municipal Civic center. He was having trouble keeping up with organizing his new tasks. He came to the acupuncture clinic interested in "smart herbs" that could improve his mental performance. When asked if he was having any other problems with organization or function in his life, he said he had always had trouble following through on tasks. "I must have five or six projects going at the same time, but I never finish them. I'm the worst procrastinator I know of." He also claimed he had always had tremendous problems focusing on reading or other activities that required sustained concentration. Despite that, with "extreme effort," he had done well in college.
- **Physical findings:** The patient was a sharp-witted Asian American male who appeared bored and inattentive several times during the interview whenever the dialogue lasted more than a minute or so. He was given a self-scoring adult ADHD questionnaire to complete and his result was moderately positive for hyperactivity and strongly positive for inattention.
- **Impression:** Possible adult ADHD
- **Plan:** The patient and his questionnaire were sent to a local psychologist known for his work with ADHD for definitive diagnosis.
- **Follow up:** The patient was sent by his psychologist to a physician skilled with alternative and conventional treatment of ADHD. He was placed on an organic, whole food diet. Food allergens, dyes, and preservatives were eliminated. Based on urinary levels of neurotransmitters a course of targeted amino acid and vitamin therapy for neurotransmitter balancing was instituted. The patient had moderately good results with these measures, but wanted a trial of a stimulant medication. He was placed on extended release methylphenidate and claimed it made "a day and night difference" in his ability to concentrate on tasks. At last check, he had received another promotion at work and was functioning smoothly.

DISCUSSION

Typical History and Symptoms

The diagnosis of ADHD in children (5-6 years old or older) is often based upon ADHD questionnaires scored by parents and teachers who score the child's behavior at home and in the classroom. Adolescents and adults can provide the requisite history on the questionnaire for adults (see Appendix C or obtain ADHD forms on the internet). The questions differ for children versus adults but the common denominator is difficulty focusing on and finishing projects, whether self-imposed or given by teachers or supervisors at work.

Left untreated, the presentation of ADHD changes through the life cycle. Hyperactivity and impulsivity drop off dramatically throughout adolescence whereas inattention rises throughout college and adulthood. A history of struggling with academic and/or occupational performance is common in all groups, even though patients with ADHD are at least as intelligent as the average population. Adults with ADHD may be high-achieving professionals, but they almost invariably give a history of having to exert a great amount of effort to focus and perform effectively.

Physical Exam Findings

The patient with ADHD typically displays problems in three major areas of function:

1. **Attention deficit:** The patient will often look dreamy and unfocused in the exam room. Gaze may wander ceaselessly around the room. Direct, repetitive, and firm questioning is often needed to obtain answers.
2. **Hyperactivity:** Children will get out of their chair, wander around the room, touch objects, and keep moving constantly. All age groups typically bounce their legs, fidget, and shift position frequently when seated.
3. **Impulsivity:** Children may blurt out answers to questions asked to their parents before their parent can answer. Adults may interrupt or change topics frequently and seem unaware of their disruption to conversational continuity.

All children and adults may exhibit some of these behaviors at times. ADHD is identified by a seeming inability to control excessive, consistent and persistent display of such behaviors except for short periods of time when they are strongly coached to settle down and focus.

Incidence and/or Prevalence

The National Institute of Mental Health's (NIMH) 1997 estimate was that two million children in the U.S. have

ADHD (3–5% of school-age children). Some up-to-date estimates rate the prevalence much higher at 7–8% of school age children and 4–5% of adults >18 years old (*Everything You Wanted to Know About ADHD...But Forgot You Wanted to Ask,* Neuroscience Education Institute, 2008). Even if we take conservative estimates, ADHD is the most commonly diagnosed disorder of childhood. It occurs three times more often in boys than girls. At least one or two children in every classroom in the U.S. have this disorder. This statistic agrees with what most school teachers tell us about their classes.

Risk Factors

The single greatest risk factor for developing ADHD is heredity. Poor parenting techniques and poor diet (high sugar content, dyes and preservatives in foods, etc.) may influence how symptoms of ADHD are expressed, but do not seem to cause it.

Mechanism Producing the Red Flag

ADHD seems to result from dysfunction with several brain pathways that run from areas of the prefrontal cortex to striated area of the brain and the thalamus and emotional centers (limbic system). The neurotransmitter imbalance seems to be an inadequacy of norepinephrine and dopamine signals in these areas.

Other Important Considerations

- A plethora of epidemiologic data indicates that ADHD and substance abuse occur together much more frequently than in the normal population. Also, co-morbidity of ADHD with bipolar or conduct disorder has a synergistic effect on the risk of developing substance abuse.
- *Untreated* ADHD patients are about *twice as likely* as treated ADHD patients to develop substance abuse.
- Since ADHD is partly genetically determined, the process of diagnosing a child with ADHD will often cause one of the parents (usually the father) to realize that he also had ADHD as a child, albeit undiagnosed.

Specific red flags:
Sudden unconsciousness followed by severe drowsiness in a previously healthy adult

Condition assumed present until proven otherwise:
Seizure

Possible consequences of missing the condition:
Disability and possible death if untreated

Stabilization, referral, and management:

1. **Stabilization:** Patients should be advised to avoid driving or performing other activities that could be dangerous if they lost consciousness until their condition can be thoroughly evaluated and stabilized.
2. **Consultation and Referral Options, Transportation:** If the patient is fully recovered and seems stable, referral can be to their PCP on a semi-urgent basis, if one is available or to an urgent care center if a PCP is not available. A PCP might be able to deal with this problem or may refer to a neurologist after some basic testing is done.

Relevance to acupuncturists: The likelihood of missing this condition is high if the history of seizure-like activity (tonic-clonic motion) is not obtained from a witness because patients will have no memory of seizure activity and will simply think they fainted. The unconscious episode is often blamed on other factors when the patient is fully recovered.

ACTUAL CASE

- **History:** A previously healthy 34-year-old male accountant came to the office with his wife for acupuncture treatment on his shoulder. He had injured it after "passing out" several days earlier. He wasn't very concerned about "fainting" because he attributed it to having no breakfast that morning and being "dehydrated." He claimed to be in good health, running 4 miles a day, 4 days a week without problems. His wife saw the episode and says her husband "passed out and shook on the floor for about 30 seconds." The patient stated that he felt extremely fatigued for several hours after awakening. There was no prior history of syncope.
- **Physical findings:** His blood pressure was 110/78 mmHg and his pulse was 65 bpm and regular. The patient was lean and appeared fit and healthy. His neurological and cardiovascular examinations were normal.

- **Impression:** New onset seizure disorder likely; cause to be determined
- **Plan:** The patient was referred to his PCP.
- **Follow up:** The patient had normal labs with his PCP and was referred to a neurologist who ordered an electroencephalogram (EEG) and MRI of the brain, both of which were negative. The cause of the apparent seizure was undetermined at that time. Years later, after the patient's marriage broke up, his ex-wife confided to the PCP that her former husband had been secretly drinking heavily and had stopped "cold-turkey" two days before the seizure.

DISCUSSION

Typical History and Symptoms

Patients with the new onset of a seizure disorder will often be unaware of seizure activity. They will, however, report the "postictal" or post-seizure state. The *postictal state* occurs after a significant seizure and lasts 5–30 minutes or longer. It is characterized by extreme fatigue, drowsiness, disorientation and sometimes headache.

Occasionally, patients have increased blood pressure in and memory deficits (including amnesia) in the postical state, which makes the diagnosis more difficult. This is another important reason that a witness should be sought out to see if seizure activity was present. Depression after a seizure is also fairly common.

Physical Exam Findings

The physical exam is often unremarkable. This is understandable when we consider that a definite cause for the new onset of a seizure disorder is undetermined in just over 50% of cases. Even if there were a definable cause present, such as a brain tumor for example, the seizure may be the first manifestation of the tumor and there may well be no neurological findings before the seizure occurs.

Incidence and/or Prevalence (Statistics from the Epilepsy Foundation)

The incidence of the new onset of a seizure in the U.S. is 300,000 people per year, 120,000 of them are under the age of 18. Up to one-third (100,000) are children under the age of five who have a febrile seizure. The prevalence in the U.S. is three million people.

Risk Factors

While specific risk factors for seizures are unclear, associations have been identified as follows:

- Mental retardation–25.8% have seizures.
- Cerebral palsy–13% of children have seizures.
- Children with both disabilities–50% have seizures.
- Alzheimer patients–10% have seizures.
- Stroke patients–22% have seizures.
- Children of mothers with epilepsy–8.7% have seizures.
- Children of fathers with epilepsy–2.4% have seizures.
- People who have had a single, unprovoked seizure–33% have further seizures.

Mechanism Producing the Red Flag

The causes for seizure are varied, but patients always have abnormal brain waves, the so-called paroxysmal "spike and wave pattern" on the EEG. Paroxysmal brain wave activity hijacks all other brain activity as it spreads across various regions of the brain.

Other Important Considerations

- The most common causes of seizures depend on the age at which they start.
- <2 years old: High fevers are the most common cause followed by temporary metabolic abnormalities such as abnormal blood glucose, calcium, magnesium, vitamin B6 or sodium levels. These kinds of seizures do not continue into later life if the conditions that cause them do not reappear. Children in this age group who do not have one of these causes are likely to have suffered a brain injury during birth or a have a hereditary metabolic abnormality or brain disorder.
- 2–14 years old: The cause is often unknown.
- 25 years old: Head injuries, strokes and tumors are common causes as is withdrawal from alcohol in a person who has been drinking heavily. The most common cause in this age group, however, is still idiopathic (>50%).
- Other causes of seizures not listed above are bleeding and infections in the brain, degenerative conditions of the brain and dementia, kidney or liver failure, use of cocaine or stimulants, stopping CNS depressants like barbiturates and benzodiazepines after long-term use and phenylketonuria (PKU), which can cause seizures in infants.

Specific red flags:
Sudden leg weakness and possible unconsciousness in elderly person when turning head

Condition assumed present until proven otherwise:
"Drop attack" from vertebrobasilar artery insufficiency (VBI). VBI is caused by significantly decreased blood flow in the vertebral artery as it courses through the transverse foramina of the cervical vertebra to supply blood to the basilar artery of the brain (see figure 2).

Possible consequences of missing the condition:
Falling episodes with possible injury or death; increased risk of stroke

Stabilization, referral, and management:

1. **Stabilization:** The patient should be cautioned to avoid extreme rotation of neck, dehydration, extreme exertion, or activities that require maintenance of posture until consult is obtained. Cervical rotation and extension to end-ranges in the elderly or patients with history of drop attacks are contraindicated, even if such manipulations are intended to relieve neck pain, because of the risk of drop attacks and strokes due to VBI. Likewise, the foraminal compression test should not be done on patients with this red flag.
2. **Consultation and Referral Options, Transportation:** Since the patient is probably safe as long as avoiding extremes of neck rotation, the referral can be timely to the patient's PCP if available or to a cardiologist if a PCP cannot be obtained. Private transport is acceptable, but the patient should avoid extreme rotation of the neck while driving.

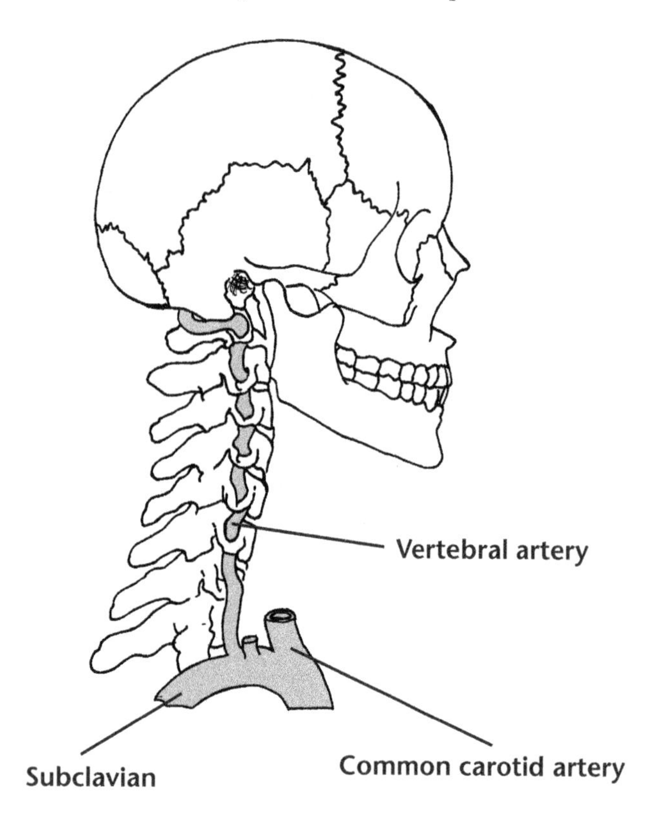

Figure 2. The vertebral artery is shown coursing through the transverse foramina of the cervical vertebra toward portions of the brain that control muscle tone. Bony spurs from arthritis can compress the vertebral artery anywhere along its course. Compression on the artery can be worsened by turning the head in extreme rotation causing a "drop attack."

Relevance to acupuncturists: This is a condition that is easy to pick up because of its interesting history and doing so may help the patient avoid dangerous falls.

ACTUAL CASE

- **History:** A 72-year-old man presented to our office for the treatment of neck pain. On review of systems he said he had a "strange problem." A few days earlier his wife was talking to him and, when he turned his head to look at her, his knees buckled and he fell. Fortunately, he did not injure himself. The only other major problem the patient had was "arthritis all over my body."
- **Physical findings:** He had a normal physical exam except for some stiffness in the low back and neck in most directions in the range of motion (ROM) exam (extreme neck rotation was avoided).
- **Impression:**"Drop attack" from VBI
- **Plan:** Patient was referred to his PCP.
- **Follow up:** The patient was found to have narrowing (stenosis) of his vertebral arteries on a magnetic resonance angiogram (MRA) and fairly severe arthritic spurs in the cervical spine area impinging upon the vertebral arteries when he turned his neck.

DISCUSSION

Typical History and Symptoms

Symptoms of VBI typically occur in the elderly, reflecting the increased incidence of cervical spine osteoarthritis and atherosclerosis in this age group. Drop attacks occasionally occur without neck rotation, however, as other factors can decrease blood flow to neck arteries. The blood pressure in the vertabral system may also fall to critical levels from dehydration, overuse of leg muscles, arteriosclerosis, or other factors that decrease blood flow.

The general risk factors for atherosclerosis are often present in patients with VBI. Patients with VBI typically experience the sensation of their legs giving way and can fall to the floor without losing consciousness.

Physical Exam Findings

Besides the patient being elderly, there may be no distinguishing physical findings. The presence of a carotid bruit would indicate the possible presence of insufficiency in the anterior circulation. This would mean that both the anterior arteries (carotids) and the posterior artery (both vertebral arteries flow to one basilar artery) may be partially blocked. A decrease in cervical ROM suggests that patient has degenerative joint disease and that osteophytes can occlude arteries as they rise through the neck.

Incidence and/or Prevalence

The exact incidence of VBI is unknown. The incidence of VBI rises as the general incidence of atherosclerosis rises. Men are twice as likely to present with VBI as women.

Risk Factors

Same as risk factors for atherosclerosis (see chest pain section). Degenerative joint disease (cervical spine osteoarthritis with facet hypertrophy) of the neck is an additional risk factor.

Mechanism Producing the Red Flag

VBI occurs because of temporary blockage of the bilateral vertebral arteries and their continuation as the basilar artery (the *posterior* circulation), which supplies blood to the middle and posterior portions of the brain, including the vision center. The temporary decrease in blood supply to centers *in the brainstem* is responsible for loss of muscle tone in the legs.

Other Important Considerations

- The maintenance of consciousness distinguishes drop attacks from true syncope and epilepsy.
- Physicians, chiropractors, osteopaths (and probably acupuncturists) have induced VBI while performing cervical manipulations intended to relieve neck pain. There have been reported minor and major strokes due to this. Care should be exercised in the elderly.
- Drop attacks can have other causes besides VBI, including carotid sinus hypersensitivity wherein carotid stimulation causes drops in blood pressure. Other causes include the vascular, cardiac, neurological, structural, metabolic, and psychological problems associated with presyncope and syncope.
- In the United States, 25% of strokes and transient ischemic attacks occur in the vertebrobasilar distribution. These must be separated from strokes arising from the anterior circulation which involves the carotid arteries.
- Patients with Meniere's syndrome can experience symptoms that mimic VBI.

▶ Specific red flags:
Loud snoring, gasping during sleep, and excessive daytime sleepiness

Condition assumed present until proven otherwise:
Sleep apnea–a significant cessation of breathing during sleep (see definitive parameters below)

Possible consequences of missing the condition:
Diminished concentration, decreased quality of life, increased risk of cardiovascular disease, and sudden death from narcoleptic accident

Stabilization, referral, and management:

1. **Stabilization:** There are no immediate stabilizing steps to take.
2. **Consultation and Referral Options, Transportation:** Referral should be to the PCP if one is available or to a free-standing medical clinic or an ENT physician if a PCP is not available. If the patient is experiencing sudden lapses into sleep during daytime, they are at high risk for motor vehicle accidents and the referral is semi-urgent, with a family member or friend serving as driver. Otherwise, the referral is on a timely basis.

Relevance to acupuncturists: Many of the complications of sleep apnea are symptoms for which patients commonly seek acupuncture care, including fatigue, insomnia, depression, headaches, generalized malaise, sexual dysfunction, weight gain, and tobacco addiction. Acupuncturists are, therefore, in an excellent position to ask questions about sleep quality during the interview.

Signs of sleep hypopnea (decreased breathing) or sleep apnea (cessation of breathing) like loud snoring, intermittent breathing and/or gasping may emerge if the patient should happen to doze off on the acupuncture table. Even seemingly minor manifestations during napping may be amplified a great deal over the course of a full night's sleep. By routinely screening for sleep apnea, a chronic, debilitating, and easily treatable disease can be identified and treated, thereby avoiding possible complications of this condition.

ACTUAL CASE

- **History:** The patient, a 45-year-old Caucasian male, came to the office for his second office visit with his wife. She was not present on the first visit. His complaint was severe fatigue and sleepiness in the afternoon. He denied taking medication, ingesting alcohol, or using other drugs, and said he was otherwise healthy. When asked about his sleep quality, he said he had no problem falling asleep and slept soundly through the night for 7-8 hours. When asked about possible snoring, he said he did not snore much, repeating what he had stated on his first office visit two weeks earlier. When he said this, his wife sat suddenly upright in her chair, looked at her husband in shocked disbelief, and blurted out, "You snore like a freight train and sound like you're going to choke to death."
- **Physical findings:** The patient looked sleepy. He was 5'6" tall, 220 pounds, most of his fat in his midsection. He also had a thick neck with a lot of fat around it. His face was broad, his palate long, and his tongue thick and beefy. His oropharyngeal opening looked small. His blood pressure was 140/90mmHg. His lungs were clear.
- **Impression:** Probable sleep hypopnea and/or sleep apnea
- **Plan:** The patient was referred to his PCP who ordered a screening test of obstructive sleep apnea (OSA)
- **Follow up:** The patient had outpatient sleep study at home with a simple finger-clip oxygen meter (oximeter), which suggested moderate severe sleep apnea as evidenced by plunging oxygen readings. A full sleep study confirmed the diagnosis and the PCP referred the patient to an ear, nose, throat (ENT) specialist. The patient was prescribed a continuous positive airway pressure (CPAP) machine for night use that pumped air into his lungs at the end of his inhalations. The patient slept with this machine for several nights, then "tossed it in the closet" stat ing he would rather have sleep apnea than sleep with it (a not uncommon reaction to the CPAP machine).

Meanwhile, his wife, desperate for some relief from her husband's snoring, scoured the internet looking for a solution. She finally ordered an oral appliance that fit into his mouth. The simple appliance cost about $100 and proved to be about 90% effective in stopping the snoring and choking sounds according to the wife. The patient was still using it as of last check. He also wears it when getting acupuncture treatments and claims he gets more benefit from his treatments since wearing it. He has not had a repeat sleep study when using the appliance, but this has been suggested by his PCP.

DISCUSSION

Typical History and Symptoms

Patients with sleep apnea are rarely aware of having difficulty breathing because they only partially wake up after episodes. It is generally the sleep partner who makes note of the problem, often complaining about their partner's snoring or "gasping for breath." Symptoms of daytime sleepiness, malaise, lethargy, and fatigue may be present and go unreported to health care providers for years or decades because the patient generally accepts these symptoms as normal.

Other tip-offs, although less specific, include morning headaches, trouble concentrating, irritability, forgetfulness, moodiness, sexual dysfunction, depression, frequent nightmares, difficulty getting up in the morning, or, perhaps most dramatically, falling asleep inappropriately during the day (see also narcolepsy red flags) or while driving.

Tip-offs for sleep apnea in children, also a serious problem, include mouth breathing and snoring at night.

Physical Exam Findings

No specific body type or gender can guarantee that a patient does or does not have sleep apnea. It can occur in children or thin young adults as well as overweight older adults. However, the majority of patients with severe obstructive sleep apnea syndrome (OSAS) are middle-aged, overweight males with thick necks and increased size of the soft palate and tongue. A receding jaw, elongated or high-arched palate, redundant peripharyngeal tissue, and enlarged uvula may also be present and not appear to allow enough room for the airway in the back of the throat. All of this can be easily noted on physical examination. In children, look for mouth breathing and large tonsils. The definitive test for sleep apnea is the polysomnogram (see below).

Incidence and/or Prevalence

Three primary types of sleep apnea are identifiable: Obstructive Sleep Apnea (OSA), Central Sleep Apnea (CSA), and mixed obstructive-central sleep apnea. OSA is the most common affecting 4.41% of the U.S. population. The frequency of CSA and mixed obstructive-central sleep apnea are not known. A reasonable estimate of overall sleep apnea, however, is one in 15 or 6.62% or 18 million people in the U.S. A male to female predominance diminishes with increasing age. Beyond age 50 years, incidence rates among men and women tend toward similarity.

Risk Factors for Obstructive Sleep Apnea

Demographic

- Middle-aged men are twice as likely to have sleep apnea as middle-age women, with the gap narrowing with age.
- Sleep apnea occurs two to three times more often in adults older than 65.

Medical history, anatomy, and health behaviors

- Excess weight
- Neck circumference > 17.5 inches. Fat deposits around the upper airway obstruct breathing.
- A congenitally narrowed airway or due to enlarged tonsils and/or adenoids.
- Family history of sleep apnea increases risk.
- Use of alcohol, sedatives, or tranquilizers relaxes the muscles in the throat, increasing the risk of sleep apnea.
- Smokers are three times more likely to have obstructive sleep apnea than nonsmokers (increases inflammation and fluid retention in the upper airway).

Risk Factors for Central Sleep Apnea

- Male sex
- Atrial fibrillation or congestive heart failure
- Stroke or brain tumors

Mechanism Producing the Red Flag

In (OSA), the respiratory effort is normal. Breathing is interrupted by a physical block to airflow. In (CSA), breathing is interrupted by the *lack of respiratory effort* because brain centers that regulate normal breathing are not functioning properly. Complex (or "mixed") sleep apnea has features of both.

OSA is caused by recurring upper airway obstruction during sleep as a result of narrowed respiratory passages, mostly in the oropharyngeal region, although nasal passages can also play a part. Decreased airway muscle tone during sleep and gravity's pull on the oropharynx in the supine position further decrease airway size and impedes airflow.

Partial obstruction leads to snoring and hypopnea. Total obstruction causes apnea. Apnea sets off a reflex struggle mechanism arousing the patient from sleep. The arousals are usually not recognized by the patient because they are partial and the patient usually quickly falls back to sleep.

The arousals do temporarily increase the muscle tone of the oropharyngeal structure until the patient falls back to sleep and the cycle repeats itself.

Other Important Considerations

- Polysomnography in a hospital has been the gold standard for diagnosing OSA. Polysomnography in a hospital is expensive, however, and not available in all locales. Home sleep studies are less costly and are becoming more popular.
- Clinically significant levels of sleep apnea are defined as five or more episodes per hour of any type of apnea (from the polysomnogram). A cessation of breathing for 10 seconds or more with either neurological arousal (measured by the EEG) and/or blood oxygen desaturation of 3-4% or greater is positive for severe sleep apnea.
- Complications of sleep apnea include: snoring, hypertension, pulmonary hypertension, cardiac disease and heart attacks, arrhythmias, stroke, sudden death, sudden death from falling asleep driving or at work, accidents, sudden infant death syndrome, and mood disorders, most clearly major depressive disorder. The chronic fatigue, sleepiness, lethargy and poor concentration from sleep apnea can lead to generalized declines in physical, social, recreational and occupational functioning, all of which can exacerbate weight gain and depression, a vicious downward spiral that can greatly decrease quality of life while increasing morbidity and mortality.
- Eliminating the obstruction usually quickly reverses the commonly associated pulmonary and systemic hypertension as well as cardiac problems. Patients successfully treated often report prompt and significant (sometimes described as "life-changing") improvements in energy, well-being, mood, concentration and functioning.
- Sudden infant death syndrome is now thought to be a result of sleep apnea.
- Treatments for OSA include weight loss, nasal CPAP and dental devices that modify the position of the tongue or jaw. Upper airway and jaw surgical procedures may be appropri-

ate in selected patients, but are invasive and expensive.

- Possible non-surgical treatments helpful for sleep apnea besides weight loss include avoidance of alcohol before bedtime, elevation of the head of the bed, sleeping on one's side, reducing bedroom allergens, avoidance of smoking, avoidance of heavy eating before bedtime, humidifying the environment, avoiding sleep aids and over-fatigue.
- Regular cardiovascular exercise has been shown to increase respiratory drive as well as improving smooth muscle tone of the airways and enhancing weight loss. Cardiovascular exercise is thus highly indicated for all types of sleep apnea (although patients with advanced cardiovascular disease should be evaluated by a physician prior to commencing vigorous cardiovascular exercise).

Specific red flags:
Excessive daytime drowsiness and sudden falling asleep in daytime without warning

Condition assumed present until proven otherwise:
Narcolepsy

Possible consequences of missing the condition:
Disability or death from falling asleep at the wrong time

Stabilization, referral, and management:

1. **Stabilization:**There are no specific stabilizing steps except to have the patient avoid situations wherein they or others could be injured or killed if they suddenly fall asleep.
2. **Consultation and Referral Options, Transportation:** The referral should be to the patient's PCP if one is available or to an ENT physician if one is not.

Relevance to acupuncturists: This is really a sleeper red flag, no pun intended. Except in the case of cataplexy (sudden collapse at moments of strong emotion), which generally gets the patient's undivided attention, narcoleptic patients often "fly under the radar" of detection by clinicians because they have learned to minimize and work around their condition with naps and other techniques. They often accept their condition as normal. The acupuncturist must keep a high index of suspicion for this disorder because the treatment is fairly simple and can make a huge impact on the patient's quality of life as well as safety.

ACTUAL CASE

- **History:** A 48-year-old unmarried professor of English literature came into the office with the complaint of "fatigue" lasting all day long. He reported sleeping 7-8 hours at night. He said that it was necessary for him to nap often during the day "to make it through." Most embarrassingly to him, however, he would sometimes fall asleep for a short while at inappropriate times, like during the middle of giving a lecture. His students attributed these incidents to his "busy teaching schedule" and the fact that the material was "sometimes dull." He just accepted that he was the "absentminded professor." His sometimes bed partner told him that he snored a little at night, but did not quit breathing or seem to gasp for air.
- **Physical findings:** The patient was a sleepy looking, but seemingly intelligent man in an old tweed sports coat and jeans. Several times during the interview he appeared to look down and dose for a few seconds, but recovered quickly each time. His neurological exam was normal.
- **Impression:** Possible undiagnosed narcolepsy, rule out OSA also
- **Plan:** The patient was referred to a neurologist because he had no PCP.
- **Follow up:** The professor underwent a sleep study which showed mild hypopnea, but no significant sleep apnea. He was eventually diagnosed with narcolepsy (everything else was excluded and it seemed the most reasonable explanation for the patient's symptoms) and put on a trial of stimulant medication that has allowed him to be alert throughout the day. The patient is exceedingly happy about this and claims the medicine has been "life changing".

DISCUSSION

History and Symptoms

It is common for narcoleptics to have more than one of the four main symptoms of narcolepsy, but rare for them to have all four.

1. **Excessive daytime sleepiness** is universally present. Patients with narcolepsy may occasionally fall asleep at inappropriate times, like while driving or talking to someone.
2. **Cataplexy** is the sudden, temporary loss of muscle tone causing collapse without unconsciousness lasting from

seconds to minutes. Mild attacks can cause slurred speech, droopy eyelids or hand weakness and dropping objects. This can resemble clumsiness. Cataplexy can be brought on by strong emotion, laughter, excitement or anger.

3. **Sleep paralysis** is the temporary inability to move while falling asleep or awakening.
4. **Hypnagogic hallucinations** are dreamlike images with falling asleep or waking up.

Approximately 60% of people with diagnosed narcolepsy have the combination of marked daytime sleepiness and cataplexy. Symptoms of narcolepsy usually begin during adolescence or young adulthood, but narcolepsy can occur at any age. Daytime sleepiness is also the earliest symptom, which is usually blamed on other problems, often delaying the correct diagnosis. *Daytime sleepiness is independent of whether or not a patient has had sufficient sleep the night before.* Narcoleptics often complain of fatigue and impaired performance at work and school.

Memory lapses and visual disturbances may be particularly upsetting to these patients. Over 50% of people with narcolepsy experience periods of memory loss caused by very short periods of sleep. During "micro-sleeps" patients may write or speak nonsense, misplace objects or even injure themselves. Patients with narcolepsy suffer from depression much more frequently than the general population, but they are also often misdiagnosed with other psychological illnesses.

Physical Exam Findings

Untreated narcoleptic patients will often appear groggy if the patient interview goes over 10-15 minutes. The neurological exam, however, is also entirely normal except for the above.

Incidence and/or Prevalence

Narcolepsy usually appears between ages 15 and 30, but the condition can appear earlier or later. Once it appears, narcolepsy is present for life. Men and women are affected equally. Narcolepsy affects at least 120,000 people in the United States.

Risk Factors

The cause or causes of narcolepsy are unknown. Many researchers postulate that multiple factors may be involved such as those listed below.

- Heredity: Narcoleptics have a 10% chance of having a close relative with similar symptoms. A genetic link involves the regulation of hypocretin.
- Infectious disease may play a part.
- People with brain injuries due to conditions such as brain tumors or strokes seem to be at higher risk.
- Contact with toxins, such as DDT and pesticides may play a role.
- Autoimmune disorders may be contributory.

Mechanism Producing the Red Flag

Narcolepsy is apparently caused by a dysfunction in the part of the brain that regulates rapid eye movement (REM) sleep because patients with this disorder go from wakefulness to REM without passing through the other normal stages to get there. Cataplexy is associated with a shortage of a brain-stimulating protein called orexin, also known as hypocretin. The sudden relaxing of muscle tone is probably the result of the brain abruptly entering REM sleep. Like cataplexy, sleep paralysis probably is related to insufficient separation between REM sleep and wakefulness.

Review What You Have Learned
Chapter 3 Altered Mental Function

1. A sustained and significant decrease in mental sharpness lasting for more than two weeks, not accompanied by a neurological deficit (like numbness or paralysis), is a general red flag for

a. Stroke
b. Vertigo
c. Neuronal hypofunction
d. Neuronal hyperfunction

2. What is true about the terms "dizziness" and "vertigo?"

a. Both can be used interchangeably to indicate near-fainting
b. Vertigo is the sensation that a person or their surroundings are spinning whereas dizziness indicates wooziness or light-headedness
c. Vertigo almost always marks a serious underlying disorder whereas dizziness seldom does
d. Dizziness is the sensation of spinning, vertigo is the sensation of fainting

3. Dementia

a. Is often reported first by a patient's family members rather than the patient
b. Is often preceded by months to years of mental decline
c. Can be caused by small strokes (lacunar state) or Alzheimer's disease, among others
d. All of the above
e. A and B

4. Mental decline in the elderly

a. Is inevitable because new neurons do not arise in the brain after childhood
b. Can often be delayed or even halted by properly designed and challenging learning tasks
c. Is often accepted as normal
d. A and C

5. Chronic, nonorthostatic dizziness (not upon standing) could be the result of

a. Severe anemia
b. Chronic heart failure
c. Chronic low blood pressure
d. All of the above

6. Patients who have severe vertigo are best referred to what type of medical doctor?

a. Cardiologists
b. Pulmonologists
c. Psychiatrists
d. Ear, Nose and Throat physicians

7. Increasing confusion over weeks to months in the elderly after minor head trauma is a red flag for

a. Epidural hematoma
b. Stroke
c. Dementia
d. Chronic subdural hematoma

8. Generalized cerebral symptoms such as confusion and weakness would be most compatible with which of the following brain disorders?

a. Slow growing brain tumors
b. Acute arterial bleeding in the brain
c. Slow accumulation of blood from venous rupture under the dura mater
d. All of the above
e. A and C

9. Severe dizziness after standing up is most common in

a. Patients with high blood pressure not on antihypertensive medications
b. Patients taking antihypertensive medications
c. Patients with low blood pressure
d. A and C
e. B and C

10. Patients with "Sick Sinus Syndrome"

a. Are not able to increase cardiac output enough to meet increasing circulatory needs of the body due to a limited heart rate
b. Are not able to increase cardiac output enough to meet increasing circulatory needs of the body due to a limit on cardiac stroke volume (% of blood pumped out with each systole)
c. Have chronic yeast infection of the sinuses
d. Often have "athletic bradycardia"

11. Attention deficit/hyperactivity disorder

a. Is more often diagnosed in girls than boys
b. Can cause life-long learning and social adjustment problems if it is severe enough and untreated
c. Should be recognized and managed regardless of treatment options with TCM, medications, etc.
d. All of the above
e. B and C

12. Severe drowsiness lasting several hours following waking from an unconscious episode

a. Is a red flag for having a brain tumor
b. Is a red flag for having had a seizure
c. Is a red flag for having had a heart attack
d. Is a red flag for having dementia

13. The vertebral arteries

a. Supplies blood to the prefrontal cerebral cortex
b. Run through the spinal canal to the midbrain
c. Flow to the basilar artery and the posterior brain circulation
d. Flow to the vertebra to nourish the disks

14. Obstructive Sleep Apnea (OSA)

a. Never occurs in children
b. Is best diagnosed with an Electroencephalogram (EEG)
c. Is common, affecting approximately 4.5-6.5% of the U.S. population
d. Is relatively rare, but dangerous, affecting approximately 0.5% of the U.S. population

15. What is true about the association between snoring, body build and OSA?

a. OSA is never found in thin individuals
b. OSA is often diagnosed in patients with thick necks who snore loudly at night
c. Snoring, weight and OSA are unrelated
d. OSA does not produce illness, but does prevent a person's bed partner from resting well

Chapter 4: ANIMAL BITES

While the main focus of this chapter is about rabies infection, there are other problems that can occur from animal bites. Patients should be monitored carefully and, if possible, the animal involved should be found and tested.

Among domesticated animals, rabies is more often found in cats than dogs. Cats and dogs, together with horses, cattle, mules, sheep, goats and ferrets, account for 90% of rabies cases in domesticated animals. Among wild animals, the disease is most often reported in skunks and raccoons, bats, foxes and rodents. The ultimate source for information concerning animal bites and risk of rabies can be easily obtained from your county health department. The following comments are a general summary of what might be included in your local health department information. It should not replace that information.

It's important for health care practitioners to recognize the kind of animal that might transmit the rabies virus so patients can be advised properly. Rabid animals are often aggressive, very sensitive to touch and vicious with stimulation. This "rabid" form of the disease is traditionally associated with mad dogs. There is also a "dumb" form in which the animal is lethargic, weak and unable to raise its head or make sounds due to paralysis of throat and neck muscles. In both kinds, death in animals so affected occurs days after these symptoms appear.

Humans exposed to the rabies virus are asymptomatic for 10 days to more than a year after exposure (average 30–50 days). After this symptom-free period they complain of malaise, loss of appetite, fatigue, headache, and fever. Over half have pain at the puncture site. They may complain of insomnia or depression. Two to 10 days later, hyperactivity and hypersensitivity, disorientation, hallucinations, seizures, and paralysis appear. Death may be sudden due to cardiac or respiratory arrest or may follow a coma that can last for months with life-support.

There is no cure for rabies, but it can be prevented by immunization after exposure because the rabies virus takes a comparatively long time to induce disease. ***A bite or scratch from a vicious or lethargic animal (or finding a bat in a room with a sleeping person)*** should be considered a general red flag for ***possible exposure to the rabies virus.*** The proper action in such cases is to clean the site with soap and water (the most valuable preventative measure) and send the patient to the nearest ED for their first dose of the vaccine within a day or two.

Specific red flags:
Cat bite of a finger with subsequent swelling and pain

Condition assumed present until proven otherwise:

Serious infection of tendon and/or bone (osteomyelitis)

Possible consequences of missing the condition:

Tendon infection with possible rupture and/or permanent injury and lifelong bone infection

Stabilization, referral, and management:

1. **Stabilization:** There are no particular stabilizing steps.

2. **Consultation and Referral Options, Transportation:** Patient should be referred to their PCP if they have one. Infectious disease or surgical consult may eventually be needed. The referral should be on a semi-urgent basis with patient or family transportation adequate.

Relevance to acupuncturists: Acupuncturists may not be the first resort for many patients with animal bites that appear severe on first inspection, but they may well be consulted for bites that seem smaller, like the types of penetrating bites we discuss in this red flag. Such bites may draw little blood and be passed off as less consequential, but we can see the inherent difficulty with them when we study this red flag. They should actually be referred to someone who can deal with the infectious possibilities before they reach the red flag stage.

ACTUAL CASE

- **History:** A 20-year-old patient came to the office with the complaint of a cat bite. She owned a "normally sweet and gentle" cat named "Dusty." One day, as she tried to restrain Dusty from hissing at another cat on her patio, Dusty suddenly dug his teeth into her finger. She treated it with washing and soaking her finger in Epson salts, but noticed that the site was swollen and red two days later. It also was very painful to move her finger.

Physical findings: The patient removed a bandage from her right index finger to reveal a red, swollen finger with central fang-type bite marks on the dorsal aspect of her middle phalanx. The finger was painful to palpation and ROM was limited due to pain and swelling. There was no discernable abscess under the skin surface. Rather, the entire finger was hot, swollen, shiny and red from the first metatarsal phalangeal joint distally.

- **Impression:** Cat bite with possible fascial, tendon, and bone infection
- **Plan:** Patient had no family physician available and an orthopedic surgeon could not be reached. She was sent to an urgent care center.
- **Follow up:** The patient was given an oral antibiotic at the urgent care center. Unfortunately, she did not improve and ended up going to the ED for continued pain and swelling in the finger. Despite IV antibiotics in the hospital, her finger became hotter and more painful over the next several days and she finally needed surgery to open the fascia (fasciotomy) to relieve pressure that had built up under it. The wound was cleansed thoroughly down to the bone. Despite this, she developed infection of the bone (osteomyelitis), which required a second operation to scrape away the infected parts of the bone. This time, her surgeon left the incision open to the bone to prevent microbes from being trapped again. Though she has a disfigured finger that must be kept covered, she has had no return of her osteomyelitis.

DISCUSSION

History and Symptoms

The symptoms listed in this red flag capture the initial history and progressive nature of infections from deeply penetrating wounds like cat bites.

Physical Exam Findings

The physical signs vary with the tissues infected. The deeper the structure, the greater the pain. An inability to move an extremity implies, that tendons are affected.

Incidence and/or Prevalence

About one million animal bites require medical attention each year. About 90% are from dogs.

Risk Factors

Patients with cats as pets.

Mechanism Producing the Red Flag

The red flag is produced by the destructive effect of deep infection and inflammation. Cat bites are deep and penetrating and the sharp fangs deliver infection deeply, but the narrow aperture from fang entry does not allow infection to escape easily.

Other Important Considerations

- Even though dog bites can do much more initial damage than cat bites because they are tearing and macerating, they are much less prone to cause the kinds of complications we've outlined for cat bites.
- This red flag points out the importance of *early and aggressive treatment of all injuries that penetrate to the bone*, even if there is little immediate swelling because the specter of chronic osteomyelitis can be so devastating to a patient.

Review What You Have Learned

Chapter 4 Animal Bites

1. The organism that produces rabies is

a. A virus
b. A bacterium
c. More likely to be encountered in dogs than cats
d. Is only encountered with bites from wild animals

2. Cat bites are more often associated with serious soft tissue/bone infection than dog bites because

a. The fangs of cats often penetrate deeper and there is less chance for infection to escape from the narrow aperture of the wound produced by fangs
b. Dogs have cleaner mouths than humans
c. Cats are more vicious than dogs
d. Cats are more likely to bite people than dogs are

3. Osteomyelitis (bone infection)

a. Can be accompanied by infection of the fascia covering muscles
b. Should be suspected by acupuncturists if signs of chronic infection are present (redness, pain, etc.) in an extremity following penetrating trauma, even if weeks or months have passed
c. Can lead to chronic, lifelong infection
d. All of the above

Chapter 5: BLEEDING FROM AN ORIFICE

The loss of blood in both Western and Chinese medicine is considered a serious, acute symptom that needs to be stopped as quickly as possible. Any of the orifices can bleed abnormally. While such occurrences can be nonserious, short-term events, they can also be symptoms of very serious disease. This chapter covers potentially serious bleeding events that warrant quick referral.

Bleeding from a body orifice is a general red flag for potentially ***serious tissue destruction***. Bleeding in general, and the amount and extent of the bleeding in particular, indicates erosion into tissues containing blood vessels. Even though there are nonserious (self-limiting) causes for bleeding from an orifice, there are enough serious causes so that ***bleeding from a body orifice*** meets our threshold for a general red flag. In other words, it is suggestive *enough* of a serious cause being present that we must assume it is present until proven otherwise.

Bleeding can be from mouth, anus, vagina, urethra, ears or nose and is sometimes accompanied by pus if infection is present. As an example, ***bright rectal bleeding in those over 45 years old***, for example, should be considered a red flag for ***possible rectal or colon cancer***, even though it often has a benign cause like hemorrhoids. Cancers bleed into the lumen of the intestine either because they become necrotic from outrunning their own blood supply, or they grow (erode) into blood vessels.

Tumor necrosis and invasion of blood vessels may combine to cause both slow oozing as well as sudden and possibly fatal hemorrhage. Cancers within hollow organs eventually bleed into the lumen and blood can be detected at the orifice. The blood isn't always bright red, however. Dark rectal blood (melanotic stool), for example, can indicate a stomach or duodenal ulcer that can eventually perforate through the stomach or the duodenum into the peritoneal cavity or an upper gastrointestinal (GI) cancer. Both can lead to sudden and life-threatening hemorrhage.

The author has personally witnessed a fatal upper GI hemorrhage in a patient with a gastric ulcer due to frequent aspirin use. This man and his doctor ignored melena (black rectal blood) as an early warning sign of upper GI bleeding. ***Melena*** is a red flag for ***upper GI bleeding*** even without the presence of abdominal pain, since pain does not always occur with ulceration.

Rectal blood is dark when there is upper GI bleeding because there is ample time for the blood to be oxidized on its way down the GI tract. In the above case, however, the bleeding was so brisk that it was vomited. ***Vomiting blood*** (hematemesis) guarantees brisk upper GI bleeding from ulceration, cancer or ruptured blood vessels. Even if ***hematemesis*** resolves and the patient survives the first episode, he or she may not survive the second.

Blood can also exit the mouth from the lung, in which case it is generally coughed up (hemoptysis). ***Coughing a significant amount of blood*** (one quarter teaspoon or more) is a red flag for ***possible lung cancer*** eroding into bronchial blood vessels or ***serious lung infection such as pneumonia***, and is especially likely in people with risk factors for cancer or infection, like smoking. The risk of permanent and serious tissue destruction associated with hemoptysis is great regardless of whether from tumor or infection.

Specific red flags:
Cough with bloody sputum in a patient without obvious respiratory infection

Serious condition assumed present until proven otherwise:
Lung cancer

Possible consequences of missing the condition:
Fatality from lung cancer

Stabilization, referral, and management:

1. **Stabilization:** There are no stabilizing steps to take
2. **Consultation and Referral Options, Transportation:** The patient should be referred to his or her PCP on a semi-urgent basis. Transport can be by patient or family.

Relevance to acupuncturists: This is not a rare red flag. An automatic assumption on the part of patient or acupuncturist that the bloody sputum is from a respiratory infection could be fatal to the patient.

ACTUAL CASE

- **History:** A 40-year-old Caucasian female presented to the office with a one-month history of cough and occasionally coughing up small amounts of bright red blood. Her cough had continued to get somewhat worse over the one-month period of time. She became alarmed when she coughed up one-quarter teaspoon of blood the morning before her visit. She denied a recent upper respiratory infection, fever, or purulent sputum.
- **Physical findings:** The patient appeared relatively well and was afebrile. Her lung sounds revealed a wheeze on the left side.
- **Impression:** Possible lung cancer
- **Plan:** Referral to patient's family physician was accomplished.
- **Follow up:** The patient did indeed have lung cancer, which was, unfortunately, fatal within two months.

Discussion

History and Symptoms

When a patient without fever or purulent sputum coughs up a significant amount of blood (> 1/4 tsp.) we must suspect that a cancer may be present. Even with signs of infection, however, we still cannot automatically assume that the blood must be due to inflection, because infection and cancer can coexist. Infection often coexists with cancer because blockage of bronchial passages by a tumor can lead to pooling of lung secretions making a patient more prone to infection. We must especially suspect lung cancer if the patient has risk factors like smoking.

Physical Exam Findings

The patient may appear normal in the initial stages of lung cancer when complete surgical excision is still possible. In later stages, the patient may have a severe, persistent cough and may already be losing weight. Ominous signs for metastatic cancer include: unintentional, unexplained weight loss, jaundiced skin (metastasis to liver), unexplained bone pain (metastasis to bone), and abnormal mentation or the presence of neurological signs and symptoms (metastasis to brain). The presence of a ***unilateral wheeze on auscultation in a person without respiratory tract infection*** is also a red flag for ***lung cancer.***

Incidence and/or Prevalence

Lung cancer was once rare. The incidence began rising sharply around 1930 when it became more fashionable to smoke cigarettes. The incidence is approximately one in 1,605 people today. It is the second leading cancer in both men and women and *the leading cause of cancer deaths in both sexes.* There is a one in 17 lifetime risk in women in the U.S. and one in 22 lifetime risk in men. The vast majority of lung cancer is related to cigarette smoking.

Risk Factors

- Smoking cigarettes
- Passive exposure to cigarette smoke
- Advancing age
- Asbestos and other carcinogenic industrial and environmental exposure
- Radon exposure
- Smoking marijuana (probable)
- Recurring inflammation
- Repeated talcum powder inhalation
- Personal and family history of lung cancer
- Vitamin A deficiency or excess
- Lower socioeconomic status

Mechanism Producing the Red Flag

The pathophysiologic mechanism that produces coughing of bloody sputum is either oozing of a necrotic bronchial cancer that has outrun its blood supply and bleeds into the bronchial passage or, more likely, growth (erosion) of a tumor into a bronchial blood vessel causing hemorrhage of that vessel, which bleeds into the bronchial passage. In both cases the blood acts as an irritant and is coughed up.

Other Important Considerations

- The percentage of patients who live five years after diagnosis (five-year survival rate) is approximately 17.5%.
- The group with the highest percentage rate of lung cancer is African-American men.

Specific red flags:
Painless, frankly bloody urination in a man over 50 (gross hematuria)

Serious condition assumed present until proven otherwise:
Urinary tract cancer (usually bladder cancer)

Possible consequences of missing the condition:
Disability and/or untimely death

Stabilization, referral, and management:

1. **Stabilization:** There are no immediate stabilizing steps.
2. **Consultation and Referral Options, Transportation:** Consult should be made to the patient's PCP or urologist if a PCP is not available, and should be on a timely basis. The ultimate consultant will be the urologist because a cystoscopic exam will be necessary.

Relevance to acupuncturists: Although the incidence of bladder cancer is not as high as many of the other red flag conditions the acupuncturist will encounter, recognizing the red flag is simple and can mean the difference between a quick cure at a stage when the cancer is removable versus a slow and agonizing death from metastatic cancer.

ACTUAL CASE

- **History:** Jack was a 51-year-old man who, one week before coming into the office, had an episode of painless, bloody urination. He called a local emergency room and said someone told him over the phone that it was "probably an infection" and to "drink lots of water and see your doctor if it reoccurs." He drank extra water and the problem cleared up.
- **Physical findings:** The physical exam was entirely normal. Jack looked quite healthy.
- **Impression:** Gross hematuria, rule out cancer of urinary tract; probably bladder cancer
- **Plan:** Jack was sent directly to an urologist at the request of his PCP.
- **Follow up:** Jack did indeed have a small transitional cell cancer of the bladder that was easily resected through a scope by the urologist. Many years later, Jack is enjoying his retirement and grandkids, living a good life that could have been cut prematurely short had the red flag not been recognized.

DISCUSSION

History and Symptoms

All patients with urinary tract cancers will eventually pass some blood, but those with bladder cancer will do so most readily. Patients with bladder cancers have no pain with urination (dysuria) unless there is an unrelated urinary tract infection.

Physical Exam Findings

The only physical finding in the early stage is the gross blood in the urine.

Incidence and/or Prevalence

The incidence of bladder cancer in men in the U.S. is 0.02%, 70,000 cases in 2009, and over 14,000 deaths. Bladder cancer is the fourth most common type of cancer in men. For the sake of perspective, we note that the incidence of kidney cancer is 0.01% and the incidence of prostate cancer is 0.07%.

Risk Factors

- Advancing age and family history of cancer
- Smoking, alcoholism
- Toxin exposure in industry. Highest risk industries are dye workers, rubber workers, aluminum workers, leather workers, truck drivers, and pesticide applicators Arylamines are most dangerous but have been largely reduced or eliminated.
- The artificial sweeteners cyclamate and saccharine have been shown to produce bladder cancer in rats in relatively high doses.

Mechanism Producing the Red Flag

The bladder mucosa is thin and vascular. Even small cancers can erode into these vessels early in their course and cause hemorrhagic bleeding.

Other Important Considerations

- Despite the fact that prostate cancer is more common than bladder cancer, it is much more likely that painless gross hematuria will indicate bladder cancer because of the much greater tendency of bleeding from the highly vascular bladder. Prostate cancer also bleeds less readily because the prostate is encapsulated.
- Bladder infection (cystitis) is uncommon in men. Therefore urinary bleeding cannot be assumed to indicate a bladder infection in men as it so often does in females.
- 85% of bladder cancer patients present with painless gross hematuria as their first and only sign.

Specific red flags: *Vaginal bleeding years after last menses*

Condition assumed present until proven otherwise:
Uterine cancer

Possible consequences of missing the condition:
Disability and untimely death due to cancer metastasis

Stabilization, referral, and management:

1. **Stabilization:** There are no stabilizing steps to take.
2. **Consultation and Referral Options, Transportation:** Referral should be in a timely manner to the patient's PCP, if one is available. If her PCP does gynecological care (aspiration of the uterus to check for cancer cells) the PCP may be able to do what is necessary. If not, the PCP may refer the patient to a gynecologist. If cancer is present, the gynecologist will be the ultimate consultant because surgery will be necessary (hysterectomy).

Relevance to acupuncturists: The importance of this red flag can be easily "explained away" by both patient and practitioner because it can be considered a normal menses. Like gross hematuria in men, however, it is often *the only early warning sign* of a uterine cancer when the cancer is curable, which can mean the difference between complete cure and an untimely and painful death due to cancer metastasis.

ACTUAL CASE

- **History:** A 53-year-old African-American female presented to the office for low back pain. Asked what she thought might have caused it, she said "I always have some back pain when I have a period." Her last prior menstruation was three years earlier. She had not taken hormones since her menopause. She said "I thought I was finished with my periods, but I must have been wrong."
- **Physical findings:** The patient's temperature was 98.8° F. Examination of her back and abdomen were normal.
- **Impression:** Postmenopausal bleeding due to *possible* endometrial carcinoma
- **Plan:** The patient's PCP was contacted and said that she could take care of the situation.
- **Follow up:** The PCP performed endometrial sampling in the office (nonpainful, small tube suction of the uterus for endometrium sampling—an office procedure). Cancer cells were found on the uterine sample. The patient was referred to a gynecologist who performed a hysterectomy and also removed the ovaries and tubes bilaterally (because the ovaries were no longer functioning and could serve as a site for further cancer).

DISCUSSION

History and Symptoms

The typical early symptom of endometrial carcinoma is vaginal bleeding in postmenopausal *and sometimes even in pre-menopausal women.* Vaginal bleeding lacks its red flag status in premenopausal women, however, because they are already having vaginal bleeding from normal menstruation. When *premenopausal women* have endometrial cancer (see incidence below) they often present with heavier than normal menstrual bleeding, bleeding between menses or abnormal discharge with blood.

Cancer must therefore be *considered* as a *distant possibility* even in younger women with abnormally heavier vaginal bleeding, even if hormonal imbalances are a much more common cause. These patients should also be referred if acupuncture/CM does not resolve their problems in a reasonable amount of time (3-6 months). At any age, later stages of endometrial cancer will eventually give other symptoms besides vaginal bleeding like a feeling of heaviness in the pelvis and possibly pain on intercourse.

Physical Exam Findings

Body temperature should be recorded to indicate whether uterine infection, also a cause for vaginal bleeding, could be present. In cases of a very large uterus an enlarged uterus can occasionally be palpable by the acupuncturist through the abdominal wall in a thin patient. An enlarged uterus can always be palpated on bimanual pelvic examination.

Incidence and/or Prevalence

The prevalence of uterine cancer is approximately 0.01% (20,400 people in U.S.). It causes approximately 7,780 deaths per year. *Endometrial cancer is the most common malignancy of the female genital tract* and is the *fourth most common malignancy in women behind breast, lung and colon cancer*. The median age at onset is 63 years. Twenty-five percent of cases, *however, occur in premenopausal women and 5% in patients younger than 40.*

Risk Factors

- Nulliparity (allows more total time for estrogen exposure)
- Early menarche, late menopause (more time for estrogen exposure)
- Obesity – 85% of patients with endometrial cancer are obese (some adrenal steroids are converted to estrogen in fat cells – adipocytes – increasing exposure to unopposed estrogen)
- Unopposed estrogen therapy – estrogen without bioidentical progesterone
- Chronic disease (including diabetes, hypertension)
- Presence of atypical hyperplasia (abnormal, but not cancerous, cells)
- Family history of gynecological cancers in female relatives

Mechanism Producing the Red Flag

The endometrium (inner lining of the uterus) will bleed early if cancerous cells are present. Without intervention, the cancer will eventually grow into the wall of the uterus and the uterus will enlarge, giving rise to symptoms of heaviness, pressure and pain. Local spread within the pelvis will worsen symptoms. Cancer can eventually fill the abdominal cavity (abdominal carcinomatosis) and be a cause of vague abdominal pain. (The author has personally seen this in two patients in acupuncture clinics.) At this point, the patient will lose weight, which will continue and accelerate when the cancer metastasizes.

Other Important Considerations

- Endometrial cancer can spread by direct extension to adjacent structures, and through trans-tubal passage, lymphatic, or vascular (hematogenous) dissemination.
- Abnormal uterine or post-menopausal bleeding is present in 90% of cases of uterine carcinoma.
- 15% of patients with post-menopausal bleeding have endometrial cancer. Other etiologies for postmenopausal bleeding include atrophic vaginitis, exogenous estrogens, endometrial polyps, and other genital tract malignancies.
- Women with inherited clotting disorders or who are on blood thinners like Coumadin® can have inadequate coagulation and more easily bleed vaginally.

Review What You Have Learned
Chapter 5 Bleeding From an Orifice

1. Bright red rectal bleeding in a person over 50 is often associated with hemorrhoids. Despite the common occurrence of hemorrhoids, what must be assumed present until proven otherwise?
a. Diverticulitis
b. Colorectal carcinoma
c. Ulcer disease
d. Cancer of the stomach

2. Melena (black bowel movements)
a. Can be an indication of upper gastrointestinal (UGI) bleeding
b. Is more common with rectal tumors than UGI bleeding
c. Does not require consideration if it only occurs once
d. Is usually caused by the passage of undigested blood

3. Bleeding is a rather late occurrence for most tumors, including colon tumors. This especially limits the sensitivity of which of the following screening techniques to reliably detect colorectal cancer in a stage wherein it is operable?
a. Colonoscopy
b. Occult blood testing of stool samples
c. Imaging the colon with barium enema
d. Sigmoidoscopy

4. What is true about bloody sputum > ½ teaspoon?
a. Infection and cancer can cause coughed blood, together or separately
b. Can always be assumed to be from infectious damage if the patient has pneumonia
c. Can be safely ignored if the patient has bronchitis from smoking Marijuana or tobacco
d. All of the above

5. A 49-year-old man wakes one morning and painlessly passes overtly bloody urine into the toilet.
a. The man should be informed that a repeat of this situation warrants referral to a urologist
b. The man should be treated for kidney weakness and told to report back if the problem recurred
c. The man should be referred to rule out bladder cancer
d. The man should be treated for bladder infection and report any further bleeding

6. Prostate cancer
a. Is more common than bladder cancer
b. Bleeds more commonly than bladder cancer
c. Bleeds less commonly than bladder cancer
d. Is the result of bladder infections

7. Postmenopausal vaginal bleeding (5 years after the last menses, for example) should be referred
a. If the bleeding is recurrent and persistent
b. Only in women who have had unopposed estrogen therapy
c. Only in women with a family history of uterine cancer
d. At the first instance of postmenopausal bleeding as described above

8. Bioidentical hormones for humans are
a. "Natural" hormones
b. Hormones with the same molecular structure as those found in the human body
c. Hormones that are not synthesized or extracted in a lab
d. Hormones extracted from humans

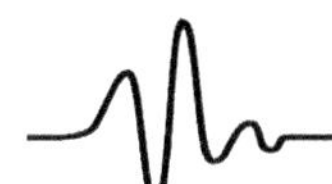

Chapter 6: BREAST PROBLEMS

A breast lump in either males or females can never be ignored and should always be referred for secondary screening and standard imaging studies.

Specific red flag:
New nipple retraction and/or fixed breast lump in a male or female

Condition assumed present until proven otherwise:
Breast cancer

Possible consequences of missing the condition:
Metastasis and death

Stabilization, referral and management:

1. **Stabilization:** There are no stabilizing steps to take
2. **Consultation and Referral Options, Transportation:** Since the likelihood for cancer is high with this red flag, referral to the PCP should be done on a semi-urgent basis. Transport can be by patient or family.

Relevance to acupuncturists: The red flag is important to acupuncturists because of the high incidence of this condition and the fact that a female (or male) patient may report the problem to you regardless of whether or not breast exams are in your scope of practice. Some timely advice and referral could save the patient's life.

ACTUAL CASE

- **History:** A 50-year-old African-American male presented to the office with the complaint of dizziness. During routine questioning, he also mentioned that he had a strange lump by his nipple. The lump did not hurt unless he pressed on it firmly. He was simply curious about it.
- **Physical findings:** The exam revealed a small pea-sized lump at the 3:00 position of the right breast that felt like a pencil eraser. It was fixed to the surrounding tissue and could not be moved.
- **Impression:** Breast cancer
- **Plan:** The patient had no PCP and was referred directly to a surgeon.
- **Follow up:** Fortunately, preliminary lab tests showed no elevation of bone or liver enzymes in the patient's serum, indicating no metastasis. A CT scan of his brain showed no metastasis there (the patient also complained of a headache). He was taken to surgery with hopes of a surgical cure. The intra-operative biopsy showed breast cancer, which was confirmed by the final biopsy reading one week later. The patient underwent removal of all breast tissue (mastectomy) and regional lymph nodes, one of which was positive for spread of the tumor. He was lost to follow up.

DISCUSSION

History and Symptoms

The typical patient is a female over 45 years old presenting with a breast mass that she or her partner discover. A new onset of nipple retraction, though not often present, makes it highly likely that cancer is present. Some women normally have somewhat retracted nipples, so this must be a new onset to be indicative of breast cancer. There is seldom any pain. Women with highly fibrocystic breasts often don't notice new lumps and sometimes even give up looking for them because they "can't tell what I'm supposed to be feeling." Less common symptoms of breast cancer include breast redness and nipple discharge or enlargement. The first symptom reported may be axillary or arm swelling in unusual cases.

Physical Exam Findings

The new onset of nipple retraction is listed as a symptom above because the patient may note it. If the examiner notes it, this makes it a sign and it carries, as we might expect, the same significance. The other very important sign, perhaps as pathognomonic as new nipple retraction, is a lump that is fixed to underlying connective tissue and relatively unmovable. This fixed property is what gives cancer its name. It is also an ominous sign. Patients who have both almost certainly have breast cancer. Patients who have such signs should also be screened for bony pain, changes in consciousness, new shortness of breath and abdominal swelling and tenderness, which are signs of bone, brain, lung or liver metastasis. Evidence of metastasis predicts a dire course for the patient.

Incidence and/or Prevalence

One in 8 women will have breast cancer sometime in their life. Three percent of all breast cancers occur in men.

Risk Factors

- Female sex
- Age > 50
- White ethnicity (although incidence in younger black women is increasing)
- Incidence higher in developed vs. developing nations (patient's origins should be considered)
- Personal history of prior breast or uterine/endometrial cancer
- Family history of breast cancer, in particular for women with mothers or sisters with a history of breast cancer, with further elevated risk if the cancer occurred before menopause or was bilateral
- Smoking, alcoholism, high-fat diet
- No pregnancies or first full-term pregnancy after age 35
- Early start of menses (menarche) and late menopause (longer total estrogen exposure)
- Use of nonbioidentical estrogen replacement therapy especially unopposed by bioidentical progesterone
- Frequent mammograms or other radiological tests when a woman is young and the breasts are most radiosensitive

Mechanism Producing the Red Flag

The lump or nodule is produced by the tumor bulk. The mechanism of nipple retraction is focal adherence of the tumor to underlying connective tissue. Cancers act this way in general due to their disrespect for boundaries, a product of their lack of contact inhibition and invasiveness.

Review What You Have Learned
Chapter 6 Breast Problems

1. A breast cancer lump would usually present, when initially palpable, as

a. An oval, hard and moveable nodule
b. A painless, fixed mass
c. A painful, fixed mass
d. Fibrocystic breasts

Chapter 7: BREATHING PROBLEMS

Difficulty breathing, shortness of breath, wheezing, coughing, or any type of insufficient respiration, if not due to a recent-onset external contraction Chinese medical pattern, may be a sign of serious illness, especially in older patients. This chapter covers red flags for hypoxia including breathing problems.

Hypoxia, the term used to connote low tissue oxygenation, has several major causes.

1. Lung conditions that block adequate absorption of oxygen from ambient air, like:
   - Chronic obstructive pulmonary disease – COPD (alveoli, the absorptive cavities of the lung, are destroyed).
   - Congestive heart failure – CHF (in CHF there is backup of fluid in the alveoli of the lungs blocking cellular respiration (02 and CO2 exchange) even in the face of normal respiratory effort and adequate ventilation.
   - Both conditions cause hypoxemia—low oxygen in the blood—leading to hypoxia at the tissue level.
2. Decrease in RBCs that carry oxygen in the bloodstream or decrease of the hemoglobin within the RBCs (different types of anemia) result in hypoxemia, leading to hypoxia at the tissue level.
3. Failure to circulate enough normally oxygenated blood around to the tissues because of pump failure of the heart (heart failure) – no hypoxemia, but hypoxia occurs.
4. Blockage of arteries stopping the delivery of blood that may be well oxygenated, but can't get to the tissues due to the blockages – no hypoxemia, but hypoxia occurs.
5. Negatively synergistic effects of combinations of the above mechanisms.

Whatever the cause, it is critical to identify the presence of hypoxia that occurs from any cause, including breathing problems, because *all causes are serious and potentially devastating.* We can survive for weeks without food and days without water, but only minutes without any oxygen delivery to tissues.

This is an excellent juncture to point out that all red flags are rather late manifesting signs and symptoms of pathophysiological problems that have run the gamut from mild to severe. Even though the main thrust of this book is to identify the end stages of physiologic processes gone awry (the red flags), the ultimate diagnostic prowess of the astute clinician is to notice the earliest stages of red flags *before* they progress to full-blown red flags.

Anyone can identify a patient with blue lips and fingernails as a hypoxic patient. The astute clinician notices earlier signs of hypoxia, perhaps even before the patient notices shortness of breath, if a breathing disorder is the cause. We want to be able to identify the advent of hypoxia as soon as subtle signs like decreased exercise tolerance, confusion, fatigue, or even minor changes in skin coloration appear. The better oxygenated the skin, the redder and healthier looking the complexion is through the "window" of the facial skin, color of the lips, nail beds, and eyelids (palpebral conjunctiva).

Although it's unlikely that patients with severe cardiopulmonary causes of hypoxia like myocardial infarction, severe pulmonary embolus, severe pneumonia or severe anemia will present first to the acupuncturist, patients in early phases of the above will. Some of these patients can go downhill fairly rapidly. In many of these cases, recognizing the red flags of low blood and tissue oxygen early on can mean the difference between life and death. As with other chapters, we also want to remember risk factors that place patients in jeopardy for hypoxia which will be reviewed along with the red flags.

Actually, superb physicians do more than pay attention to skin color and hue for purposes of making a diagnosis. They often present it as evidence to patients that, even though patients with early evidence of hypoxia may feel "normal," they're on a slippery slope to what may become life-threatening hypoxia if they continue the same activities that are causing the problem, like smoking.

Wise clinicians might also use the appearance of pale,

sweaty skin to not only advise patients to stop negative health behaviors, but also to start positive ones like doing exercise and antianxiety activities like yoga, meditation, or simply taking a walk on a beach or through their neighborhood. These seemingly simple "lifestyle measures" are actually lifesaving strategies to reduce the chance of serious future hypoxia with all of its accompanying problems. With that said, we now present the only general red flag in this section below.

General red flags: *Blueness of the lips (peri-oral cyanosis) and nail beds (nail bed cyanosis)*

This is a red flag for ***advanced hypoxia***. It's included as a general red flag in this book because there are no nonserious causes of hypoxia that reaches this level and also because it can come on so slowly in some patients that it can be ignored by patients who become accustomed to a decreased level of function. Smokers with chronic obstructive pulmonary disease (COPD) typically present this way, for example. They may be only "a little short of breath" while, at the same time, having subtle cyanosis of the lips and nail beds.

Specific red flags: *Sudden shortness of breath (SOB) in the middle of the night, cough, bilateral ankle swelling*

Condition assumed present until proven otherwise:

"Paroxysmal nocturnal dyspnea" (PND) from congestive heart failure (CHF) – PND from CHF is an episode of severe SOB that awakens patients from sleep and forces them to sit or stand up. It usually starts 1–3 hours after lying down when the pooled blood in the lower extremities is returned to the heart. It resolves in 10–30 minutes after standing.

Possible consequences of missing the condition:

Disability and/or sudden death from CHF (see also red flag for "swelling, ankles")

Stabilization, referral and management:

1. **Stabilization:** The stabilizing advice to give the patient is to caution against exercise until consultation can be made and to avoid heavily salted foods or adding salt to table food to prevent the fluid retention that comes from excess sodium in the vascular system. It's also important to advise the patient to take any heart or blood pressure medications already prescribed if they've missed doses for some reason, which is common. Many of these medicines, such as diuretics, can have significant short-term effects and might take a patient out of heart failure within minutes to hours until further stabilization can be accomplished.
2. **Consultation and Referral Options, Transportation:** This depends upon the severity of symptoms, but the patient with PND was, by definition, decompensated enough at the time it happened so that even the small amount of additional blood returning to the heart from the lower extremities was enough to overwhelm the heart's ability to pump it out. PND should be considered at least a semi-urgent situation for this reason. Because the patient may be in a different (improved or worsened) state of compensation than they were at the time of their PND, however, every case should be evaluated individually when they present to you.
   - Patients with chest pain, moderate to severe SOB, pallor, sweating, an anxious facial expression, or in some extreme cases, blueness around the mouth or nail beds should trigger a call to 911.
   - Absent any of these, the patient can go on a same day basis to their PCP or an urgent care center if no PCP is available. It would be prudent to have a family member transport the patient to his or her consultant due to the small risk of a heart attack while driving.

Relevance to acupuncturists: Heart disease and its sequelae, heart failure (the inability to pump enough blood out of the heart into circulation to meet the needs of the body) and congestive heart failure (same as for heart failure, but also with congestion of blood trying to get into the heart, are common problems. Acupuncturists will often care for many patients with heart failure and CHF. Most of these patients will be well-compensated and have little or no symptoms, making it all the more important to be able to recognize those who are decompensated by knowing the red flags for PND and CHF in general.

ACTUAL CASE

- **History:** A 57-year-old Caucasian male with a previous history of asthma and a heart attack 10 years earlier presented to the office with a history of SOB that woke him at night several hours after going to bed. He would feel like he was being smothered or "fighting for air" and would have to immediately sit up. The only other complaint was some new ankle swelling in both ankles, some mild shortness of breath when he walked fast and a little weight gain from "eating too much." He denied fever, chills or wheezing. He had been prescribed a diuretic for blood pressure and "ankle swelling" by his PCP, but had stopped it because he had been "feeling fine" until recently.
- **Physical findings:** The patient appeared slightly anxious and pale. His blood pressure was 140/88mmHg. There was no cyanosis of lips or nail beds. His heart sounds were normal and his lungs were clear to auscultation with a stethoscope. He had 1+ pitting edema on the ankles bilaterally.
- **Impression:** Probable PND from CHF
- **Plan:** Referral was made back to his PCP and patient was advised not to exercise strenuously and to resume his previously prescribed blood pressure and diuretics medications.
- **Follow up:** The patient resumed his medication. He lost three pounds over two days, and his ankle swelling resolved by the time he saw his PCP two days later. He had no further episodes of PND and his medications were adjusted. He is currently doing well.

DISCUSSION

History and Symptoms

The typical symptoms and history for PND is well covered by the actual case and the red flag in this chapter. The symptom of fatigue, exercise intolerance, shortness of breath and notice of ankle swelling are the symptoms most often presented by patients in stages of heart failure and CHF leading up to the appearance of PND.

Physical Exam Findings

Whether the Eastern or the Western clinical eye is applied, patients in heart failure tend to look pale and sometimes even ashen. Additional symptoms, as mentioned in the referral section above, include sweating, moderate to severe SOB, an anxious facial expression (from catecholamine release), or, in extreme cases, blueness around the mouth or nail beds. They may well have some bilateral ankle edema, which can be massive in extreme cases. If the failure is bad enough, the observant acupuncturist may even see elevation in the height of the blood column in the jugular vein.

Incidence and/or Prevalence

Although we could find no reliable incidence statistics on PND alone, the prevalence of CHF in the U.S. is five million people, 6–10% of people over 65 have some amount of CHF. The incidence is 500,000 new cases annually. CHF results in one million admissions to hospitals/year making it the most common reason for hospital admission in patients over 65.

Risk Factors

The typical history and risk factors for PND are the same as those listed for CHF because PND is a rather late manifestation of CHF. It's useful to think of them in five general categories of etiology of CHF: (1) coronary artery disease (2) hypertension (3) valvular heart disease (4) cardiomyopathy (5) conduction and rhythm problems. These are listed below, followed by their risk factors.

1. Risk factors for heart failure from coronary artery disease (CAD)

- Positive family history
- Male sex
- Smoking
- Abnormal lipids
- High C-reactive protein (CRP)
- Sedentary lifestyle
- Diabetes mellitus
- Also see also risk factor in chest pain section for angina

2. Risk factors for hypertension

- Renal arterial disease
- Advancing age
- African-American > Caucasian
- Family history of high blood pressure
- Obesity
- Sedentary lifestyle
- Cigarette smoking (nicotine use)
- Too much salt (sodium) in the diet
- Potassium deficiency

- Vitamin D deficiency (probable)
- Too much alcohol
- Stress
- Idiopathic

3. **Risk factors for heart failure from valvular disease and dysfunction**

- Congenital valvular disorders
- History of a severe sore throat when young (causing rheumatic heart disease as autoantibodies to streptococcus attack the valves)

4. **Heart failure from cardiomyopathy (primary disease of the heart muscle itself)**

- Alcoholism
- Diabetes mellitus
- Viruses

5. **Heart failure from conduction and rhythm problems**

- Same as for the above four conditions

Mechanism Producing the Red Flag

Again, the mechanisms of the red flag are listed according to which of the five etiological categories they belong to.

1. **Heart failure from coronary artery disease (CAD)**

Blockage by plaque and/or emboli within coronary arteries (atherosclerosis) reduces the flow of oxygen carrying RBCs to heart muscle cells (myocytes), weakening the heart and decreasing cardiac output.

2. **Heart failure from hypertension**

High blood pressure causes backward pressure against the blood ejected from the left ventricle, decreasing the cardiac output as the heart muscle pumps against a gradient.

3. **Heart failure from valvular heart disease**

Aortic and/or mitral valves that are either too loose or too tight can cause decreased cardiac output either by allowing too much regurgitation backwards into the heart or not allowing enough blood flow outward, respectively.

4. **Heart failure from cardiomyopathy**

Damaged heart muscle decreases cardiac output and leads to the signs of heart failure and then CHF as the weakness progresses.

5. **Heart failure from arrhythmias and conduction problems**

Many arrhythmias can lead to acute heart failure, but some can lead to slower onset CHF. "Sick sinus syndrome," for example, is caused by a sick pacing node in the atrium causing a slow heartbeat (bradycardia) that will not respond to increasing exercise demand. (Its red flag is listed in this book under dizziness.) At other times, heart failure can be the result of abnormal (aberrant) conduction or blocked conduction across the AV node of the heart.

Another Important Consideration

- PND generally occurs somewhere along the spectrum from mild failure with some decreased exercise tolerance all the way to severe failure with massive edema and almost no exercise tolerance.

Specific red flags:
Cough with severe episodic shortness of breath and expiratory wheezing

Condition assumed present until proven otherwise:
Moderate to severe chronic asthma (spasm and decreased caliber of bronchial tubes caused by reaction to allergens —"extrinsic" or "intrinsic" asthma)

Possible consequences of missing the condition:
Disability and death

Stabilization, referral and management:

1. **Stabilization:** The patient should be instructed to avoid obvious inciting allergens until referral and stabilization has been accomplished.
2. **Consultation and Referral Options, Transportation:** All patients with moderately severe asthma, even if recurrences are infrequent, should consult with a family physician or pulmonary medicine specialist. Moderately severe asthmatics should be followed by the consultant because all asthmatics with moderately severe asthma have the

potential for dramatic decompensation under certain circumstances (allergen exposure, bronchitis, pneumonia, etc.). The urgency of referral, who to refer to and the transportation to use, depends on the degree of decompensation of the patient. We suggest the following grading system to use for the patient who presents with wheezing.

Grade 1: Patients with mild wheezing and no significant shortness of breath as well as no history of ED visits or hospitalization for asthma in the past, can be referred to their PCP on a semi-urgent (day or two) basis unless they advance to further grades below. Patients can drive to their visit.

Grade 2: Patients with mild to moderate wheezing and mild SOB and history of ED visits or hospitalization for asthma, can deteriorate rapidly and should be referred on a same day basis to their PCP or a pulmonary medicine specialist if a PCP is not available. Someone else should drive if possible.

Grade 3: Patients with moderate wheezing and moderate SOB and history of prior ED visits or hospitalization for asthma should be sent to their PCP if the PCP has an office nebulizer to use for the patient or to an urgent care center. If these options are not available, the patient should be sent to ED of a hospital. Private transportation is acceptable with someone other than the patient driving.

Grade 4: Patients with severe wheezing, severe SOB, bluish discoloration of lips and chest tightness should be sent directly to a hospital ED by medical transportation (911).

Relevance to acupuncturists: Due to the high incidence and prevalence of asthma (see below), acupuncturists will see many patients with this condition. In many, asthma can lie dormant. In some cases, asthma will appear aggressively without obvious provocation. Clinicians who have dealt extensively with asthma understand the necessity for early recognition and treatment. Preventing a full-fledged outbreak is definitely preferable to treating it after it develops. By under- standing and acting on this red flag, acupuncturists can be in the position to guide such patients and keep them out of trouble.

ACTUAL CASE

- **History:** A 38-year-old Iranian man presented to the office complaining of mild and occasional shortness of breath in the preceding two weeks, with some infrequent cough. He wanted to try acupuncture for his problems because he "didn't like the side effects" of Western medication. He denied chest pain, fever, or bloody or purulent sputum. He had a past history of asthma, however, that had landed him in the ED on several occasions. He had previously been on "inhalers," but had stopped them several weeks prior to this visit because he was "doing well." The remainder of his PMH was unremarkable.
- **Physical findings:** The patient did not appear short of breath. His temperature was 99.0° F and his blood pressure was 120/78mmHg. His lungs were normal at resting respirations but positive for wheezing on forced expiration. His heart sounded normal.
- **Impression:** Mild asthmatic episode with history of ED visits and hospitalization
- **Plan:** Due to the patient's prior history of decompensation, he was advised to see his PCP. The patient indicated that he did not want to do so and said he would take his chances with herbs and acupuncture. The patient was treated, but our advice for consultation was noted in his chart.
- **Follow up:** The patient had a severe asthmatic attack that night and was found unconscious on the kitchen floor by his nephew, who called 911. The patient was found to be hypoxemic in the ED. Oxygen and IV bronchodilators were started and the patient recovered after four days in the hospital. He met a young doctor in the hospital that he thought he could trust and was started on medication that did not cause side effects. As of last check, he was doing well and had no future severe attacks over several years time.

DISCUSSION

History and Symptoms

The most obvious symptoms with active asthma are SOB and dry cough. Less often, patients complain of wheezing. Their report of how much wheezing they have, however, is not as reliable in estimating the severity as their report of how SOB they are. Wheezing *is* a valuable sign to the clinician in estimating the severity of the episode.

The past history of a patient's asthma is very predictive of what may happen to them in the future and needs to be strongly considered in making decisions about referral. We must always remember that an asthmatic patient's current state can change dramatically in a very short time and that the patient will often get worse toward the evening. A patient who is struggling to breathe in the morning or afternoon can end up in the ED that night.

Another factor to consider in judging how ill an asthmatic patient might be is to ask if an infection is also present. It is fine and good to discuss bronchitis and asthma in the academic world as separate conditions, but in the real world, the two conditions often coincide, giving rise to the term "asthmatic bronchitis." Each adds to the severity of the other. Thus, a patient with a history of purulent sputum and fever in addition to bronchospasm is going to be sicker than a person without these symptoms.

Physical Exam Findings

The physical findings advance as the grades of asthma advance. At first, the patient appears mildly SOB. At this point, they will often have mild wheezing with mostly dry cough. The wheezing is best appreciated by listening with a stethoscope high on the anterior chest wall bilaterally. Sometimes, if the condition is mild, little wheezing is heard with normal respirations. Occult or subclinical tendency toward bronchospasm, however, can be exposed by asking the patient to forcefully exhale after a deep inhalation, as if trying to blow out a fire.

This maneuver, seldom performed in my experience, is extremely helpful in bringing out subtle bronchospasm that may get worse later. It is very indicative of how much hidden bronchospasm is present and may correlate better with how sick or unstable the patient is than a cursory exam with the patient taking normal respirations only.

As asthma progresses the patient's wheezing will *usually* get worse. If the patient has had asthma for quite a while this is not always the case, however, repiratory efforts can diminish and the wheezing may become less prevalent. This quiet spot in a sea of wheezing is an ominous sign because patients who wheeze less, yet are more SOB, are often on their way to prolonged hospitalization.

If high fever and purulent sputum are also present, the patient may have pneumonia as well as bronchospasm.

The end point of severe asthma, with or without infection, will be a patient who appears extremely SOB, exhibits audible wheezing and air hunger, and eventually cyanosis and unconsciousness.

Incidence and/or Prevalence

The prevalence of asthma (as indicated by SOB and wheezing episodes) in a 1996 study was 6.6% of the US population. Asthma affects 14-15 million in the US including five million children. Asthma causes 5,000 deaths per year.

Risk Factors

- Personal or family history of asthma
- History of atopy and nasal allergies
- History of airway hyperreactivity to noxious substances
- Cigarette smoke exposure and environmental pollutant exposure
- Obesity (38% more common in the obese, BMI > 25%)
- History of frequent bronchial inflections

Mechanism Producing the Red Flag

Both wheezing and shortness of breath in asthma are caused by a decreased caliber of bronchial passages. Just as a reed in a wind instrument partially blocks the airway of the instrument to produce a musical note, so also wheezing is caused by partial spasm and constriction of airways in asthma. The wheezing is primarily expiratory.

Bronchospasm isn't the only thing that can decrease the airway caliber. A bronchitis component can do so also by adding mucous blockage. When the bronchospasm combines with mucous, as it often does in "asthmatic bronchitis," the combination is synergistic. The sensation of dyspnea is generated by tissue hypoxia. These signals make their way through interneurons of the spinal cord to the brain along with signals from stretch receptors in around the lungs that are hyperstimulated by increased respiratory effort to cause dyspnea.

Other Important Considerations

- Asthma is called "extrinsic" if obviously caused by external allergens and "intrinsic" if it is not, although the two types probably coexist and overlap one another.
- Extrinsic asthma (also called atopic asthma) usually begins in childhood and is often accompanied by other signs of atopy (type I, immunoglobulin E mediated allergy) such as eczema and allergic rhinitis.
- Intrinsic asthma is usually caused by respiratory infections, noxious fumes, changes in endocrine status, temperature and humidity, or drugs like aspirin and other NSAIDs as well as tartrazine, a yellow food dye. Exercise and anxiety may also produce an asthma attack in those so disposed.

Review What You Have Learned
Chapter 7 Breathing Problems

1. What is true regarding tissue hypoxia (low tissue oxygen) and hypoxemia (low oxygen in the blood)?

a. Hypoxia is always the result of hypoxemia
b. Hypoxia has other causes in addition to hypoxemia
c. Cyanosis is an early sign of hypoxemia
d. A and C

2. Persistent cyanosis (blueness) of the lips and fingernail beds is a general red flag for tissue hypoxia. What is true about this situation?

a. There are many causes of tissue hypoxia
b. Many, if not all, causes of tissue hypoxia are serious
c. Cardiopulmonary causes of tissue hypoxia are common
d. All of the above

3. Paroxysmal nocturnal dyspnea

a. Can mimic a sudden asthma attack
b. Shares the same risk factors as congestive heart failure
c. Is generally improved by increasing sodium in the diet
d. All of the above
e. A and B

4. Which of the statements listed below about asthma is true?

a. History of prior hospitalizations add little information about possible severity of future attacks
b. The words "bronchospasm" and "asthma" can often be used synonymously
c. Intrinsic asthma is more often associated with eczema than extrinsic asthma
d. Asthmatic episodes are seldom associated with infections like bronchitis

Chapter 8: CHILDREN'S PROBLEMS

Children become ill differently from adults and very young children may be unable to articulate their experience to caregivers. This chapter covers several unusual conditions, from possible child abuse to cross-eyes, as well as what to ask about and do in each case.

Specific red flags:
Unexplained or poorly explained trauma or failure to thrive in a toddler or young child

Condition assumed present until proven otherwise:
Child abuse and/or neglect

Possible consequences of missing the condition:
Severe psychological, sexual and/or physical trauma or death

Stabilization, referral and management:

1. **Stabilization:** There are no specific steps to stabilize the situation except to approach it in a nonjudgmental way that allows the truth to emerge and protects the child.
2. **Consultation and Referral Options, Transportation:** The recommended referral is to the department of child protective services in each county. The phone call should be made by the practitioner on a semi-urgent, same day basis, if possible. Child protective service will protect the anonymity of the reporter.

Relevance to acupuncturists: All clinicians share in the responsibility to detect child abuse, a surprisingly common condition that puts innocent patients at risk for harm, lifelong disability and possible death. This is another one of those instances where a small amount of recognition and intervention may make a huge difference.

ACTUAL CASE

- **History:** A mother brought her 6-year-old son in for acupuncture for "hyperactivity" because a friend's daughter had benefitted greatly from acupuncture for similar symptoms. A conservative needling treatment was begun. After the needles were in, the mother indicated that she wanted to talk privately. Out of hearing range, the mother told us that she suspected that the child's father (they were divorced) had physically abused their son when the boy stayed with him but "she couldn't prove it." The boy only said that his father "spanked me" and the father denied hurting the boy when confronted by the mother.
- **Physical findings:** The boy was exceptionally shy and seemed to wince several times when we approached him. We noticed two palm-shaped bruises on his back, which we showed to the mother after his treatment. We advised that the department of child protection should be contacted to evaluate the situation. She hesitated, finally saying that she couldn't do that because "they may suspect my new boyfriend if I call and he just gotten out of jail."
- **Impression:** Child abuse likely
- **Plan:** After her visit, the child's protection agency was contacted and the information was given.
- **Follow up:** The boy was lost to follow up.

DISCUSSION

History and Symptoms

The child is often unable to supply the history if he or she is very young, so attention should be paid to the presence of risk factors outlined in the risk factors section below and poor explanations for physical findings.

Physical Exam Findings

In addition to injury patterns, take note of whether or not a child appears withdrawn, unhealthy or morose. Although these are general signs, they can point the clinician in the right direction. Physically abused children may wince when you approach them as if fearing assault. Occasionally, an abused child can also present with a "dreamy" affect and an unusual amount of isolated fantasy play.

Injuries that occur in physical abuse often do not make sense, or sometimes they are downright incriminating. Cigarette burns on a child are highly unlikely to be the result of childhood play. Unusual and severe trauma such as broken femurs, ankles or other fractures should have witnessed explanations. Sometimes bruises in the shape of palm prints are noted. Vaginal bleeding and vaginal lacerations may be present in cases of sexual abuse to young girls. If abuse is suspected, the injuries should be carefully documented.

In infants and toddlers, failure to thrive (specifically meaning the lack of normal weight or length gain) may be present in instances of neglect, maternal ignorance or severe mental health issues in the mother.

Incidence and/or Prevalence

Childhood abuse (maltreatment) and neglect are common problems, more common than heart attacks or just about any other malady known to mankind. According to an article in *JAMA* (Prevalence of Child Physical and Sexual Abuse in the Community. 1997; 278(2):131-135) childhood physical abuse occurs more often in males (31.2%) than females (21.1%) and sexual abuse is more common in females (12.8%) than males (4.3%). Severe physical abuse was reported in similar proportions of males (10.7%) and females (9.2%). A greater percentage of females reported a history of severe sexual abuse (11.1%) compared with males (3.9%).

Risk Factors

- Personality and psychopathology in parents: lack of internal locus of control, poor impulse control, depression/anxiety, low tolerance for frustration, insecurity
- Parental immaturity and unrealistic expectations about child behavior
- Young parental age and unmet parental emotional needs
- The stresses of child care, economic stress and high general stress levels
- Domestic and spousal violence and high parental conflict
- Drug or alcohol use in parents
- Insecure attachment with own parents and childhood history of abuse in parents
- Family structure—single parent, high number of children in household
- Social isolation, lack of support, dangerous/violent neighborhoods, parental unemployment, homelessness, low socioeconomic status, lack of social services
- Separation/divorce, especially high-conflict divorce
- Poor parent-child interaction, negative attitudes and attributions about child's behavior

Mechanism Producing the Red Flag

Direct trauma and neglect produce the patterns we considered in the red flag.

Other Important Considerations

- There is often a temptation to turn away from suspecting abuse, especially if a parent seems pained by the situation. This temptation must be avoided. A parent can protect the abuser thinking it will never happen again, or the parent may be the abuser. *It is not the duty of the practitioner to completely sort out every situation, but to act to protect the abused as soon as possible and allow the protection agencies to sort through the situation.* Health care practitioners are required by law to report *suspicion* of abuse, not certainty.

Specific red flags:
Noncentering of reflected light in one pupil, crossed eye

Condition assumed present until proven otherwise:

Strabismus – a misalignment of one eye in relation to the other

Possible consequences of missing the condition:

Permanent loss of vision in the misaligned eye

Stabilization, referral and management:

1. **Stabilization:** There are no particular stabilizing steps to take.
2. **Consultation and Referral Options, Transportation:** Consultation should be on a timely basis to the child's PCP or pediatrician. Ultimate referral will be to a pediatric ophthalmologist. Early intervention will prevent vision loss.

ACTUAL CASE

- **History:** A mother brought in her 3 1/2-year-old daughter for infant massage and mentioned in passing that her child seems to have "cross eyes" at times.
- **Physical findings:** The child appeared to be seeing people in the room and following their movements well. When the child was asked to look directly at a pen light, however, the light reflex was in the center of one pupil and not centered in the other.
- **Impression:** Strabismus
- **Plan:** Referral to pediatrician who referred to a pediatric ophthalmologist.
- **Follow up:** The patient was seen by the pediatric ophthalmologist and was immediately started on various types of vision therapy. She was doing well and had normal vision with no eye crossing at last contact.

DISCUSSION

History and Symptoms

The child may be too young to complain of episodes of double vision but the parent, guardian or practitioner may note the crossing of one or both eyes. Adolescents and adults with strabismus will invariably complain of double vision.

Physical Exam Findings

The red flag captures the only reliable sign of strabismus. When the examiner tells the patient to look directly at a light held in front of the patient's face, the light reflection will be centered in one of the patient's pupils and will be off-center in the other. The noncentering of may be slight, but it will be definite. Warning: The noncentering may come and go. Repeat exams may be warranted if you suspect the condition.

Risk Factor

- Hereditary seems to be predisposing for the condition, but many patients have no family history. Male to female ratio is equal.

Mechanism Producing the Red Flag

The exact cause of the misalignment is not fully understood, but involves a defect in the way the six eye muscles of each eye coordinate with each other to line up both eyes on a single target (binocular vision).

Incidence and/or Prevalence

Strabismus is more common than most people realize. It affects as many as 5% of children to some degree or another. Although more common in children, it can occur at any age.

Other Important Considerations

- *Strabismus is the most common cause of vision loss in children, more common than all other causes combined.*
- The misalignment causes amblyopia or "lazy eye", a condition wherein the brain doesn't fully acknowledge the vision from the affected eye. The brain will eventually not recognize images from this eye, leading to blindness.
- Adults will have a much more difficult correction process, which is why this common condition must be detected as early as possible.
- Unlike some other red flag conditions, in which tragically little can be done to save the patient, blindness is 100% preventable if strabismus is picked up early and referred to experts in treating it.

Specific red flags:
Child with defective language skills, self-isolating behavior, repetitive non-useful motions

Condition assumed present until proven otherwise:

Autism – a disorder of neural development characterized by impairment of language, communication skills and social interactions and also showing restricted and repetitive behavior starting before age three.

Possible consequences of missing the condition:

Lifelong isolation and lack of the ability to live independently as an adult, family stress

Stabilization, referral and management:

1. **Stabilization:** There are no immediately stabilizing effects
2. **Consultation and Referral Options, Transportation:** Referral should be made to the patient's PCP (pediatrician or family physician) on a timely basis. Further referrals will be made to subspecialists and autism diagnosis and referral centers.

   Relevance to acupuncturists: Autism is fairly common.

Early intervention is associated with much better outcomes than in children for whom intervention is delayed. For this reason, the first clinician to notice the condition should prime the entire system for the holistic response that will be necessary to effectively treat these children. Acupuncturists may well become more and more involved with treating this problem as awareness of it increases.

ACTUAL CASE

- **History:** A 32-year-old mother brought her 4-year-old son to the acupuncture clinic for *tui na* massage due to "hyperactivity." She said the child was always "fidgeting around" and said very few words. The child had never seen a pediatrician because the mother did not want any immunizations given, so he had been treated for minor infections at a local urgent care center. His last visit there was at age 2.
- **Physical findings:** The 4-year-old boy isolated himself in the corner of the exam room, rocking and occasionally banging his head into the wall. It was difficult to get his attention. When spoken to firmly by his mother, he looked up briefly, but returned to his rocking movements moments later.
- **Impression:** Autism
- **Plan:** The patient was referred to a local pediatrician skilled with autistic children.
- **Follow up:** The pediatrician confirmed the diagnosis of autism. The patient was also found to have otitis media, which was further impairing the child's ability to listen. Several significant food allergens were identified and eliminated and only organic foods were allowed. He was started on dye free vitamins and mineral supplement and herbs were given to relieve his constipation, which he was assessed to have on his first visit. Foods containing gluten were removed from his diet after a food sensitivity panel showed he was reactive. The patient's language skills improved by approximately 20% after these measures according to the mother.

He was referred to a tertiary care center for a comprehensive evaluation and further suggestions. The diagnosis of autism spectrum disorder was confirmed and the child was started on an ABA (applied behavioral analysis) program and one-on-one tutoring. The parents were taught skills for bringing the child out of his isolating behaviors and made significant progress with these additional interventions. By his fifth birthday, he was much more communicative (with the verbal skills of a 3.5-year-old) and his isolating behaviors were much diminished. He moved from the area and was lost to further follow up.

DISCUSSION

History and Symptoms

The diagnosis of autism is based on signs and the mother's report of their child's lack of normal language and social skills. It is sometimes surprising that the mother isn't more concerned about what can appear to be glaring developmental delays by the time of diagnosis. It is not unusual, however, for the mother to have brought such concerns up to treating physicians only to be told that the child's development was "within normal limits." This, together with a mother's acceptance that all children are "a little different from one another" and possibly some denial, can result in a delayed recognition of this potentially devastating developmental disorder. This situation will probably change as more and more clinicians and parents educate themselves about the signs of autism and how to spot them at the earliest possible stage.

Physical Exam Findings

The red flag signs above are typical of autism, but it can be somewhat difficult to identify this disorder before language skills are normally expected. By three and four, children should be saying several words and even some simple sentences. They should also exhibit an eagerness to interact with parents and siblings, rather than isolate themselves with material objects and exhibit repetitive motions, like rocking or banging their head against objects, also typical of autistic children.

Incidence and/or Prevalence

Autism is not uncommon. The prevalence of autism is about 1–2 per 1,000. The prevalence of the broader category of autism spectrum disorder – ASD (see discussion section below) is about 6 per 1,000 (4:1 male to female ratio). The number of people diagnosed with autism has increased dramatically since the 1980s, at least partly due to changes in diagnostic awareness. The question of whether the actual incidence has increased is unresolved at this time.

Risk Factors

Risk factors are difficult to elucidate because it appears that autism probably has multifactorial causes.

Known influences

- Hereditary – Twin studies show a high concordance for autism and even higher for Asperger syndrome. Siblings of autistic children have a 25% greater chance of autism. The exact genetic mechanisms are not fully known and autism cannot be traced to a single gene mutation or to a single chromosomal abnormality like Fragile X syndrome (a chromosomal abnormality that can cause autistic features).
- Exposure to teratogens in the first eight weeks of pregnancy

Suspected risk factors

- Pollutants: heavy metals, prenatal stress, PCB's etc.
- Food allergens

Factors with disproven or possible minimal risk factors

- Mercury-free modern immunizations

Mechanism Producing the Red Flag

The exact way information processing in autistic brains produces its signs is unknown, but there must be abnormal regulation of cross-signaling neural pathways and neurotransmitter imbalances at specific loci.

Other Important Considerations

- Autism spectrum disorders belong to the general category of pervasive developmental disorders (PPD). PPDs are characterized by widespread abnormalities of social interactions and communication and severely restricted interests, as well as highly repetitive behavior.
- Asperger syndrome, a disorder in the autism spectrum, is perhaps the closest to autism in signs and likely causes, but language skills and cognitive development are not as impaired as in autism. It is also not unusual for Asperger patients to have areas of very high function (with numbers, for example).
- Rett syndrome, childhood disintegrative disorder and PDDs not otherwise specified (PDD-NOS) round out the list of the other PDDs.
- Not many children with autism live independently after reaching adulthood, though some become successful. This is changing with early intervention programs.

Specific red flags: *Child with sore throat, high fever (>102° F), inspiratory stridor, drooling*

Serious condition assumed present until proven otherwise:

Acute epiglottitis – Inspiratory stridor is the term used for a harsh and croup-like sound on inspiration. (Expiratory sounds are more consistent with bronchospasm.)

Possible consequences of missing the condition:

Respiratory arrest and death

Stabilization, referral and management:

1. **Stabilization:** There are no stabilizing steps to take, but an attempt to look at the tonsils with a tongue blade is contraindicated because it can cause laryngeal spasm that can worsen respirations.
2. **Consultation and Referral Options, Transportation:** This is a medical emergency. The patient should be transported to the nearest ED by the quickest transportation possible. If there is no cyanosis or extreme air hunger it is not necessary to call 911. With these signs, it is. A call should be made to the triage person at the ED because a team needs to be ready to possibly place a breathing tube past the swollen epiglottis and treat the condition with appropriate antibiotics.

Relevance to acupuncturists: Children with end stage acute epiglottitis will probably not be coming into acupuncture clinics, but as always, we must all be alert to conditions like these in early or milder stages. The presence of *any* inspiratory stridor, especially if it is consistent in a child with a high fever and throat pain qualifies for full red flag status.

ACTUAL CASE

- **History:** A 5-year-old female child was being evaluated at the pediatric acupuncture clinic for frequent illnesses to see what herbs might be appropriate to boost her immunity. The mother said she was going to cancel the appointment because her child was complaining of a sore throat that morning, but she decided to bring the child in to show us "how bad she gets." The child reportedly had a fever of 102.5° F earlier that day. The child was not immunized.

- **Physical findings:** The young girl looked quite ill. Her temperature was 103° F. She was not talking and was drooling a little. She was making a croup-like sound on some of her inspirations. There was no cyanosis.
- **Impression:** Possible early acute epiglottitis.
- **Plan:** The patient was sent to the ED with her mother driving. We called the ED to explain the situation.
- **Follow up:** The child did have acute epiglottitis at the ED. She was started on oxygen, aerosolized fluids, other medications and was watched closely. Fortunately, she did not need intubation and resolved over the next few days and is now doing well.

DISCUSSION

History and Symptoms

The child will often have a history of an upper respiratory infection preceding the epiglottitis. The history of a very sore throat is always present. Drooling is common as is the reluctance to talk or swallow fluids or food. Malaise will always be present and the child will appear quite ill.

Physical Exam Findings

The child looks ill, has a high fever, inspiratory stridor and is often drooling. The skin between the ribs may appear to be pulling in with each respiration (retractions). If the air passage is sufficiently narrowed there may be the bluing of the lips (peri-oral cyanosis), an ominous signs indeed.

Incidence and/or Prevalence

Acute Epiglottitis occurs most often between the ages of 3 – 7 years of age. Before routine immunization for *Hemophillus/Influenza* type B (a bacterium, not to be confused =with the influenza virus), there were 5,000 deaths yearly in the U.S. due to acute epiglottitis.

Risk Factors

- Age 3-7 years
- Prior upper respiratory tract illness
- Other sick children with sore throats in the family
- Immunocompromised children from drug therapy or congenital immune deficiency
- Unvaccinated children

Mechanism Producing the Red Flag

Narrowing of the space between the epiglottis and the trachea causes the noise called "stridor" much as the reed in a wind instrument causes a high pitched tone as air is blown across it.

Other Important Considerations

- Acute epiglottitis is a true medical emergency of the highest magnitude occurring as the result of infection by *Hemophillus/Influenza (H. influenza)*, Beta-hemolytic strep, and *pneumococcus*.
- Viral croup can cause inspiratory stridor also, but there isn't a significant fever with viral croup while there is with acute epiglottitis. Furthermore, exposure to moist air will "break" a croup attack, but will not stop acute epiglottitis.
- A child under seven years old has a sore throat and croupy type respirations and the parents may report fussiness, a high fever and drooling. Risk factor is lack of *Hemophillus/Influenza* vaccination.
- The stridor of acute epiglottitis brings to our attention the importance of problems with the inspiratory phase of respiration. Whereas problems with expiration, as found in asthma, can be serious and even life-threatening, problems with inspiration, heralded by stridor, are even more urgent whether from epiglottitis or aspiration of a foreign body, which can produce sudden death.

Specific red flags:
Crying child holding flexed arm against body with hand pronated

Condition assumed present until proven otherwise:

Nursemaid's elbow (dislocation of the elbow)

Possible consequences of missing the condition:

Extreme pain

Stabilization, referral and management:

1. **Stabilization:** There are no immediate stabilizing steps to take
2. **Consultation and Referral Options, Transportation:** Referral should be made to a family practitioner, pediatrician, orthopedic surgeon or physician in urgent care center familiar with the method to reduce nursemaid's elbow

Relevance to acupuncturists: Nursemaid's elbow is common. Although it is unlikely that a child with nursemaid's elbow will be seen first by an acupuncturist, this red flag is so characteristic that is well worth knowing.

ACTUAL CASE

- **History:** A four-year-old girl resisted leaving her house to come to a pediatric *tui na* treatment. On the way out of the door, she threw herself to the floor in a temper tantrum while her father held onto her hand to prevent her from falling. Moments afterwards she was crying and holding her arm to her side, unwilling to move it.
- **Physical findings:** The child was whimpering in pain when she reached the office. She was holding her arm against her body with her elbow flexed and her hand pronated. (Palm flat against her body) She resisted any movement of it.
- **Impression:** Possible partially dislocated elbow (nursemaid's elbow)
- **Plan:** The patient's pediatrician was not available. A physician adept at reducing nursemaid's elbow was located at a nearby urgent care center and the patient was referred there.
- **Follow up:** The reduction was accomplished easily (easy if you know how to do it) by the urgent care physician and the child had almost instant relief of her pain.

DISCUSSION

History and Symptoms

The history listed in the actual case is typical. Sometimes the injury is sustained when the child is being held by the hand and twirled in play, but it happens most commonly when a child is falling and the individual holding the hand doesn't let go. The pain is nearly immediate and the child is inconsolable except when the hand and arm are held in the characteristic posture previously noted.

Physical Exam Findings

The pronated posture (palm down position) of the hand with the elbow slightly flexed is invariant.

Incidence and/or Prevalence

We were unable to locate estimates of incidence of nursemaid's elbow except for frequent mention of it being "common" in children younger than four years-old.

Risk Factors

- More common in girls than boys
- More often on the left side than the right
- Usually between 1-3 years of age and rare after age 5

Mechanism Producing the Red Flag

Nursemaid's elbow is an interposition of the annular ligament into the radial-humerus joint. The annular ligament normally passes around the proximal radius just below the radial head. With traction on the extended arm, the annular ligament slides over the head of the radius into the joint space and is trapped, producing pain and decreased range of motion. Pronation is maintained for comfort. Supination (palm up) of the hand is resisted, even though this is the very motion that will reduce the radial head in the hands of an expert.

Review What You Have Learned
Chapter 8 Children's Problems

1. Child abuse is a harmful phenomenon that is remarkably common. What statement is true regarding child abuse in the U.S.?

a. Physical abuse occurs in 31.2% of males and sexual abuse occurs in 12.8% of females
b. It can be tempting for the clinician to turn away from child abuse for a variety of reasons
c. Child abuse is more likely to occur in high stress marriages where drug abuse is present
d. Health care providers are required by law to report instances of suspected child abuse
e. All of the above

2. Strabismus is an eye disorder that

a. Is more common in adults than in children
b. Can lead to partial blindness if not detected and referred early
c. Occurs most commonly in young adults than children
d. Is self-correcting in almost all circumstances

3. What statement is true about autism

a. Autism is a problem of neural development wherein severe problems are noted with language and social interaction, and restrictive and repetitive behavior is also present
b. Autism is convincingly associated with modern mercury-free immunizations
c. It is a minor problem that usually self-corrects by seven years old
d. All of the above

4. Which statement(s) is (are) true regarding inspiratory stridor or expiratory wheezing that might be encountered in ill children?

a. Expiratory wheezing is a more immediate emergency than inspiratory stridor
b. High fever is a particularly ominous finding in expiratory wheezing, but not in inspiratory stridor
c. Acute epiglottitis more commonly produces expiratory wheezing than inspiratory stridor
d. Immunizations against the bacterium Hemophillus influenza Type B (HIB) have drastically reduced the incidence of acute epiglottitis in the U.S.

5. Nursemaid's elbow, a common injury in toddlers, is

a. Dislocation of the radius at the radio-humeral articulation causing the child to hold their forearm in a pronated position
b. A dislocation of the navicular bone of the wrist causing anatomic snuff-box tenderness
c. A rare injury of children more common in girls than boys
d. Usually caused by a direct blow to the elbow

Chapter 9: NEW ONSET CONSTIPATION

While often relatively benign and not difficult to treat with Chinese medicine, if constipation is of new onset, the patient is relatively older, and there are any other potentially serious symptoms such as unexplained weight loss, this common symptom deserves more scrutiny.

Specific red flags:

New onset of constipation and unexplained weight loss in a person over 40

Condition assumed present until proven otherwise:

Carcinoma of the colon (and rectum)

Possible consequences of missing the condition:

Debilitation and death from metastatic colon cancer

Stabilization, referral and management:

1. **Stabilization:** There are no specific stabilizing steps to take
2. **Consultation and Referral Options, Transportation:** Referral can be to the patient's PCP who will refer to a colorectal surgeon, or directly to a colorectal surgeon if there is no PCP available. Private transportation for this timely consult is appropriate.

Relevance to acupuncturists: This red flag is important for acupuncturists because colon cancer is a common problem and because it can only be cured if detected and treated early. Since the complaint of bowel habit changes are so common in all primary care practices, including acupuncture practices, and routine screening is still relatively uncommon in many people, early stages of colon and rectal cancer are often missed by health care providers and is one of the most common causes of malpractice litigation.

ACTUAL CASE

- **History:** A 52-year-old male presented to the office with a history of new onset of constipation for six weeks. He had also lost five pounds in the prior two months. He was not able to explain his weight loss on the basis of diet or change in exercise patterns.
- **Physical findings:** The patient had a regular pulse at 70 bpm. His other vital signs and general exam were normal, including his abdominal exam.
- **Impression:** Possible colon cancer
- **Plan:** Referral to the patient's PCP, who referred the patient for a colonoscopy.
- **Follow up:** The patient was found to have a large cancer of the descending colon. On surgery, however, the only spread of the cancer was to one regional mesenteric lymph node which was removed with the cancer. There has been no recurrence of cancer in the last three years.

DISCUSSION

History and Symptoms

The red flag captures the essence of only one type of patient with colon cancer, namely one with a fairly advanced cancer of the descending colon. The red flag includes a significant weight loss, perhaps 8-10 pounds, and a significant length of time for the constipation, perhaps several weeks. It's important to know that the most common symptom of early colon cancer, unlike the patient in the actual case, is no symptom at all. This is because the colon is so distensible that a tumor can grow quite large before there are significant symptoms.

Possible earlier symptoms than those noted in our red flag are variable, but include:

- Any persistent change in bowel habits. Tumors may be irritative to the colon and may release substances that promote loose stools. Diarrhea may therefore precede constipation. That is why any change in bowel habits for more than a few weeks may be an early warning sign for colon cancer.
- A persistent feeling of incomplete defecation, especially if the tumor is near the rectum

- Bright blood in stool or dark melanotic stool
- *Persistently* narrower or thinner stools than normal. A tumor at the rectal verge, for example, can produce flattened stools. (The narrowing of stools in irritable bowel syndrome, in contrast, comes and goes.)

If symptoms like this are present, watching and waiting are not appropriate options. It's also important to realize that symptoms vary with the location of the tumor. Those near the rectum and in the descending colon (left-sided tumors) are more likely to produce obstruction than those near the cecum (right-sided tumors)

Interestingly, abdominal pain is rare with colon cancer except in cases where there is a tumor spread outside of the colon throughout the abdomen, a dreadful condition called "peritoneal carcinomatosis." Additional systemic effects like fatigue, weakness, and unexplained anemia are also likely to occur in later stages of colon cancer.

Physical Exam Findings

The physical exam may be entirely normal, or the patient may look emaciated as the cancer progresses. A colon tumor has to be very large and/or the patient very thin, to be palpable on abdominal exam. So this sign cannot be relied on to help detect colon cancer.

Incidence and/or Prevalence

The incidence rate of colon cancer is 0.05%. In 2009, 146,970 men and women in the U.S. (75,590 men and 71,380 women) were diagnosed with colon cancer. Of these 49,920 people died from it. The median age at diagnosis for cancer of the colon and rectum was 71 years of age, but 12.0% were between 45-54. Lifetime risk: one in 26 women and one in 17 men will develop colorectal cancer during their lifetime. (Australia)

Risk Factors

Genetic and demographic risk factors

- Risk elevates significantly after age 45. Patients > 50-years-old are at greatest risk.
- Personal history of colorectal polyps or colorectal cancer
- Personal history of inflammatory bowel disease (ulcerative colitis and Crohn's disease)
- Family history of colorectal cancer
- Inherited syndromes (familial adenomatous polyposis can have hundreds or thousands of colonic polyps), hereditary non-polyposis colorectal cancer
- African-Americans have the highest colorectal cancer incidence and mortality rates of all racial groups in the United States. Jews of Eastern European descent (Ashkenazi Jews) have one of the highest colorectal cancer risks of any ethnic group in the world.
- Type 2 diabetes mellitus

Lifestyle-related factors

- Diet high in animal fat and red meats and low in fruits, vegetables, and fiber
- Sedentary lifestyle
- Obesity
- Smoking
- Alcoholism

Mechanism Producing the Red Flag

Colon cancer is caused by changes to cellular DNA of the cancer cells, as in all types of cancer. Constipation is the result of blockage of the colonic lumen by the cancer's sheer bulk. Because the colon is quite distensible, a malignancy may grow quite large before the lumen is narrowed enough to produce constipation. Thus, constipation from a colon tumor is an ominous symptom, as is weight loss because it indicates a fairly large tumor that has possibly already metastasized. An early site for metastasis would be the liver.

Other Important Considerations

- It would obviously be better to detect colon cancer at an earlier stage than that represented by this red flag. Although expensive, colonoscopy, which explores the entire extent of the colon from rectum to cecum, has the strongest evidence basis for helping find colon cancer and has the most favorable risk/benefit ratios of any screening tests currently available. It is the gold standard for colon cancer screening because it directly observes the left (descending) colon, the transverse colon, and the right colon to the cecum and allows for biopsy or removal of precancerous lesions at the same time as the exam.
- Because about 40% of malignancies lie beyond the reach of the 60 cm sigmoidoscope, many authorities recommend routine barium enema every 5-10 years in addition to sigmoidoscopy for those over 50 years old who are not undergoing colonoscopy.
- Routine annual fecal occult blood testing and sigmoidoscopy every five years starting at 50 is still advised for those not undergoing colonoscopy even though the positive predictive value of fecal occult blood testing is < 10%.

- Virtual colonoscopy (the patient swallows a pill-shaped camera that photographs the GI tract all the way through) has some appeal due to its ease of use, but does not allow biopsy of detected lesions.
- The discovery of hemorrhoids in patients with rectal bleeding, a more common cause of rectal bleeding than malignancy, does not preclude the search for a higher malignancy that might be causing the rectal bleeding in those over 40-45.
- All screening procedures should begin earlier than 50 for those with risk factors.

Review What You Have Learned

Chapter 9 Constipation

1. What is the best advice to give a 50-year-old patient with the new onset of constipation, 15-pound weight loss over several months and a small amount of rectal bleeding?

a. Increase fiber in the diet, use herbs and acupuncture to obtain relief

b. As in "choice a" above, but also instruct patient to test for blood in the stool (the test kit can be obtained in drug stores)

c. As in "choice a" above, but also refer patient to a gastroenterologist for barium enema test

d. As in "choice a" above, but also refer to the patient's PCP for possible colonoscopy

2. The above patient does not heed your advice and sees you five months later. He incidentally mentions that he did not go to a consultant because he found a protruding, bleeding hemorrhoid in his anal area. Your advice would now be

a. The discovery of a hemorrhoid doesn't preclude a higher lesion, so refer as before

b. The discovery of a hemorrhoid is sufficiently reassuring to avoid referral at this time

c. Whether hemorrhoids are present or absent, the patient's age alone warrants some type of screening for possible colorectal cancer

d. All of the above

e. A and C

Chapter 10: DIARRHEA

This common clinical condition can be due to many things both in Chinese and Western medicine. While acupuncturists may immediately consider spleen qi vacuity or damp heat, both persistent unexplained diarrhea or acute bloody diarrhea with concomitant fever are important to refer for medical screening. This chapter explains why.

Acupuncturists are frequently faced with patients who have bowel complaints, including loose stools. Because many such cases are self-limiting, vigilance must be maintained for instances of diarrhea that are red flags for serious conditions. This can easily be done in the case of acute diarrhea, which is presented as a specific red flag in this chapter. Before going into the specific red flag, however, we first need to examine diarrhea presenting as a general red flag, as it does in the case of ***persistent unexplained diarrhea (> 3-5 loose stools daily) over months to years.***

Not all, or perhaps even most, cases of chronic diarrhea are the result of serious illnesses, but enough are that we must consider the above as a red flag for ***some type of parasitic enteritis or significant malabsorption syndrome.*** Infectious causes of chronic diarrhea include protozoa like *Entamoeba histolytica and Giardia lamblia* as well as helminths (worms) like whipworm (trichuriasis). In the case of malabsorption, the substance that is poorly absorbed and produces symptoms is generally a carbohydrate or fat.

We must distinguish malabsorption from food allergy. Malabsorption is not food allergy. True food allergy involves antibody reactions to protein components of food that can subsequently damage the bowel wall. An example is gluten enteropathy. In some cases of food allergy, sufficient damage can occur to the mucosal lining of the intestine that malabsorption of vital nutrients can occur as a secondary result, but the fact remains that food allergy and malabsorption are different entities that can coexist.

Persistent unexplained diarrhea is a general red flag because there are many possible explanations for the problem and because it can mark illnesses that can result in chronic malnutrition, developmental stunting and even eventual death in some cases. Fortunately, we get clue when such disorders are afoot. Although a complete description of all possible individual causes and presentations are beyond the scope of this book, we can make some generalizations that help us recognize patients with significant malabsorption syndromes and parasites.

With malabsorption, we get clues because nonabsorbed substances are either fermented by bowel bacteria that produce methane gas (as in lactose intolerance), or transit the bowel and generally produce loose stools. In many cases malabsorption produces gas and loose stools. Patients with fat malabsorption may present with nutritional deficiencies of fat soluble vitamins and with multiple loose, greasy, floating stools (steatorrhea).

With parasites, it's a different story. While some chronic infections are fairly well tolerated, many are not. In addition to loose stools, parasites can cause bloody diarrhea, debilitation from severe anemia, blindness, malnutrition and cognitive delays. In fact, the shocking truth about intestinal parasites is this. If we add up the numbers of all those infected and suffering significant ill effects around the world from parasites, we see that intestinal parasites have an estimated global impact as great as HIV or malaria.

Consider the following. *Ascaris lumbricoides* is the most common intestinal parasite in the world, infecting an estimated one billion people. It is also the largest roundworm, reaching 16 inches and the thickness of a pencil. The female produces an enormous number of eggs (about 27 million a year), which are expelled in feces but can live for up to seven years in warm soil. Collectively, roundworms infect more than 1.6 billion people yearly, killing two million and debilitating many others.

People with an amoeba infection may experience nausea, loose stools, weight loss, abdominal tenderness and occasional fever. Rarely, the parasite will invade the body beyond the intestines and cause a more serious infection, such as a liver abscess. And we aren't just talking about third world countries here. *Entamoeba histolytica* is the primary cause of amoebic dysentery or amebiasis, infecting between 1.5-

30% of the U.S. population depending on the region studied.

Giardia, a protozoan organism can give rise to similar symptoms. According to the FDA Bad Bug Book, the overall estimated incidence of *Giardia* infection in the U.S. is 2% of the population – 2.5 million people annually. It is the most frequent cause of nonbacterial diarrhea in North America and is more prevalent in children than adults, possibly because many individuals seem to have lasting immunity after infection. It is implicated in 25% of gastrointestinal disease cases.

Patients with these types of problems can be referred in a timely manner to medical doctors, acupuncturists, naturopaths or other licensed practitioners with experience in ordering and interpreting comprehensive stool tests (some of the best labs do not require an MD license). If testing has already identified pathogens that require medication (*Giardia*, etc.), or if the patient is unstable, losing weight or malnourished, they should be semi-urgently referred to a gastroenterologist experienced in dealing with parasites, as should patients with significant malabsorption syndromes.

Specific red flags: *Acute bloody diarrhea (> 6–8 loose stool/day) and fever >101.5° F*

Condition assumed present until proven otherwise:

Serious enteritis (gastroenteritis if vomiting is present in addition to diarrhea)

Two types:

1. **Acute infectious enteritis** from viruses, bacteria or parasites (some parasites can cause acute as well as chronic diarrhea).
2. **Inflammatory autoimmune bowel disease** such as ulcerative colitis or Crohn's disease.

Possible consequences of missing the condition:

Serious disability and/or death from dehydration and electrolyte imbalance

Stabilization, referral and management:

1. **Stabilization:** Patients should frequently drink small amounts (1 oz or less) of clear fluids only and not eat solid foods until referral can be accomplished.
2. **Consultation and Referral Options, Transportation:** Patients can be referred to their PCP on a semi-urgent, same-day or next-day basis by private transportation. Activation of medical transport may be necessary if the fever is very high and the patient appears very frail, ill, and/or stuporous, or has a racing pulse and low blood pressure.

Relevance to acupuncturists: Acupuncturists are frequently faced with patients with bowel complaints, including frequent loose stools. They, and other clinicians, can be lulled into a false sense of complacency about acute diarrheal disease because so many cases are self-limiting. This makes it all the more important to be able to recognize instances of diarrheal illnesses that are red flags for serious causes.

ACTUAL CASE

- **History:** A 36-year-old Chinese American exchange student came to the office complaining of diarrhea. Asked how often, he said "too many times to count." He denied vomiting. He had a temperature of 101.5° F the night before and twice there was blood in his stool. He denied history of hemorrhoids.
- **Physical findings:** The patient appeared tired. His temperature was 102°. F.
- **Impression:** Probable bacterial enteritis
- **Plan:** We were able to contact the PCP and the patient was seen the same day.
- **Follow up:** Patient had positive white blood cells (WBC) on his stool smear and culture and sensitivity for stool pathogens had results pending. (Having WBC in stool is suggestive of bacterial enteritis.) The next day, the patient got suddenly worse with profuse watery diarrhea and with fever to 103° F. He was admitted to the hospital for fluid and electrolyte support and his stool culture grew campylobacter jejuni. He was treated with appropriate antibiotics and made a smooth recovery over the next several days.

DISCUSSION

History and Symptoms

Symptoms of enteritis or gastroenteritis can occur at any age. Most patients with florid cases of gastroenteritis with profuse vomiting, diarrhea and prostration (exhaustion) go directly to the ED. Acupuncturists and other primary care providers are likely to see early cases of what will eventually be severe diarrhea. Asking about the number of stools daily and the presence of blood in the stool and fever will allow you to pick up potentially dangerous cases.

Ascertaining the number of stools/day is important because it can help us estimate how much fluid and electrolytes may be lost. This alone cannot be relied on to predict the possible danger to the patient, however. Vigorous diarrhea *without blood and fever* (often due to a virus) may be dangerous in a young child due to dehydration alone. The presence of fever and blood marks the presence of an organism of higher pathogenicity (often a bacterium) which can be dangerous regardless of number of stools/day.

This actual case we cite is typical of acute diarrhea from a bacterial cause. Noninfectious enteritis from inflammatory bowel disease (Ulcerative colitis or Crohn's disease) generally presents with less diarrhea and more abdominal pain than bacterial diarrhea, but is included here because it can also present with fever and blood. The distinction between diarrhea from infection and inflammatory bowel disease is not as important to us here as is the recognition that all serious enteritis presents with fever and blood in the stool.

Physical Exam Findings

If the acupuncturist sees visible blood in the stool and records a temperature greater than 101.5° F, these *confirm* the symptoms of serious bowel inflammation from infection or autoimmune disease. Hyperactive bowel sounds (increased borborygmi) and generalized abdominal tenderness to palpation, especially if found over the area of the descending colon in the left lower quadrant, may be further confirmatory signs of severe enteritis, but may also occur with other disorders.

Incidence and/or Prevalence

Globally, acute infectious diarrheal illnesses from viruses, bacteria, amoeba and other parasites have a devastating effect on health, especially in children. Acute infectious diarrheal diseases (most often contracted from drinking infected water) caused 4% of international mortality and the demise of 2.2 million people worldwide in 1998, mostly children (WHO, 2000). Diarrhea is still a threat in the U.S., causing 54,000 – 55,000 children to be hospitalized every year. Of these, approximately 3,100 die, usually of dehydration and electrolyte imbalances. The incidence of the other major cause of fever and blood in stool, autoimmune inflammatory bowel disease (Ulcerative colitis or Crohn's disease), is much lower than that of infectious enteritis, but is still sizable at 0.2% of the U.S. population, with a death rate of five per million. Though not generally as lethal in the short term, these illnesses can be quite debilitating or even deadly in the long term. Ulcerative colitis, for example, may necessitate removal of large portions of the colon and is associated with a higher rate of colon cancer.

Risk Factors for Infectious Enteritis

- Age < 5 years
- Residence in a third world or economically poor country or poor section of a country
- Travel to above
- Known exposure to unclean water or food
- Lack of hand washing in kitchen staff after bathroom use
- Lack of hand washing in households with infected individuals

Risk Factors for Inflammatory Bowel Disease (IBD)

- Cigarette smoking – risk factor for Crohn's
- Family history of IBD
- Jews and Caucasians > African-Americans, Asians, Hispanics or Native Americans

Mechanism Producing the Red Flag

The organisms that cause acute diarrhea have a direct toxic effect on the mucosal surface of the bowel. The diarrhea is an intense discharge of fluids from the intestinal walls intended to wash the pathogen out. Like other protective effects of the body, however, the diarrhea can cause harm, in this case dehydration and loss of vital electrolytes like sodium and potassium. In contrast, the ultimate cause of inflammatory bowel disease, like many autoimmune diseases, is unknown. Whatever the cause is, the result is damage to the mucosal surface and severe inflammation of the intestinal wall – enteritis, with subsequent bleeding, pain and discharge of fluids into the lumen as in infectious enteritis.

Another Important Consideration

- The threat of fluid and electrolyte loss in gastroenteritis is even greater than with enteritis alone because of the additive loss of fluids due to vomiting.

Review What You Have Learned
Chapter 10 Diarrhea

1. The most common intestinal parasite worldwide is

a. Giardia

b. Entamoeba histolytica

c. Ascaris lumbricoides (roundworm)

d. Trichuriasis (whipworm)

2. Acute diarrhea is a common occurrence. What factors make it a red flag for serious enteritis?

a. The degree of cramping and stools greater than 5 per day

b. Vomiting and cramping

c. Fever and blood in the stool

3. The difference between enteritis and gastroenteritis is

a. There is no difference

b. In gastroenteritis, there is often vomiting with diarrhea

c. Enteritis is common, gastroenteritis is rare

d. None of the above

4. Inflammatory bowel disease (like Ulcerative colitis) is caused by

a. Poor digestion

b. Food allergies

c. Infection

d. Autoimmunity

Chapter 11: FATIGUE

Fatigue is a bread and butter complaint in acupuncture clinics worldwide. While it may be easily explained as a short-term secondary symptom, as a chronic symptom it can be a marker for several quite serious medical conditions that requires swift medical intervention.

Fatigue is among the most common problems presenting to acupuncturists as a secondary complaint, if not the primary one. Acute fatigue is often easily explained by simple factors like lack of sleep, pregnancy, temporary illnesses and stress, etc. Chronic fatigue (fatigue every day for at least three months), is less easily explained and often indicates serious underlying illness. It also has a long list of possible diagnoses associated with it. It doesn't make for a long chapter in this book, however, because conditions with fatigue as one component of a red flag are often listed under other symptoms.

Chronic fatigue with shortness of breath (SOB) and/or chest pain is a general red flag for *significant cardiopulmonary disease* like coronary artery disease (CAD) resulting in decreased blood flow (perfusion) to the brain or lung problems like pneumonia that decrease oxygen to the brain. The common pathophysiologic mechanism in all cases of cardiopulmonary fatigue is decreased oxygen delivery to neurons (hypoxia), which the brain interprets as SOB and fatigue. Many of these situations are also covered under the chapter dealing with altered mental function and SOB.

This is a semi-urgent to urgent red flag because *all* cardiopulmonary causes of fatigue are serious and potentially life-threatening. If the patient seems unstable, with a crescendo pattern of chest pain, falling blood pressure, faintness, and/or acute respiratory distress, emergency medical services should be activated with a call to 911. If the patient has mild SOB or a history of mild chest pain, the patient can go to the ED of a local hospital by private transport (but should not drive).

Referral to the patient's PCP on a same-day, semi-urgent basis is also appropriate if the patient is stable and the symptoms are mild. The PCP may then refer to a cardiologist if the heart is the primary suspect or a pulmonary specialist if the lungs are suspect. Please refer to the chapter on angina section for more differentiation of an unstable vs. a stable patient.

Chronic fatigue with enlarged lymph node(s) and/or abdominal mass is a general red flag for the *possibility of widespread cancer, either primary lymphatic cancer or cancer that is metastatic from other sites* (like lung, breast or prostate). There can also be widespread distribution within an area of the body like "abdominal carcinomatosis." In any of these cases, the discovery of a *hard (indurated)* and *rooted nodule* in a patient with chronic fatigue is an ominous finding because it may be one of many autostatic lesions.

Patients with this extent of cancer often have other symptoms and signs such as weight loss, jaundice and pallor, for example. Even though this presentation seems extreme, I have personally seen patients with these kinds of findings walk into acupuncture clinics completely unaware of the seriousness of their condition.

These patients should be referred on a semi-urgent basis to their PCP. The ultimate consultant will be a cancer specialist (oncologist), but most oncologists will only see patients referred by their PCP because they want to get as much past medical history as possible. For this reason it is often wisest to first refer to a patient's PCP, even if you know the PCP will then refer to the oncologist(see the referring patients section in Chapter 2).

Chronic fatigue in a patient with jaundice and/or an enlarged liver is a general red flag suggesting the possibility of either *serious liver diseases, a primary liver cancer or cancer metastatic to the liver.* The liver diseases include various types of liver inflammation (hepatitis) like hepatitis from alcohol, viral, or other causes. Whatever the etiology, the combination of hepatic findings and chronic fatigue generally indicates a very serious problem and should spur a referral on a semi-urgent basis to the patient's PCP.

Chronic fatigue with unintended and unexplained weight loss is a general red flag for *cancer*, just as unexplained and unintended weight loss by itself is also a red flag for *cancer*. It should be handled in the same way outlined in the section for unexplained weight loss in the weight loss chapter.

Chronic, debilitating fatigue, weakness, muscle pain and sleep disturbance is a general red flag for *chronic fatigue syndrome (CFS)*, which qualifies as a serious medical condition because CFS patients often function at a substantially lower level of activity than normal people. Although controversy surrounds the diagnosis of CFS, most authorities agree that profound fatigue is the one indispensible symptom for the diagnosis. Impairment of short-term memory or concentration, recurrent sore throat, tender lymph nodes, and headache are also common.

The prevalence of CFS in the U.S. has been reported at 1.8%, but some authorities estimate that 80% of cases remain undiagnosed, at least partly because of the fact that there is no specific lab test available to verify its presence. The NIH estimates that there are 500,000 cases of CFS in the U.S. Those of us who work with CFS think this estimate is also much too low. We also believe that a disproportionate number of CFS patients eventually seek treatment from "alternative" practitioners because of a paucity of solutions from many medical doctors. Acupuncturists certainly see many patients with CFS.

While the acupuncturist may indeed have much to offer patients with CFS, it may be prudent to refer patients with debilitating symptoms or those unresponsive to Chinese medicine to physicians skilled in the treatment of CFS from a multidisciplinary approach. Such physicians are often known by word-of-mouth in a community. They may be family practitioners, rheumatologists, osteopaths (DOs), or naturopaths (NDs), possibly with specialization in functional medicine.

Physicians with special interest and skills in dealing with patients who have CFS may also be identified through CFS support groups and on-line sources. Acupuncturists lacking specific interest or training in CFS may also wish to consider referral to acupuncturists who do specialize in treating CFS. One caveat is in order here. Occasionally, CFS patients will be found to have a perfectly conventional diagnosis that has simply been missed, like hypothyroidism or adrenal failure.

Review What You Have Learned
Chapter 11 Fatigue

1. Chronic fatigue with shortness of breath and chest pain is a general red flag for

a. Chronic fatigue syndrome
b. Mononucleosis
c. Some type of serious cardiopulmonary problem
d. Some type of serious neurological problem

2. What are the most important signs and symptoms for the diagnosis of chronic fatigue syndrome and the often overlapping problem of fibromyalgia?

a. Fatigue in the afternoon, shortness of breath, joint pain
b. Fatigue, weakness, muscle pain and sleep disturbance
c. Depression, muscle pain and poor skin turgor
d. General fatigue, thyroid problems, adrenal hyperfunction

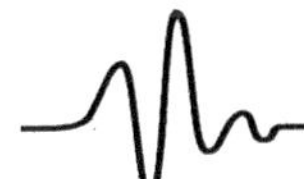

Chapter 12: FEVER

Not all fever is bad. In fact, fever up to approximately 101.5° F increases the competence of the immune system. **A fever above 105° F**, however, is a general red flag in its own right regardless of etiology because temperature over this range can cause ***brain damage*** if not brought down promptly. High fevers can also trigger febrile seizures in children. Any patient with a fever of 105° F should be immediately taken to urgent care, regardless of the suspected cause.

Persistence of a fever 101.5° F for > two weeks is also a general red flag, even in the absence of other signs or symptoms. Such a fever is commonly called "fever of unknown origin" (FUO) by allopathic physicians, and is a red flag for ***occult infection, metabolic, or autoimmune disease.*** FUO must be aggressively worked up to find its cause so that proper treatment can be rendered.

It doesn't take much additional information to make fever a *specific* red flag. For example, a **fever > 103.5° F plus severe sore throat** is a red flag for the *possible* presence of a ***streptococcal throat infection*** (strep throat). The concern is not so much about the sore throat, which is self-limiting, but rather the possible sequelae of heart valve or kidney damage as a result of an autoimmune response attacking the body's own tissues even after the bacteria are gone. Other specific red flags including fever are found in their respective sections in this book.

Review What You Have Learned

Chapter 12 Fever

1. Fever of unknown origin—FUO (temperature > 101.5° F > two weeks is a red flag for

a. Occult infection and/or seizure disorders
b. Occult infection, depression, chronic fatigue syndrome
c. Occult infection, metabolic disease, autoimmune disease
d. All of the above

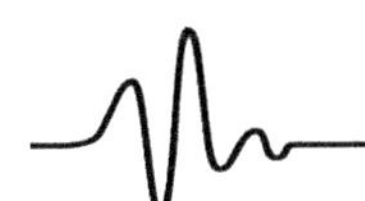

Chapter 13: HEARING AND BALANCE

Negative symptoms involving our hearing and/or balance almost always involve the brain or neurological system. Acupuncture may be helpful, but serious symptoms should be ruled out with a thorough neurologic exam and appropriate testing when necessary.

Specific red flag:
Progressive unilateral loss of hearing and balance

Condition assumed present until proven otherwise:
Acoustic neuroma (AN)—a benign tumor of cranial nerve VIII (vestibulocochlear) that does not have "benign" consequence for the patient

Possible consequences of missing the condition:
Permanent deafness, loss of balance and severe disability

Stabilization, referral and management:

1. **Stabilization:** There are no stabilizing steps to take
2. **Consultation and Referral Options, Transportation:** These are often slow growing tumors so the referral can usually be made in a timely manner to the patient's PCP or a neurologist if the patient does not have a PCP.

Relevance to acupuncturists: This is another problem that can present with subtle symptoms that seem trivial to patients and practitioners and can be easily overlooked or explained away as being "normal" in aging. It is another situation in which early recognition can make a huge difference to the patient, especially because of advances in treatment of small tumors available today (see other important considerations section below).

ACTUAL CASE

- **History:** A 37-year-old Caucasian shoe salesman presented to the office with difficulty making out the words people were saying to him and a feeling of being "off balance". Both problems were progressively getting worse. His PCP told him that his trouble making out words was due to normal hearing loss secondary to aging, and because the patient had played in a "rock and roll" band when he was younger.

  The patient was not satisfied with this explanation and was seeking acupuncture for the problem. He said his hearing was only getting worse in one of his ears, his left ear.

- **Physical findings:** The patient had a normal physical exam except for slightly diminished hearing in the left ear compared to the right (tested by seeing if the patient could hear the sound of fingers being rubbed together outside of the ear canal on each side).
- **Impression:** Possible early acoustic neuroma
- **Plan:** The patient did not want to return to his PCP. The acupuncturist tried to arrange a visit with a neurologist, but was unsuccessful. He was sent to a freestanding medical clinic and was urged to ask the medical doctor he saw there for a referral to a neurologist or ENT physician and was eventually referred to an ENT physician.
- **Follow up:** The patient had an audiogram done by an audiologist that showed a significant diminution of hearing on the left side. The right side was normal. He was referred to a neurologist by the ENT and an MRI confirmed the presence of a small acoustic neuroma on the left. The tumor was treated with a Gamma Knife's 201 beams of cobalt radiation and the patient has had complete resolution of his symptoms for the last five years.

DISCUSSION

Typical History and Symptoms

The usual patient with an AN is middle-aged or older. Because ANs tend to enlarge unpredictably, the presentation can be different in different patients. The first symptom usually noticed is unilateral loss of hearing, but some patients may first present with "balance problems."

Since some hearing loss often accompanies aging, and because there is no pain associated with early ANs, patients may delay seeking medical attention for some time.

The point of distinction between normal aging and AN is that the hearing loss is unilateral in AN. (*see exception below in incidence section*) Also, normal aging doesn't usually affect balance to the degree that AN does. The history of balance difficulties and unilateral hearing loss in a middle-aged person, therefore, is highly suggestive of AN. The hearing loss usually worsens slowly, but can occur suddenly in about 5% of cases, sometimes months or years prior to the tumor's discovery. It can be triggered by head trauma or vigorous physical exercise.

Vertigo may appear early with AN, but may get better as the central nervous system adapts the loss of balance information from the affected ear. As the tumor enlarges, pressure upon the facial nerve may result in facial weakness. It can eventually also press on other nerves like the trigeminal nerve (CN VII), which controls facial sensation, causing facial tingling and numbness. Larger tumors can press upon sensory fibers of the dura mater causing unilateral headaches that may radiate to the neck or head. Untreated, AN can eventually press on the brain stem with resulting severe neurological effects.

Physical Exam Findings

The only initial sign of an AN is unilateral hearing loss, best determined on the audiogram, but which may also be picked up on gross testing in the office by whisper detection from a distance or finger rubbing tests. Later cases can have obvious dysequilibrium and obvious facial muscle weakness on inspection, with inability to draw up the corners of the mouth, and decreased ability to close the eyelid or hold the eyelid down firmly (facial nerve signs).

Incidence and/or Prevalence

There are two types of ANs, the unilateral "sporadic" type that usually starts at middle age or older, and those associated with Neurofibromatosis Type II (NF-II), which occur in younger people and are usually bilateral. (NF-II is a rare, inherited disorder.) Sporadic ANs, the subject of this red flag, are responsible for 95% of cases. NF-II causes the remainder.

The average person has a 1/1000 chance of developing an AN sometime in their life. ANs comprise about 6% of all intracranial tumors.

Risk Factors

Heredity and Genetics

- Bilateral ANs in NF-II patients are thought to result from the functional loss of a tumor suppressor gene localized to the long arm of chromosome 22.
- In more than 95% of patients the disease is unilateral and results from somatic mutations that are not associated with hereditary risk.

Mechanism Producing the Red Flag

ANs arise from cranial nerve VIII, the vestibulocochlear nerve. This nerve transmits information about a person's position in space from the inner ear to the brain as well as information for hearing. The word "benign" usually implies a less than severe prognosis, but this is unfortunately not the situation with AN because there is little room for unusual growths within the hard confines of the bony skull. ANs compress vital structures already discussed causing hearing loss and balance problems.

In some patients, other mechanisms responsible for balance can compensate for a while (visual, etc), and balance can stabilize. Additionally, some of the information for balance is preserved by the intact inner ear signals from the nonaffected side. Most patients lose hearing gradually over many years, but progress to total deafness on the side of the tumor. The loss mainly involves the higher frequencies of sound at first affecting speech discrimination.

Other Important Considerations

- It is widely, but not universally, accepted that open microsurgical resection is the treatment of choice for larger tumors. This procedure can be lifesaving, but has a fairly high incidence of complications like facial paralysis.
- For the vast majority of patients with smaller ANs, stereotactic radiosurgical ablation using a Gamma Knife's 201 beams of cobalt radiation directed toward the neuroma has a better than 98% chance of success.

Review What You Have Learned
Chapter 13 Hearing and Balance

1. A patient presents to an acupuncturist's office with a history of balance problems and progressive unilateral hearing loss occurring over several months. The most likely diagnosis is

a. Generalized anxiety disorder

b. Transient ischemic attack (TIA)

c. Cerebrovascular accident (CVA) – stroke

d. Acoustic neuroma

Chapter 14: INDIGESTION AND NAUSEA

Patients presenting with either acute or chronic indigestion may respond very well to acupuncture treatment. When symptoms do not abate as expected or if they worsen, a timely referral can prevent serious consequences. This chapter covers what we need to know.

Indigestion and nausea are some of the most common and nonspecific symptoms presenting to all primary care clinicians. These problems present commonly to acupuncturists because many patients have heard through word-of-mouth that acupuncture works with these types of problems beyond, or in addition to, what can be offered by Western medicine. This is probably at least partly due to acupuncture's ability to influence smooth muscle motility, excretion and other subtle functions of the gastrointestinal (GI) tract.

To take one common example, the influence on needling of ST-36 on sphincter function is well-documented in the literature. Gastroesophageal reflux is also handled nicely by the experienced acupuncturist through acupuncture and herbal remedies. The effect on GI motility is an area where in Western medicine struggles for success. This remedial effect of acupuncture can be extended throughout the entire GI tract, from swallowing to elimination. It is therefore important for an acupuncturist to recognize red flags within this symptom category.

It is also an area that overlaps considerably with other symptoms presented in this text. For example, the red flags for gallbladder disease could well have been placed under the pain section because gallbladder disease eventually produces pain in many cases. Patients often complain of "bad digestion" or "indigestion," however, before they complain of pain. So the red flag for gallbladder disease is in this section even though it would have been placed in the pain chapter.

Specific red flag:
Indigestion, right upper abdominal pain, feeling of fullness under diaphragm following a meal

Condition assumed present until proven otherwise:
Acute gallbladder inflammation (acute cholecystitis)

Possible consequences of missing the condition:
Possible bowel paralysis (ileus) from stone passage or gallbladder infection (empyema) and sepsis (infection in the blood), which can lead to death

Stabilization, referral and management:

1. **Stabilization:** There are no specific stabilizing steps in the throes of a full-blown attack, but the patient should not take anything by mouth.
2. **Consultation and Referral Options, Transportation:** The urgency of referral depends on the stage of gallbladder disease and will often be obvious from the patient's clinical course and level of pain. An asymptomatic patient with a history of mild attacks in the past, for example, could be referred to their PCP in a timely manner. Patients with persistent symptoms and those in extreme pain will need to be taken by the fastest available means to the ED of a local hospital. Emergency vehicle transportation is usually not necessary unless there are cardiopulmonary signs or symptoms like chest pain, SOB, falling blood pressure, etc.

Relevance to acupuncturists: Indigestion is a common symptom which may be a chief complaint or may arise during the course of routine questioning about diet, appetite, and digestive function. The lack of severity of the symptoms of early gallbladder disease may mislead patient and acupuncturist into underestimating the potential to develop dangerous complications noted in this chapter.

ACTUAL CASE

- **History:** A 38-year-old Caucasian female presented with a history of recurrent "indigestion" that occurred several times a year lasting for 10 minutes following a heavy meal. She also describe an uncomfortable "pressure" under her diaphragm and a feeling of being "overly full." The episodes had been getting worse in the prior several months.

- **Physical findings:** The patient was mildly obese. Her temperature was 98.8°. F. She had mild tenderness to palpation in the right upper abdominal quadrant.
- **Impression:** Subacute cholecystitis with a history of acute flare-ups.
- **Plan:** The patient was sent to her PCP for a next day visit.
- **Follow up:** The patient was found to have stones in her gallbladder on sonography. The walls of the gallbladder were also thickened, suggesting some inflammation. She was scheduled for elective surgery due to the gradual worsening of her condition, but had a severe attack with fever before the elective surgery could be done and had to have emergency surgery for acute cholecystitis and an infected gallbladder.

DISCUSSION

History and Symptoms

Many patients with acutely inflamed gallbladders (acute cholecystitis) have a known history of gallstones (cholelithiasis). The stones may be asymptomatic for many years (silent cholelithiasis) and may have been detected serendipitously on a plain film of the abdomen or chest. A significant number of patients with cholelithiasis, however, eventually develop acute cholecystitis.

Patients with acute cholecystitis often experience right upper abdominal fullness and discomfort described as just under the diaphragm. The pain can radiate to the tip of the right scapula. Symptoms occur most reliably after a fatty meal, but in advanced cases they can occur with almost any food intake and become quite severe, persisting for hours. They may then resolve completely, or not at all, in which case emergency surgery is needed. Vomiting occurs in some patients and may be followed by temporary symptom relief. Patients with advanced disease and those who have infected gallbladders, rather than merely inflamed gallbladders, will report fever and severe systemic symptoms like prostration as well.

Physical Exam Findings

The typical patient with gallbladder disease is an overweight woman in her 40s, but acute cholecystitis can occur in an adult of either sex, and rarely in children and teenagers. The patient who is having a gallbladder "attack" will usually have right upper quadrant abdominal tenderness and muscle guarding to palpation directly over the gallbladder (Murphy sign), but some patients have diffuse midepigastric tenderness. Both may worsen on release of palpatory pressure (rebound tenderness), indicating peritoneal inflammation as well as gallbladder inflammation.

Fever is common if the gallbladder is infected. These patients will appear very ill. Tachycardia from fever will probably be present in these cases. A palpable gallbladder or fullness is present in approximately 30% of patients. Blockage of the cystic duct by a stone will lead to jaundice in approximately 25% of patients. Elderly patients and/or those with diabetes may have fewer signs.

Incidence and /or Prevalence

An estimated 10-20% of Americans have gallstones, and as many as one-third of these people develop acute cholecystitis. Cholecystectomy for either recurrent biliary colic or acute cholecystitis is the most common major surgical procedure performed by general surgeons, resulting in approximately 500,000 operations annually (usually laparoscopic). Gallstones are 2-3 times more frequent in females than in males.

Risk factors

- Prior personal history of gallstones and/or gallbladder disease, cirrhosis of the liver, Crohn's disease, or insulin resistance syndrome and diabetes mellitus
- Family history of gallbladder disease
- Age > 40 years
- Female sex
- High-fat diet, hyperlipidemia, sedentary lifestyle, obesity
- History of rapid weight loss
- Pregnancy (elevated progesterone in pregnancy may cause biliary stasis)
- Use of oral contraceptives, female hormone replacement therapy, or clofibrate, octreotide, ceftriaxone medications

Mechanism Producing the Red Flag

The pain from gallbladder disease occurs when the inflamed and tender gallbladder walls contract down the irritating stones as it tries to squeeze bile out of the gallbladder. Pain can occur from small stones escaping the gallbladder and getting stuck in the cystic duct or lower down in the common bile duct (see figure 3). Fatty meals produce the greatest pain because the gallbladder contracts most vigorously in response to fats.

Other Important Considerations

- Gallstones (cholelithiasis) and cholecystitis usually go

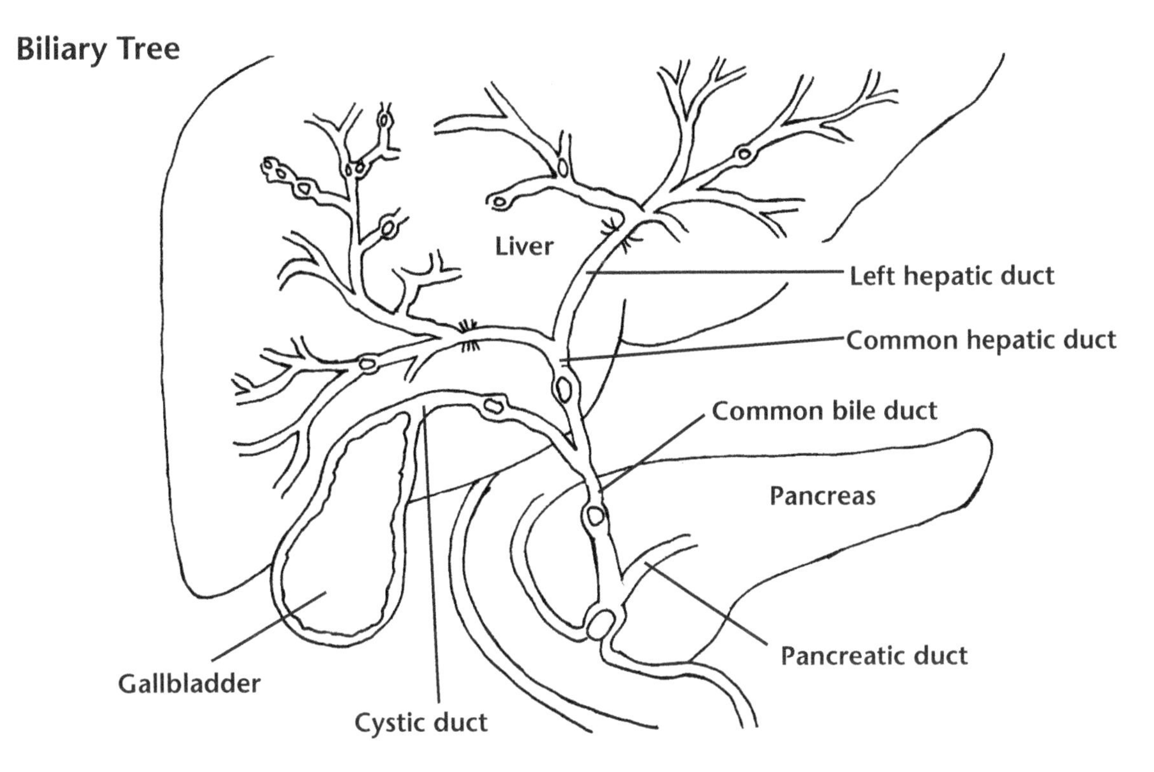

Figure 3. The ducts of the "biliary tree" are shown in this illustration. Blockage can produce extreme colicky pain. The cystic duct leading from the gallbladder and the common bile duct are often the sites of blockage.

hand in hand causing "calculous cholecystitis" –in 90% of cases. Cholecystitis can occur without cholelithiasis (acalculous cholecystitis) in 10% of patients.

- Ninety percent of cases of cholecystitis occur when a gallstone gets stuck in the cystic duct.
- Although fifty percent of gallstones remain asymptomatic throughout a person's lifetime, we should always be more vigilant for cholecystitis in people who have known cholelithiasis because an asymptomatic disease can turn symptomatic without warning.
- Most patients with acute cholecystitis have a complete remission within 1-4 days, twenty-five percent of patients require surgery or develop some complication.

Review What You Have Learned
Chapter 14 Indigestion and Nausea

1. What is true about acute gallbladder inflammation?

a. Cholecystitis is usually accompanied by cholelithiasis (gallstones)

b. Cholecystitis can have fatal consequences

c. Cholecystitis and pancreatitis can coexist

d. All of the above

Chapter 15: MENSTRUAL PROBLEMS

In both Western and Chinese medicine, a lack of menstruation or very scanty menstruation is considered abnormal. Chinese medicine is able to treat most menstrual disorders successfully, but the long-term health of patients with chronic amenorrhea may be improved with Western screening and treatment as well.

Small fluctuations in the timing, flow, or discomfort associated with menses are common and do not represent serious problems in most patients. Large fluctuations can signal serious disease. Significant menstrual fluctuations (excluding complete absence of menses – amenorrhea) come in three varieties:

1. The menses can be too heavy
2. The menses can be too light
3. The timing of menstrual cycles can be irregular

It is also common for combinations of these abnormalities to occur. We've already encountered red flags associated with heavy flow or vaginal bleeding after menopause. It remains for us to consider in this chapter implications of infrequent menses and menses that are too light.

Menses that are scant and infrequent may not seem like a problem to many people and may even be welcomed. The concern, however, is not because light flow itself is a problem, but because of what light flow and infrequency might signal —a seriously low serum estrogen level (hypoestrogenemia). If severe enough, hypoestrogenemia can produce bothersome, serious short term problems like hot flashes, insomnia, depression and severe vaginal dryness. Additionally, the long term consequence of osteoporosis can lead to disabling fractures and death from complications due to fractures.

Clinicians often identify these kinds of problems in elderly females, but are often less inclined to recognize them in young females. Yet, the result of hypoestrogenemia is no less devastating for young women as it is for older women. For these and other reasons, the significance of abnormal menstruation (abnormally scant menstruation in this chapter) must be understood and acted upon by acupuncturists and other health care professionals. To be able to do this, acupuncturists who deal with menstrual problems must thoroughly understand the physiology of the cycle and be able to obtain a stellar menstrual history.

The first general guideline is this: *It is absolutely imperative to get a good menstrual history*. This may seem like a no-brainer, but it is often omitted or done in a cursory manner by many clinicians. Taking a good menstrual history means ascertaining the age of menarche and the postmenarche menstrual pattern *before* a patient went on oral contraceptives (OCs), if she did. A great deal of attention must be paid to a woman's natural pattern so we can estimate how hormones may be unbalanced.

We must also ascertain the menstrual history when women are at the peak of the reproductive years, between approximately 18-30 years of age. If the menses *aren't* normal in this menstrual window, they will probably never be normal. We can estimate what hormones are likely to be deficient or excessive in relation to one another from this history and whether or not this means the patient is at risk.

As mentioned, anyone who hopes to do a decent job in this area must thoroughly understand how the menstrual cycle works in terms of hormone release, and the regulation by the pituitary, ovulation, and the effect on the endometrium (the inner lining or the uterus). With these two pieces of information in hand, a knowledge of the patient's menstrual history and a firm knowledge of the basic science of the menstrual cycle, we are ready to determine what too light, too heavy, or irregular menses mean to the patient's health.

The first generalization we come to is this: **a history of no menstruation or late menarche with skipped menses and extremely light menstrual flow thereafter** is a general red flag for ***inadequate estrogen in the blood*** (hypoestrogenemia). This can have all of the consequences that result from hypoestrogenemia, including osteoporosis, extreme vaginal dryness, hot flashes, and depression. Age is not an absolute protector, as young women with premature ovarian failure (POF) know very well. If estrogen is low, problems associated with hypoestrogenemia are the result, regardless of age.

Specific red flag: *Amenorrhea, anorexia and athleticism in young women*

Condition assumed present until proven otherwise:
Female athletic triad – a syndrome in family and sports medicine

Possible consequences of missing the condition:
Women with the female athletic triad can develop life-long osteoporosis from hypoestrogenemia. Indeed, they may already have it, as well as other symptoms and signs of hypoestrogenemia. If full-blown anorexia nervosa is also present, the considerable risks from these eating disorders should also be factored in (see red flag for anorexia under the symptom of weight loss).

Stabilization, referral and management:

1. **Stabilization:** The patient should be educated about the necessity to eat enough and decrease exercise enough to allow for normal menses to occur. It is also helpful to let patients know that the majority of bone mass in women is laid down before the age of 26, and it is often not possible to "catch up" later if estrogen deficiency is too extreme during adolescence and early adulthood.
2. **Consultation and Referral Options:** This red flag doesn't necessarily need referral if hormone supplementation is not necessary and if the acupuncturist understands the importance of early intervention and knows how to advise such patients and follow them to ensure a favorable outcome. On the other hand, a consult can be made to the patient's PCP in a timely manner. If anorexia nervosa is present, the patient will usually need referral to a specialist in eating disorders as well as her PCP.

Relevance to acupuncturists: Acupuncturists who care for young athletic patients will undoubtedly see girls with the female athletic triad. Many will be otherwise healthy and might be surprised to know that, in their enthusiasm to be competitive and eat right, they are laying the groundwork for significant osteoporosis later in life. The right kind of education about this problem is essential for the patient, and the patient's parents, if the girl is still in grade or high school.

ACTUAL CASE

- **History:** A 16-year-old female cross-country star for a local high school was treated in the office for ankle pain that lingered after a recent stress fracture. She described herself as a vegetarian and said she had a "healthy diet," which consisted of a lot of salads and few meats. Her menarche was at age 14. She only had two light periods before starting cross-country training. Her parents described her as "highly motivated" and said she ran extra mileage compared to the rest of the team. She was the fastest runner on the team. She was also an excellent student and played flute in an orchestra.
- **Physical findings:** The young woman was bright and articulate, 5'5" and 110 pounds, and had little body fat.
- **Impression:** Amenorrhea, athleticism, anorexia – the female athletic triad
- **Plan:** The young lady had only seen a pediatrician in the past. They chose a family doctor who had extra sports medicine training.
- **Follow up:** The patient was diagnosed with the female triad and a bone density scan showed osteopenia (the stage before osteoporosis). Once the patient understood that she was putting her future health at risk, she cut back on her mileage and added meat in her diet. She added some speed work to her routine and decreased her total mileage. Her running times actually improved. She began having light menses, which have continued. She is now a college athlete and doing well in school and in track. She is being followed for osteopenia and will be stopping her running after the current semester.

DISCUSSION

History and Symptoms

The history in the actual case is typical, but the patient can be any age. The author has seen this in several women in their 40s and 50s who belonged to runner's clubs. Dietary issues are not always the biggest issue. It can be excess mileage. The presence of anorexia nervosa at any age should be gently probed for.

Physical Exam Findings

These patients are often lean and percent body fat can be in the single digits, which is too low for women to make adequate additional estrogen in fat cells where adrenal hormones are converted to estrogen. Extremely thin women or those with an obvious body image disorder should be considered to have anorexia nervosa until proven otherwise.

Incidence and/or Prevalence

The exact prevalence of the female athlete triad is unknown, but some studies have reported disordered eating in 15-62% of female college athletes. Amenorrhea occurs in 3.4-66% of female athletes compared to 2-5% of women in the general population.

Risk Factors

- Competitive athletics
- Sports that involve maintaining a certain weight
- Poor social support due to sports demands
- Excessive exercise, more than required for the sport
- High expectations by coaches and parents to win at any cost

Mechanism Producing the Red Flag

Estrogen and progesterone are both important for bone density. Women who have very low estrogen generally have low progesterone as well. This is because they don't ovulate as often and hence do not form a corpus luteum (the corpus produces progesterone). Women who do not menstruate, therefore, are probably deficient in both important female sex hormones and are prone to early osteopenia (weak bones) and osteoporosis (de-mineralized bones).

Other Important Considerations

- Many authorities list osteoporosis as part of the female athletic triad (amenorrhea, anorexia, and osteoporosis). The original formulation of the female triad, did not include it, however. I see osteoporosis as a possible consequence, rather than part of the triad itself and prefer the original triad because osteoporosis isn't always present when young girls first present with this syndrome.
- Some young women may not get their menses with adjustment of exercise level and dietary change. Some of these patients will need supplemental hormone therapy and should be referred.

Review What You Have Learned
Chapter 15 Menstrual Problems

1. What is the significance of uncovering a history compatible with the "female athletic triad"?

a. It can be predictive of future bone strength in a woman

b. It can be predictive of athletic performance

c. It can lead a clinician to an estimation of whether or not a woman has low estrogen in the blood

d. All of the above

e. A and C

2. The presence of secondary amenorrhea (no menstruation after having started menstruation)

a. Is suggestive of a prolactin hormone problem

b. Could indicate premature ovarian failure (POF)

c. Is suggestive of hypoestrogenemia (low estrogen concentration in the blood)

d. All of the above

e. B and C

Chapter 16: PAIN

Pain is probably the most common symptom seen in acupuncture clinics worldwide. While many patients have already been seen by their Western medical care providers before they get to our clinics, this chapter can help us consider which patients with which types of pain require more screening or Western medical intervention.

Pain is the body's most immediate and common alarm signal of impending harm and is the most common reason that patients seek acupuncture care. Because of this, the subject of pain deserves and receives special attention in this chapter. Pain is complex by its very nature because it is an interpretation involving our thoughts and emotions. Pain can be a *general* red flag that can suggest the presence of many possible disorders in many possible anatomical regions, or it can be part of many specific red flags.

The timing of pain as a factor in red flags

Pain that worsens progressively over weeks to months is a general red flag for ***ongoing tissue damage***. The timing of pain is often given less attention in Chinese medicine than its severity, quality (colicky, sharp, dull, etc.), radiation and palliative/provocative factors (heat vs. cold, movement vs. rest, etc.). While severity, quality, radiation and palliative/ provocative factors are useful for differentiating *Chinese Medicine* patterns like stagnation of *qi* vs. blood, these factors may not be as valuable in red flag analysis, by themselves, as the timing of pain.

Nonserious pain is generally short-lived, episodic, and stable over time. Acute, severe pain, for example, may accompany temporary colicky spasm of the intestine or temporary misalignment of a vertebral facet of the spine. Though vexing, neither is life-threatening and both resolve spontaneously. **Pain that steadily increases in severity over weeks-to-months**, however, indicates a ***threat of irreversible tissue damage*** from serious medical conditions like cancer, nerve damage, post-traumatic or post-surgical pain syndromes, or inadequate blood supply to tissues (ischemia).

We can understand how timing plays a role in general red flags by looking at the way cancer produces pain. Cancer cells lack "contact inhibition." Their growth is not impeded, as is the growth of normal cells, when they grow into other tissues. Since the growth is relatively slow, as compared to acute trauma, the pain may have a gradual onset, but because cancer never retreats, the pain is almost always progressive and eventually becomes constant.

Increasing pain can signal a host of serious medical conditions in addition to cancer like nonunion of fractures, necrotizing bone, internal bleeding or infections, development of scar tissue pressing on nerves, failure of surgical implants or devices, and onset of "complex regional pain syndrome" (CRPS—see general red flag for CRPS below).

Acupuncturists also deal with postsurgical pain. Those who do and expect "healing crises" or assume routinely poor outcomes from surgery or injections are at risk of wrongly accepting progressively worsening posttraumatic or postsurgical pain as "normal." In fact, **progressively worsening pain after surgery** *is never "normal" and should always be considered a red flag.* An acupuncturist can prevent possible permanent pain, disability, or even death by noting abdominal pain pattern and referring the patient back to the surgeon.

We cannot be reassured, however, if ongoing and increasing pain or tingling (paresthesia) is replaced by complete numbness. Since pain is carried along sensory neurons, an **increasingly painful area that turns numb** is a red flag for ***total sensory nerve destruction*** as seen in advancing cases of median nerve compression (carpal tunnel syndrome) or spinal radiculopathy. Such total sensory disruption can rapidly lead to irreversible loss of strength and function in the limb.

Finally, we should also mention that **worsening of any stable chronically recurring pain** is also a general red flag for ***new tissue necrosis or injury***, as in the case of a worsening headache pattern. Recognizing this general red flag for a change in the patient's condition, even without knowing what is causing the change, can save the patient's life.

Pain in inflamed joints

The four classical signs of inflammation in a joint are swelling, redness, pain, and heat. A **persistently inflamed joint** is a general red flag because, regardless of the cause, diseases that cause severe inflammation will invariably cause ***permanent joint and soft tissue damage*** if left untreated.

One group of diseases, autoimmune diseases like rheumatoid arthritis (RA) and lupus arthritis, can also cause life threatening systemic attacks on vital tissues like the kidney and heart. This is especially true of systemic lupus erythematosus (SLE). The life expectancy of SLE patients has improved from an approximate 4-year survival rate of 50% in the 1950s to a 15-year survival rate of 80% today, but it is still a significant cause of death in the U.S.

Bacterial infections and crystal deposition diseases also cause inflammatory arthritis. Bacterial infections of joints can spread to the bloodstream (sepsis) and lead to death. Even crystal deposition diseases like gout (uric acid crystals deposited in joints) and pseudogout (calcium crystals), though unlikely to cause death, can leave the patient with significant deformity and disability. In fact, **persistent inflammatory arthritis** is somewhat unique among general red flags in that the list of possible diagnoses includes *only serious conditions.*

This is all relevant to acupuncturists because inflammatory arthritis is common. RA alone has an incidence of 1% in the U.S. (over 3 million people). While not all RA patients will have disastrous outcomes, consultative comanagement with a rheumatologist may be wise for inflamed patients who do not respond adequately to Chinese medicine to prevent permanent joint damage.

To summarize and add a few points:

1. Acute joint pain and/or inflammation following surgery should be considered an urgent and serious medical condition. *This is particularly true if there are open, purulent lesions at the joint, or redness is traveling proximally along a limb.* Generalized sepsis and death can result within 24 hours if the infection is not controlled.
2. Joint inflammation without recent surgery or trauma is less urgent in the short run, but still requires prompt referral because again, there are no non-serious explanations. Acute joint inflammation can permanently deform and damage joints.
3. Persistent and chronic joint inflammation can worsen quickly at times and become acute. Acute flare-ups can lead to permanent destruction of bone, cartilage, and tendon rupture. A rheumatology consult is indicated to direct appropriate therapy before destruction occurs.

Pain and trauma in degenerative joints

Progressive, *noninflammatory* joint pain with or without abnormal joint motion and/or swelling is another general red flag for ***serious joint deterioration.*** In this case the decision to refer may be based on the progression and severity of a patient's symptoms (and/or unresponsiveness to acupuncture), rather than its mere presence. Noninflammatory joint pain can be divided into traumatic versus degenerative disorders. The two can often coexist, however.

Traumatic disorders like rotator cuff tears of the shoulder or major meniscal and ligament tears in the knee often become more painful over time because too much or too little joint motion, or loose fragments, can irritate the joint. When a stabilizing ligament like the anterior cruciate ligament (ACL) of the knee is torn, for example, abnormal laxity can cause the knee to wear out prematurely from too much motion. Loose piece of meniscus can not only produce pain, but also damage the joint surface.

Traumatic injuries within joints can happen at any age and are more frequent in degenerative joints because collagen at the ends of long bones is less abundant and resilient.

The term "osteoarthrosis" is more accurate than "osteoarthritis" when referring to degenerative joint surfaces because the primary cause of swelling and dysfunction is wear and tear rather than inflammation, even though the two terms are often used interchangeably. Although a little inflammation may be secondarily present in degenerative joints, it is not a primary causative factor as in diseases like RA.

Swelling secondary to osteoarthrosis is typically "cold" and "bony," rather than hot and inflamed. It corresponds well to painful, cold predominant phlegm and blood stasis, and bone types of impediment (painful obstructive syndromes) conditions in Chinese medicine. Bony swelling and stiffness increase along with pain as osteoarthrosis progresses. Swelling can't be seen in joints buried deep within the body such as the hip or vertebral facets of the spine, however.

In deep joints like the spine, we can infer that degeneration is present without seeing the buried joint because other signs associated with degenerative joints like stiffness and pain are often present. The bony swelling, stiffness and decreased ROM come from abutment of enlarged and cartilage denuded joint surfaces with inadequate gliding motion.

Just as *too much* motion and loose joint fragments can cause joint damage and progressive pain, a *loss of motion* can also increase the speed of further degeneration because proper motion of the joint is necessary for optimal lubrication and neuromuscular function of the joint (supply of blood, fluids, and qi in Chinese medical terms). Inadequate joint motion, by depriving the joint of lubrication and inhibiting neuromuscular function around the joint, contributes to further degeneration, a vicious cycle that underlies the degenerative nature of osteoarthrosis.

Although less urgent than inflammatory joint pain, progressively severe joint pain and abnormal motion and/or swelling may contribute to a generalized decline in physical and social activity in many patients. Sometimes, depression and weight gain secondarily occur with their adverse effects on all body systems, including the joints themselves. This degenerative cascade makes it important for acupuncturists to refer patients with progressive joint pain that is unresponsive to acupuncture for coevaluation and comanagement.

Although acupuncture can be very effective, sometimes as a stand-alone treatment for joint pain, we nonetheless advise that patients with severe pain or functional limitations be referred to physicians for consultation, particularly if not satisfactorily responding to acupuncture care. The patient's primary care physician can determine whether physical or injection therapies are indicated to help manage the pain, possibly slow joint degeneration and help the patient adapt to the disability, or whether surgery may be eventually indicated.

Progressive and unremitting bone pain

This is another red flag symptom that can occur anywhere in the body and is a general red flag for bone cancer. Although it is unlikely that patients with advanced bone cancer will present to the acupuncturist as a first resort, early stages will present, as will established cancer patients for adjunctive care. Like all cancer pain, bone cancer pain may begin gradually and be initially underestimated.

The periosteum of bone is richly innervated with pain fibers. Malignant invasion of the periosteum disrupts this sensitive tissue and produces the pain that is so characteristic of bone cancer. Patients with bone cancer typically report the pain as dull, progressive, and eventually constant. Bone cancer may also generate pain in areas not usually affected by other conditions. For example, the pain might occur at the midshaft of the femur rather than at the knee joint.

Bone cancer can be primary (originating in bone), or more commonly, metastatic from cancers in other regions. In men, primary cancers metastasize to bone from, in descending order of frequency: prostate, lung, bladder, stomach, rectum, and colon. In women, they metastasize from, also in order of frequency: breast, uterus, colon, stomach, rectum, and bladder. Whenever bone cancer is suspected, a history screening for general cancer risk factors and symptoms suggesting cancer in other locations should be taken.

When bone cancer is primary, the likely culprits are: osteosarcoma (about 35% of all primary bone cancer), chondrosarcoma (about 26% of primary bone cancer) and Ewing's tumor, which usually affects children and adolescents (about 16% of primary bone cancer). Not included in the above is the multiple myeloma, (0.02%). To know the true incidence of both primary and metastatic type cancers, we would have to put together the frequencies of all types.

Bones with cancer are weak and more prone to break ("pathological fracture") than normal bones. Since osteoporosis also results in easy fracture, the temptation might be to blame fractures that occur with minimal trauma on osteoporosis. The presence of bone cancer should also be considered in these cases, however. It follows from this that **an unexplained fracture caused by minimal or unidentified trauma** is another general red flag for some type of ***pathological deterioration of bone***, whether from osteoporosis, cancer, Paget's disease or some other bone weakening disease.

Pain or loss of function after trauma

The appearance of **severe immediate pain, numbness, weakness and/or loss of function after trauma** is a general red flag for ***fracture or disruption of a vital structure.*** This remains a red flag *even if the pain gets a little better over time.* Any trauma severe enough to produce exquisite pain at the time of injury can also seriously damage tissues. It is included here to highlight ideas that aren't covered elsewhere.

I vividly remember a patient who had *severe* neck pain *immediately* following a motor vehicle accident. The pain was greatly diminished by the time she was examined in the ED. The patient was found to have a neck fracture by an alert physician, even though she claimed to be "much better." The tipoff was the history of the *initial* intensity of the pain. This fracture, undetected, could have allowed a slippage of vertebral elements that could have caused paralysis had the fracture not been detected and stabilized.

How to use pain as a sign for the presence of fracture

This is an appropriate time to point out a common fallacy about fractures: the fallacy that a patient cannot move an extremity if a fracture is present. While this can be true in certain circumstances, and a patient may well be *hesitant* to move a fractured extremity due to pain, it is *not invariably* true. There is often enough continuity of ligament, tendon and perhaps even periosteum to allow movement of fractured extremities.

If the statement that "a patient cannot move a fractured extremity" isn't reliable (therefore not a red flag), what *can* we count on to help us detect the presence of a fracture? The answer is that we can count on the fact that fractures are *always* painful to careful palpatation. This is because periosteum covering bone is richly innervated with pain fibers and is invariably disrupted when a fracture occurs. Palpation of this disrupted periosteum is always painful and is a reliable sign of fracture.

The patient referred to above, in fact, had exquisite palpatory tenderness of the vertebral facets of C-6. In addition to the history of severe initial pain at the time of the injury, this guides us to the presence of a fracture. We cannot make palpatory tenderness over a suspected fracture site a *specific* red flag for fracture, however, because there may be other tender nonbony structures under the examining hand, but *its absence is reliable to help us rule out fracture.*

Pain and immediate swelling

Severe pain and swelling in a joint immediately after trauma is another general red flag, for ***ruptured arterial or arteriolar vessels.*** Venous tears don't produce as much swelling as arterial tears because there is much less pressure in veins. Arterial tears will bleed into a joint until the backward pressure from the swelling equals the 120 mm of mercury pumping out of the ruptured artery. The history of immediate and severe swelling after trauma therefore indicates the possibility of torn arteries or arterioles, which often accompanies tears of major ligaments and/or tendons.

Other pain that can turn chronic

Intense pain and **skin changes persisting many weeks after trauma** is a general red flag for ***complex regional pain syndrome (CRPS).*** CRPS is sometimes also called "causalgia" or "reflex sympathetic dystrophy," the latter term capturing some of the essence of this often baffling and painful disorder; dysfunction of the sympathetic arm of the autonomic nervous system (ANS). CRPS is most likely to occur as the result of major trauma in an extremity. We have seen it often enough in people with seemingly insignificant trauma and after surgery, however, to make us suspicious for early signs of CRPS even in the slightly injured.

The literature agrees with this, noting that approximately 10% of cases occur without identified cause. A small minority of cases appear after stroke or herpes zoster infections as well. Regardless of cause, the consequences of untreated CRPS, which has a poor prognosis even with treatment, can be devastating. It can cause chronic excruciating pain, total disability of the affected limb, severe anxiety and depression, a general decline in health status, localized and bodywide osteoporosis, substance abuse disorders, and suicide.

Although the literature is inconclusive about whether or not early intervention of CRPS can help, we think that it can help for reasons we'll cite below. *We also strongly think that acupuncture is a restorative modality that, with other methods, should be attempted early in the course of CRPS, rather than as a last resort, which is usually the case.*

Since there are no good studies to refute the idea that we

can influence the course of CRPS with early intervention, we'll explore ways to recognize very early stages.

Currently recognized stages of CRPS

Although signs and symptoms of CRPS can vary somewhat from case to case, most authorities agree with something like the following three stages of CRPS. These three stages, all of which include pain, as well as a "prestage" we'll describe later, are based on clinical observations. We'll use the example of CRPS following trauma to an extremity when describing these stages.

Stage one: The first generally recognized stage can last from two weeks to three months after injury. It is characterized by severe (often burning) pain at the site of injury spreading proximally, muscle spasm, joint stiffness, sometimes fast hair growth, changes in the color of the skin (usually toward a reddish or red-purple hue), and changing temperature of the skin (usually warm). A light touch from clothing may feel like a scalding or "wire brush" sensation. This stage is already a fairly established stage of the problem.

Stage two: The second generally recognized stage starts at about three months after the injury. It is characterized by intensifying pain, swelling, decreased hair growth, and changes in the nails that include cracking, brittleness, grooving, or spotting. The skin can go through a cold, pale stage, and look taut, smooth, or even glassy. It is also often moist and sometimes sweaty. Osteoporosis at the ends of bones in the area of the CRPS commonly occurs (localized osteoporosis on plain films) as does joint stiffness and weak muscle tone.

Stage three: The third generally recognized stage begins after the above. By this time there are irreversible changes in skin, joints, and bones. Pain is unrelenting, often involving the entire limb. The skin can be dry, sometimes scaly and mottled. The nails can be thick and ridged. There is often atrophy of the extremity and limited mobility of joints. Neurological dysfunction of the motor nerves is evidenced by tremors (50% of CRPS patients). We occasionally see involuntary contractions of the muscles and contorted and deformed limbs.

As we've discussed with other processes that occur in stages, clinicians should try to detect early stages of the red flag for CRPS. Just as we want to recognize pallor in a patient's complexion without waiting for blueness of the lips as a sign of hypoxia, so we also want to identify an earlier stage for CRPS when therapy might be optimally beneficial. To see if we can do so, we need to reexamine the issue of the timing of pain that we opened this chapter with.

Specifically, we want to look at normal timing of pain resolution versus abnormal timing to see if we can find the earliest point at which a person starts to veer from normal healing to faulty healing.

Using the timing of pain to detect early stages of CRPS and other chronic pain syndromes—the pain trajectory

Injuries that eventually develop into CRPS start out just like other injuries and should resolve like them unless some factor(s) interfere with normal healing. Recognizing the earliest *pre-stage* of CRPS, or any chronic pain syndrome for that matter, is possible by identifying when the normal progression of pain resolution veers off the track.

Although there is always some individual variation, the healing process and accompanying decreasing of pain experienced is remarkably consistent among patients with injuries. The progression of healing and pain resolution can be easily followed by grading and documenting the pain at every visit.

Students are often trained to do this, of course, but we find that they sometimes do not chart or keep up with these scores on a long-term basis or don't remember the pain score from visit to visit. In the busy and sometimes stressful circumstance of practice, we need to force ourselves to grade and document the timing of pain resolution. We can easily graph the progress.

We expect that the injury will "hurt like crazy" for a time and then gradually get better in a "peaks and valleys" pattern over a week or two, eventually crossing a line (pain threshold) under which no significant pain is perceived. Any particular peak along this curve may be higher than a preceding valley, but *a line drawn across the tops of the peaks clearly shows a decreasing slope (trajectory) compatible with normal healing.*

The patient who veers off into a chronic pain condition like CRPS follows a different course. After some initial healing, a factor or set of factors (presence of pathogenic factors or lack of beneficial factors) interferes with normal healing. By two weeks after the injury, even though some of the valleys may dip below the pain threshold, a line drawn across the peaks clearly shows that the trajectory begins increasing, rather than decrease at point C. The point at which the slope changes from a negative (decreasing) slope to a positive (increasing) slope is the crisis point, a danger point for the development of some type of chronic pain.

We can use this crisis point as a signal to initiate aggressive treatment to circumvent the patient's progression toward chronic pain—to remove and/or help a patient remove obvious physical and psychological pathogenic influences (including negative thinking and desire for secondary gain) and/or strengthen beneficial influence, including proper circulation factors as well as energetic and neurological factor. The longer a clinician waits, the more likely it is that a chronic pain condition will develop. The pain trajectory can be an extremely valuable aid to both clinician and patient in understanding the healing process and motivating patients to participate fully in their recovery.

Causes and incidence of CRPS

There is much debate about what causes CRPS, but the symptoms and signs alone tell us that there must be dysfunction of at least three major systems: the neurological, endocrine and immunological. Dysfunction of the sympathetic nervous system must play an important role in the skin changes like sweating and abnormal circulation since the autonomic system regulates such changes. Hormones like epinephrine and norepinephrine (which are also neurotransmit- ters) must also be dysfunction. Finally, inflammation secondary to immune system involvement is also dysfunction.

The best estimate of CRPS incidence can be found in the 1996-2005 "Integrated Primary Care Information (IPCI) project," a general practice research database with electronic patient records of 600,000 patients in the Netherlands. The estimated overall incidence rate of CRPS was 26.2 per 100,000 person years with females affected at least three times more often than males and the highest incidence occurring in females in the 61-70-year-old range. The upper extremity was involved more frequently than the lower and a fracture was the most common precipitating event (44%). Postmenopausal woman were at highest risk for CRPS.

Abdominal pain as a general red flag

Abdominal pain is a common problem in primary care, accounting for 2.5 million office visits and eight million ED visits yearly. Although it may not be as common in acupuncture practices as back pain or anxiety, it may frequently present itself as "digestive problems." Gallbladder disease, for example, can cause both digestive problems and abdominal pain. (Gallbladder red flags are presented in the Indigestion symptom section in this book.)

Most patients with abdominal pain have minor causes, but a surprisingly high percentage, approximately 20%, are eventually admitted to the hospital for evaluation and treatment. Although most acute abdominal pain situations will not be seen first by acupuncturists, patients with serious abdominal pain may present to acupuncturists in subacute phases or between acute attacks, or abdominal pain may be mentioned of as a symptom in patients presenting with different chief complaints.

There are many serious conditions that can cause **abdominal pain and rigidity of abdominal muscles**, but whatever their specific etiology, they all have the same common mechanism for producing this *general red flag – **irritation of the inner lining of the abdominal peritoneum from blood and/or pus***. The irritation causes the abdominal muscle to go into spasm in an attempt to protect the abdominal contents from jostling and further irritation, resulting in the characteristic rigid abdomen.

This condition is sometimes also called an "***acute abdomen***," or a "***surgical abdomen***" to indicate, in the first case, its urgency and, in the second case, the probability that surgery may be necessary. Many beginning students have some difficulty differentiating a true rigid abdomen from a well muscled, tense abdomen. The distinction should be simple, however, because a muscular abdomen can be relaxed at will and an acute abdomen cannot and is also accompanied by extreme pain on palpation.

The blood and/or pus that irritate the inner lining of the peritoneum can come from either from a solid or hollow organ or blood vessels associated with organs. Penetrating injuries like knife and bullet wounds or sufficient blunt trauma can cause hemorrhage of solid organs, particularly the spleen and liver. Hollow organs are less likely to bleed from blunt trauma due to their flexibility, but are susceptible to infection. Both types of organs can ooze pus and/or blood into the peritoneal cavity causing abdominal muscle splinting.

The solid organs: pancreas, liver, spleen, and kidneys are susceptible to being infected through dissemination of pathogenic organisms in blood. This does not generally happen as often with hollow organs because the infection is washed away. It can happen, however, if the opening of the organ becomes blocked, as with appendicitis. To determine which specific hollow organs can become blocked, inflamed, infected, or can bleed we need to ask ourselves what "tubes" are present within the abdominal cavity. Here is a list of candidates:

a. **Stomach.** The stomach isn't generally a source of infection probably because it is churning and full of digestive enzymes and stomach acids, discouraging the growth of many organisms. Ulceration through the stomach can occur, however.

b. **Gallbladder.** Any viscous organ with a narrow orifice that can be blocked by stones or swelling or some combination of stones or fecal matter and infection is susceptible to blockage and abscess formation. The GB duct is one such orifice that can become blocked causing oozing through the GB wall.

c. **Appendix.** The appendiceal orifice that empties into the cecum is prone to blockage with fecal material and swelling causing stasis in the appendix with the buildup of pressure and oozing of pus through the appendiceal wall into the peritoneum.

d. **The fallopian tubes.** The salpinges (fallopian tubes) can be infected by a number of organisms from the female genital tract. If the infection and oozing are bad enough, there may be severe lower pelvic pain. Although this doesn't commonly cause a rigid abdomen, it can cause "pelvic inflammatory disease" (PID)."

With these general concepts in mind, let us proceed to the specific red flags under pain, starting with abdominal pain and continuing through all categories of red flag pain.

Specific red flags: *Upper abdominal (midepigastric) pain and vomiting blood*

Condition assumed present until proven otherwise:
Upper GI hemorrhage from inner lining of stomach and/or esophagus

Possible consequences of missing the condition:
Possible death due to massive bleeding from upper gastro-intestinal tract

Stabilization, referral and management:

1. **Stabilization:** If the vomiting is finished *and the patient is no longer nauseated,* they may be offered anti-emetic acupuncture and herbal medicine as well as over the counter acid reducers. These can be important to help stabilize the patient until referral and future diagnostic workup are accomplished.
2. **Consultation and Referral Options, Transportation:** In the situation of *relatively* stable patient described above, semi-urgent referral should be made to the PCP if one is available or an urgent care center if not. Transport can be by private vehicle with a friend or family member driving unless cardiopulmonary support is needed. If the patient is vomiting blood and is unstable from a cardiopulmonary point of view (see chest pain), 911 should be called.

Relevance to acupuncturists: The common symptom of upper and mid- abdominal pain may be a chief complaint or may arise during the course of routine questioning about diet, appetite, and digestive function. Although the presentation in this red flag can be acute and severe, most cases have milder presentations and may mislead patient and acupuncturist into missing a potentially dangerous condition.

ACTUAL CASE

- **History:** A 30-year-old male patient with a history of drinking a six-pack of beer a day and taking Ibuprofen daily for headache was seen in the office for upper abdominal pain. During the interview, the patient became nauseated and began retching. He then threw up some visible blood with stomach contents.
- **Physical findings:** The patient appeared generally healthy, but in obvious pain, holding his abdomen. His blood pressure was 110/70mmHg and pulse was 85bpm and regular. The abdomen was non-obese and fairly soft. There was significant midepigastric tenderness to deep palpation.
- **Impression:** Probable gastric mucosal bleeding, but also possible bleeding as from esophageal varices due to alcoholism.
- **Plan:** Since the bleeding had stopped and the patient was not nauseated and appeared stable, the patient's father was called to transport his son to the ED of a nearby hospital.

- **Follow up:** The patient began vomiting blood profusely once he arrived at the ED. His blood pressure dropped to 100/60mmHg. A nasogastric tube was promptly placed to empty the stomach and he was given fluids intravenously and two units of packed RBCs because his hemoglobin was 7.0 (14-16 normal). The patient was taken to surgery where an ulcer was excised from his stomach and the defect repaired. He had a long and stormy postoperative course, but was eventually discharged from the hospital and has done well since then.

DISCUSSION

History and Symptoms

The history of abdominal pain during GI hemorrhage is almost universally present, but some patients have surprisingly little pain leading up to hemorrhage, making it very important to keep the risk factors identifying those *likely* to suffer GI hemorrhage in mind. Additionally, reports of previous melanotic stools should serve as a marker for possible prior upper GI bleeding. Reports of prior "indigestion" or epigastric fullness and burning sensations or nausea are also symptoms that may be suggestive of underlying gastritis. If heartburn symptoms are noted, we must remember that the upper GI tract is one continuous tract and that gastric inflammation and esophageal inflammation may well coexist. In the alcoholic, esophageal varices (swollen esophageal veins) may be present.

Physical Exam Findings

There may be no physical exam findings other than vomiting. The clinician who suspects upper GI bleeding should check for midepigastric tenderness (the midepigastrium in the *region of the abdomen just beneath the zyphoid process of the sternum)* with careful palpation. Any significant blood pressure fall (systolic > 20 points) or shock signs (low BP, cerebral dysfunction, rapid and weak pulse, etc.) would indicate an extreme situation with possible circulatory collapse.

Incidence and/or Prevalence

Gastritis, esophagitis and gastric ulcer disease serve as the backdrop for upper GI hemorrhage and are extraordinarily common. Gastritis is the beginning stage of inflammation. When discreet defects of the gastric mucosa develop, the disease has entered the peptic ulcer disease (PUD) state. Approximately 10% of Americans eventually develop PUD, and about 10% of patients presenting to the ED with abdominal pain are diagnosed with PUD. NSAID and aspirin use has become the most common cause of gastrointestinal mucosal damage and bleeding in Western countries. It is estimated that up to 30% of *regular* NSAID users have one or more ulcers.

Risk Factors

- Previous history of ulcers or gastritis
- Male gender
- Overuse of aspirin or other NSAIDs
- Cigarette smoking
- Psychosocial stress or skipped meals
- Heavy alcohol use is a risk factor for gastric ulceration
- Heavy alcohol use is also a risk factor for cirrhosis of the liver and esophageal varices (see mechanism producing red flag section of this red flag)

Mechanism Producing the Red Flag

Bleeding into the esophagus or stomach causes nausea and vomiting. Erosion of blood vessels by the gastric inflammation can cause rupture and fatal hemorrhage. The trauma of retching may break other fragile vessels and cause more vomiting resulting in a vicious cycle of vomiting and bleeding. Esophageal varices may also rupture with continued retching. Varices are swollen veins in the esophagus formed by backpressure from the scarring of liver cirrhosis due to alcoholism.

Other Important Considerations

- The incidence of PUD
- PUD, as the final stage of gastritis related illness, is increasing in the industrialized world.
- The presence of the organism H. pylori is associated with an increased incidence of PUD.
- Not covered in this red flag, but important, is the other possibly disastrous complication of PUD. An ulcer may penetrate through the stomach lining into the abdominal cavity leading to sepsis, shock, and death if not treated promptly treated.

Specific red flags:
Daily heartburn for many years

Condition assumed present until proven otherwise:

Chronic esophagitis

Possible consequences of missing the condition:

Barrett's esophagus (precancerous) or esophageal cancer

Disability and untimely death

Stabilization, referral and management:

1. **Stabilization:** The patient should be instructed to avoid overeating just prior to lying down and to avoid foods that cause reflux (chocolate, coffee, alcohol, mint, tomatoes, fatty, and spicy foods) until the consult can be accomplished. Over the counter stomach acid reducers can be taken as needed to quench the acidity.
2. **Consultation and Referral Options, Transportation:** Patients with chronic esophagitis should be treated to relieve the condition completely. Chinese medicine is certainly effective, but the patient with long standing problems should also be checked for H. pylori infection and should possibly have endoscopy. These can be accomplished through a referral to the patient's PCP, who will likely refer to a gastroenterologist. Although the risk of Barrett's esophagus (the cellular precursor to esophageal cancer) and esophageal cancer is substantial with chronic heartburn, the disease progresses slowly so the referral is only timely. No special transportation is required.

Relevance to acupuncturists: Chronic heartburn is a common symptom which may be a chief complaint or may arise during the course of routine questioning about diet, appetite, and digestive function. Heartburn is so common and the risk of developing esophageal cancer from chronic heartburn is so little known that patients and acupuncturists may miss the potential of this lethal condition developing. At the very least, spotting this red flag and understanding its importance is strong motivation to treat chronic heartburn aggressively.

ACTUAL CASE

- **History:** A 55-year-old male CEO presented with a history of moderate to severe "heartburn" almost every day for at least 20 years. He reported smoking one pack per day of cigarettes and drinking two glasses of wine every night, the latter to "keep my heart in good shape."
- **Physical findings:** Examination revealed a mildly over weight Caucasian male with a normal exam except for moderate positive midepigastric tenderness
- **Impression:** Chronic reflux esophagitis
- **Plan:** Referral to gastroenterologist
- **Follow up:** The gastroenterologist performed an upper GI endoscopy and biopsy on abnormal appearing mucosal tissue in the esophagus, which turned out to be Barrett's tissue (precancerous). The patient, when faced with the facts and the possible bleak prognosis, complied with advice to quit smoking and to decrease alcohol con sumption. He was also placed on proton pump inhibitors and is currently asymptomatic, but is on a heightened surveillance program of every other year endoscopy to check for possible progression to malignancy.

DISCUSSION

History and Symptoms

The typical symptoms are burning reflux pain in the central chest, occasionally with bitter/sour/acidic wash into the back of the throat or mouth ("water brash"). Interestingly, some people with fairly severe esophagitis (as proven by endoscopy) never have the symptom of severe heartburn, so a high index of suspicion must be maintained for chronic esophagitis if risk factors are present.

Physical Exam Findings

There is often midepigastric tenderness to deep palpation, but sometimes no physical findings are present.

Incidence and/or Prevalence

A 1999 study in the New England Journal of Medicine states that up to 9% of the population has daily heartburn. Esophageal cancer risk is nearly eight times higher in this group. Esophageal cancer is not the most common type of cancer, but it is particularly dangerous. This is not only due to its intrinsic malignant potential, but also because most cases are not detected until the cancer has metastasized to regional lymph nodes. The U.S. incidence is 12,500 cases yearly, of which 12,000 are fatal. Like most other cancers, it is most common in people over 50.

Risk Factors

Risk factors are the same as those for reflux esophagitis

(Gastroesophageal reflux disease— GERD).
- High fat diet
- Heavy meals before lying down
- Cigarette smoking
- Alcohol ingestion
- Obesity
- Family history of GI cancer

Mechanism Producing the Red Flag

- Chronic inflammation can be a cause of cancer in many areas of the body, as it is in the esophagus.

Specific red flags:
Severe abdominal pain (better with leaning forward) with nausea and vomiting

Condition assumed present until proven otherwise:

Acute pancreatitis – Inflammation of the pancreas due to autodigestion by pancreatic enzymes

Possible consequences of missing the condition:

Severe pain and possible fatality

Stabilization, referral and management:

1. **Stabilization:** There are no specific stabilizing steps. Patient should not ingest anything during a full-blown attack because they will invariably vomit it. They should not consume alcohol if they are between acute attacks.
2. **Consultation and Referral Options, Transportation:** Patients with acute pancreatitis should be directed to the nearest ED of a hospital because they will need admission. The quickest means available should be taken. A 911 call is not necessary unless there is cardiopulmonary or neurological compromise (falling blood pressure, irregular pulse, unconsciousness, etc.).

Relevance to acupuncturists: Although patients in the throes of severe acute pancreatitis are unlikely to walk into your office, those in early stages or between acute attacks will. Knowing the red flag for this painful and potentially deadly problem will help you refer those in the beginning stages and identify those between attacks so you can counsel them about how to avoid future attacks (see risk factors).

ACTUAL CASE

- **History:** A 40-year-old African-American female had an episode of severe abdominal pain that had landed her in the hospital several months before coming in for acupuncture treatments. She described the episode as extreme abdominal pain. She did not have a known history of gallstones (one of the causes of pancreatitis), but did have a history of drinking two six packs of beer on most weekends.
- **Physical findings:** The patient had a normal physical exam.
- **Impression:** Probable pancreatitis, now asymptomatic
- **Plan:** The patient was counseled about the link between alcohol and pancreatitis and was also given the name of a PCP that she could consult for future therapy should it recur.
- **Follow up:** The patient did not follow up with the PCP consulted. She had another episode one month later. In the ER, she had high serum amylase and lipase levels in her blood. A nasogastric tube was placed to empty the stomach due to continuous vomiting. The patient was given fluids and pain meds intravenously. A sonogram of the gallbladder was negative.

  The presumptive cause for her pancreatitis was alcohol abuse. She had surgery to remove a necrotic area in her pancreas. The patient was eventually discharged from the hospital in good condition. Unfortunately she continued to drink alcohol and had a repeat admission two months later for the same diagnosis. After her second discharge, she joined A.A. and is now in recovery. She has had no further episodes of pancreatitis.

DISCUSSION

History and Symptoms

The main symptom of acute pancreatitis is abdominal pain in the upper left side or middle of the abdomen. The pain is persistent and worse when lying flat on the back, which is the reason we so often find these patients leaning forward. The pain may radiate to the back or below the left shoulder blade and may be worse immediately after eating, especially foods with a high fat content, and resemble cholecystitis patients in this regard. They are also worse after drinking alcohol. Drinking alcohol may well set off an acute attack, as in our ACTUAL CASE. They invariably have nausea and often severe vomiting. Other common symptoms may include anxiety, fever, mild jaundice, and sweating. Mild or early cases may present as" indigestion."

Physical Exam Findings

Patients with acute pancreatitis will invariably look very ill and can go into shock, i.e., blood pressure can fall to unsafe levels and vital signs can be unstable. The patient may look ashen. On abdominal exam we note exquisite abdominal tenderness with distension, guarding, and rigidity. They often also have fast heartbeat (tachycardia) and breathing (tachypnea), fever, and mild jaundice

Incidence and/or Prevalence

The yearly incidence of acute pancreatitis is 20-40 per 100,000 people. Males are affected more than females. Mild edematous pancreatitis occurs about 80% of the time, and the mortality rate is below 1%. Severe acute pancreatitis occurs in about 20% of presentations, with a mortality rate reaching 30%.

Risk Factors

In adults, 40% of cases are due to cholelithiasis, 40% are due to alcohol abuse, and the remaining 20% are due to causes including:

- Drugs: especially estrogens, corticosteroids, thiazide diuretics, and azathioprine
- Trauma: Some types of bile duct surgery, pancreatic surgery, or severe blow to abdomen
- Viral and bacterial infections: including mumps, Coxsackie B, Mycoplasma pneumonia, and Campylobacter
- An abnormal structure of the pancreas
- Complications of cystic fibrosis
- Genetic factors (hereditary pancreatitis)
- High lipid levels in the blood (hypertriglyceridemia)

In children, this disorder may be associated with:

- Abdominal trauma
- Cystic fibrosis
- Hemolytic uremic syndrome
- Kawasaki disease
- Mumps
- Reye syndrome
- Some medications
- Various viral illnesses

Mechanism Producing the Red Flag

The mechanism of injury to the pancreas due to gallbladder disease is the passage of a gallstone into the common bile duct where it enters the duodenum. The pancreatic digestive enzymes that are normally excreted to aid in digestion cannot get past the stone and back up through the pancreatic duct into the pancreas, where they "autodigest" pancreatic tissues (see figure 3) . In the case of alcoholism, the injury to the pancreas is due to a direct toxic effect of alcohol, as it is with other drugs.

Other considerations

- Acute pancreatitis tends to be recurrent as long as the causes are not addressed.
- Patients with silent pancreatitis may have gallstones removed to decrease their risks of acute severe pancreatitis. In all cases, treating the condition that caused the problem can prevent recurrent attacks.
- In some cases, radiologic or endoscopic therapy is needed to drain fluid collections in or around the pancreas, remove gallstones or blockages of the pancreatic duct. In the most severe cases, surgery is necessary to remove dead, infected pancreatic tissue.

Specific red flags:
Mid-abdominal pain followed by vomiting then pain moving to right lower abdomen

Condition assumed present until proven otherwise:

Acute appendicitis

Possible consequences of missing the condition:

Infection in the abdominal peritoneal cavity (peritonitis), possible generalized blood infection (sepsis) and death

Stabilization, referral and management:

1. **Stabilization:** There are no specific outpatient stabilizing steps to take. The patient will usually have little interest in eating or drinking, and should not attempt it.
2. **Consultation and Referral Options, Transportation:** Patients in whom appendicitis is suspected will need to go the ED to rule it in or out because surgery is invariably necessary for acute appendicitis. They can go by family transport, if they are stable enough, which they usually are. As always, patients unstable from a cardiopulmonary point of view should have emergency transport via a 911 call.

Relevance to acupuncturists: It would be unlikely that an adolescent in the peak of acute appendicitis would go first to an acupuncturist's office, but patients in early stages may. Also, older adults may have much less dramatic symptoms and may come for acupuncture treatments.

ACTUAL CASE

- **History:** Joey was a 16-year-old male brought to the office by his mother with a history of waking with pain above his umbilicus. He vomited shortly thereafter. His temperature was 99.0° F orally at home.
- **Physical findings:** The patient appeared to be in moderate pain. He was most comfortable when lying still. Shaking the acupuncture table accidentally caused an increase in his pain (positive jar sign). His right lower abdomen was painful, rigid, and exquisitely tender on palpation. There was positive rebound tenderness. Bowel sounds were absent.
- **Impression:** Possible acute appendicitis
- **Plan:** The patient was sent to the ED at a local hospital, transported by his mother.
- **Follow up:** The patient was seen by the ED physician who concurred with the possibility of appendicitis. A WBC count of the blood was elevated to 15,000 and a CT scan of the abdomen showed a swollen appendix. An infected appendix was removed in surgery and the patient recovered nicely.

DISCUSSION

History and Symptoms

The classical appendicitis presentation of **mid-upper abdominal (midepigastric) pain followed by vomiting, then the pain moving to the right lower abdominal quadrant (RLQ)** only occurs in 50% of cases. Appendicitis can be easily missed, because not all presentations are classical. Another common symptom not mentioned earlier is absence of appetite (anorexia). Variations in the position of the appendix around McBurney's point, age of the patient, and degree of inflammation make the clinical presentation of appendicitis notoriously inconsistent.

Migration of pain from the midepigastric or periumbilical area to the RLQ is the most discriminating feature of the patient's history and has a sensitivity and specificity of approximately 80%. When vomiting occurs, it nearly always follows the onset of pain. Vomiting that precedes pain is suggestive of intestinal obstruction. Diarrhea or constipation is noted in as many as 18% of patients and should not be used to discard the possibility of appendicitis.

Physical Exam Findings

RLQ tenderness is present in 96% of patients. Rarely, left lower quadrant (LLQ) tenderness is the major manifestation in patients with the abdominal organs in reverse position (situs inversus) or in patients with a long appendix that extends into the LLQ. The most specific physical findings are rebound tenderness (worsening of pain when the examining hand is pressed firmly on the abdomen and suddenly removed), pain on percussion, rigidity, and guarding. Bowel sounds are invariably absent. The patient's pain is worsened with shaking the abdomen or the table upon which the patient is lying (jar sign). Fever may be completely absent or is low grade *unless there is rupture of the appendix* (see next red flag).

Incidence and/or Prevalence

Appendicitis has a yearly incidence of 1.1 cases per 1000. The incidence gradually rises from birth, peaks in the late teens then gradually declines. 3% of women and 2% of men older than 50 years old are affected. Although rare, neonatal and even prenatal appendicitis has been reported.

Risk Factors

- Age < 30, but can occur at any age.
- Some familial predisposition exists.

Mechanism Producing the Red Flag

The appendix is an anatomical blind pouch. Obstruction of the appendiceal opening (lumen) causes appendicitis. The most common obstructing factors are fecaliths and lymphoid hyperplasia. Obstruction is less commonly associated with parasites (*schistosomes*, for example), foreign material like tongue studs, tuberculosis, and tumors. Whatever the cause of obstruction of the appendiceal lumen, the result is distension of the appendix due to accumulation of intraluminal fluid.

The inability of debris to exit the appendix causes intra-appendiceal pressure to build that forces blood and pus out through the inflamed walls into the abdominal cavity where they act as irritants to the peritoneal lining. This irritation causes a reflex spastic constriction of the overlying muscles in an attempt to "splint" the abdomen from further harm. Inflammation of the intestine also leads to paralysis of the intestines (adynamic or paralytic-ileus), which causes lack of appetite (anorexia) and vomiting. This explains not only the anorexia and sometimes vomiting in appendicitis, but also the absence of gurgling bowel sounds (borborygmi) on exam.

The initial midepigastric pain that occurs in classic cases is probably a reflex pain radiating from the appendiceal irritation to the midepigastrium. The fever in appendicitis is minimal because the body contains most of the pus within the abscessed appendix.

Other considerations

- Acute appendicitis doesn't "smolder" over years, a theory I occasionally hear advanced by students when considering obscure causes of lower abdominal pain. Long-term abdominal pain near the appendix is much more likely to be irritable colon, intestinal volvulus ovarian cysts in women, or even a trigger point in the psoas muscle rather than appendicitis.
- Spasm of the abdominal muscles causing a rigid abdomen is typical of all conditions in which blood and/or pus irritate the peritoneal lining – whether from the appendix, a ruptured ovary or a penetrating ulcer. This always produces **abdominal muscle rigidity**, which has already been mentioned as a general red flag for *peritoneal irritation.*
- Mortality rate from appendicitis rises above 20% in patients older than 70 years. This increase is thought to be due to diagnostic and therapeutic delay. An overall mortality rate of 0.2-0.8% is generally due to complications of the disease, rather than surgical intervention.
- Perforation (rupture) of the appendix rate is higher among patients < 18 and > 50 years old and is thought to be due to delays in diagnosis. Appendiceal perforation is associated with a sharp increase in morbidity and mortality rates (see next red flag).

Specific red flags:
Sudden lessening of appendicitis symptoms, followed by later worsening of pain and fever

Condition assumed present until proven otherwise:
"Honeymoon" from decreased pressure in appendix, then peritonitis

Possible consequences of missing the condition:
Generalized sepsis, precipitous fall in blood pressure (shock) and death

Stabilization, referral and management:

1. **Stabilization:** There are no stabilizing steps to take.
2. **Consultation and Referral Options, Transportation:** The patient should be sent directly to the ED of a hospital by the fastest means available. A call should be made before the patient reaches the ED about the patient's imminent arrival and what you suspect. If the patient is not in shock and vital signs are stable, transport can be by private vehicle with friend or family member driving, otherwise 911 should be activated.

Relevance to acupuncturists: It would be unlikely that a patient in the peak of acute appendicitis would present to the acupuncturist first, but it is not unreasonable to think that a patient in the midst of the relief phase from appendiceal rupture would present for treatment.

ACTUAL CASE

- **History:** A 16-year-old male patient was brought to the office by his mother for previously scheduled treatment of headache. She was going to cancel because symptoms of vomiting and abdominal pain had occurred when they were getting ready to come to the office but it suddenly improved, so she decided to keep the appointment.
- **Physical findings:** The patient initially appeared only tired, but as the interview progressed he became more and more distressed and complained of increasing abdominal pain. His temperature was 102.9° F. His abdomen was rigid with rebound tenderness in the right lower quadrant. He began to have chills and sweating and his complexion became ashen.
- **Impression:** Ruptured appendix
- **Plan:** The patient was sent directly to the ED of a nearby hospital with his mother driving and the ED doctor was called to inform him of the situation.
- **Follow up:** By the time the patient arrived at the ED the physician there had alerted a surgeon about the impending arrival of the patient with a possible ruptured

appendix. The patient was supported with IV antibiotics and fluids. A ruptured appendix was removed in the OR within the hour. The patient made a full recovery.

DISCUSSION

History and Symptoms

Patients who experience a rupture of an infected appendix generally feel better for a while after release of pressure in the swollen appendix. The "honeymoon" is fairly short, however, because infected material is released into the abdominal cavity causing peritonitis. Symptoms of high fever, shaking chills, vomiting, and nausea replace the relief. These symptoms are then accompanied by intensification of the abdominal pain. Soon it is obvious the patient is getting much worse rather than better.

Physical Exam Findings

The patient will appear to be in less pain after an appendix rupture, but the exam remains positive for a rigid abdomen even as the symptoms improve, a tip off that the problem has not passed. Soon the patient's general appearance will worsen as the complexion becomes ashen, the pulse more rapid and fever increases. The patient will eventually go into shock and die if the situation is not addressed by surgery as soon as possible.

Incidence and/or prevalence

The incidence of appendicitis is 1.1/1000 per year. An unknown percentage of these cases suffer from rupture.

Risk factors

- Appendicitis symptoms, as outlined previously
- Patient younger than 30

Mechanism Producing the Red Flag

As mentioned, the buildup of pressure in the appendix is suddenly relieved as the appendix ruptures, relieving symptoms associated with intra-appendiceal pressure, but ushering in those associated with peritonitis.

Other considerations

- Parents have been known to "turn the car around" after a honeymoon like this en route to the ED, only to redirect even more urgently as the patient suddenly worsens again, becomes ashen, and goes into shock.

Specific red flags:
Mid to lower abdominal colicky pain, vomiting, constipation, abdominal distension

Condition assumed present until proven otherwise:
Bowel obstruction

Possible consequences of missing the condition:
Death

Stabilization, referral and management:

1. **Stabilization:** The only stabilizing step is to not let the patient attempt to eat anything.
2. **Consultation and Referral Options, Transportation:** The situation is an emergency. The patient should be sent to the nearest ED and the physician on duty or triage nurse should be notified. If the patient is showing unstable vitals, shock or cardiopulmonary compromise, emergency transport should be summoned via 911. Otherwise, private transport with non-patient driver is adequate.

Relevance to acupuncturists: Early cases of bowel obstruction can present self-diagnosed by patients as "stomach flu" or "food poisoning." The phrase "bowel obstruction" is also commonly misused by patients and some clinicians to mean various conditions of bowel slowdown or constipation, adding to the confusion. True bowel obstruction, however, is a medical emergency that must be recognized and acted on promptly by the acupuncturist.

ACTUAL CASE

- **History:** A 75-year-old otherwise healthy Caucasian female came in to the office complaining of constipation and greatly decreased appetite (anorexia) and mild abdominal pain. There was prior history of gallbladder removal (cholecystectomy) and appendix removal (appendectomy). Before the patient could finish her intake history, she became ill and vomited. Her abdominal pain grew progressively worse.
- **Physical findings:** The patient initially looked rather ill, but she looked much worse after vomiting. Vital signs were stable.
- **Impression:** Probable bowel obstruction
- **Plan:** While we were contemplating whether or not the patient's sister could take her to the ED, that patient also began to complain of chest pain. A call was placed

to 911 and the patient was transported to the ER.

- **Follow up:** The patient was placed on nasogastric suction in the ED after an abdominal film showed loops of gas filled bowel above an area of presumed obstruction. She was supported by IV fluids and her pain lessened somewhat. An emergency colonoscopy showed no cancer or diverticulitis disease. Possible surgery was anticipated, but it was called off when the section of colon that had been kinked over intra-abdominal scar tissue (from the prior surgeries) released itself spontaneously. The patient's symptoms resolved completely. She has not had a recurrence to date.

DISCUSSION

History and Symptoms

In "acute" small bowel obstruction, pain appears first, followed by vomiting, distension and constipation. In large bowel obstruction, constipation is followed by distension, pain and vomiting. Either way, persistent vomiting is a key feature of true bowel obstruction (as opposed to bowel slowdown – ileus).

Physical Exam Findings

A distended abdomen is always present. The abdomen can be tapped on to reveal air in the bowel (tympanic sounds). Bowel sounds on auscultation with a stethoscope often have a crescendo-like quality as peristaltic waves rush up to the obstruction only to stop, causing the tone to rise.

Incidence and/or Prevalence

Obstruction of the large or small bowel is a major health problem for the elderly accounting for 12% of abdominal pain cases.

Risk Factors for Small Bowel Obstruction

- Internal abdominal scarring (adhesions) due to prior surgery
- Cancers
- Neoplasm
- Hernias

Risk Factors for Large Bowel Obstruction

- As above
- Colon carcinoma
- Diverticulitis
- Sigmoid volvulus

Mechanism Producing the Red Flag

What cannot go down must come up. True bowel obstruction invariably produces vomiting. The distension of the abdomen is caused by air that gets caught in the swollen loops of bowel just proximal to the obstruction.

Another Important Consideration

- Nasogastric suction in the hospital gives a chance for the obstruction to relieve itself without surgery.

Back Pain
Introductory remarks

Low back pain is the most common condition sending patients to seek acupuncture in the U.S. It is therefore crucial for acupuncturists to be able to identify the urgent presentations of this ubiquitous and usually non-serious condition. More than 80% of people will have significant back pain sometime in their life. Ninety percent will resolve within 4-12 weeks regardless of therapy. The remaining patients whose symptoms don't resolve still represent a huge number of patients.

Many sources divide back pain into two categories based on etiology: mechanical and nonmechanical. While this is somewhat helpful, it is also arbitrary and limited because the two conditions often overlap. For example, back pain from nonmechanical causes (tumor, inflammation, etc.) is sometimes exacerbated by mechanical factors like lifting and bending, and mechanical back pain can be complicated by nonmechanical factors such as psychological depression. We prefer to distinguish back pain based on severity of signs and symptoms along with specific anatomy and etiology.

Before we go to the specific red flags under back pain, please note that the type of back pain that usually ends up being serious is back pain with neurological complications. These complications fall into two general categories: spinal cord compression syndrome and nerve root radiculopathy. Compression on the cord causes bilateral neurological signs and symptom. Compression on nerve roots where they exit the neuroforamina cause unilateral signs and symptoms (radiculopathy). Rarely there can be simultaneous bilateral radiculopathy.

Specific red flags:
Low back pain with progressive leg numbness, tingling, and weakness

Serious condition assumed present until proven otherwise:
Compression neuropathy from pressure on lumbar nerve roots (radiculopathy)

Possible consequences of missing the condition:
Permanent numbness, weakness and loss of function of lower extremity, especially the feet.

Stabilization, referral and management:

1. **Stabilization:** The patient should be advised about postures and positions that can be used to rest the back and about avoidance of activities that risk exacerbation (forward flexion, lifting and carrying, prolonged bed-rest).
2. **Consultation and Referral Options, Transportation:** Referrals can be guided by grading radiculopathies into 4 stages, with different degrees of threat at each stage. The grading of radiculopathy is based upon an understanding that the anatomy of major nerves that carry both motor and sensory fibers. Major nerves have sensory fibers on the outside of the nerve trunk and motor fibers on the inside, so that sensory symptoms appear before motor signs if a nerve is impinged upon from the outside of the nerve, like pressure from a ruptured disc. This is the reason that the presence of motor symptoms and signs always indicates greater threat to these types of nerves, because motor symptoms and signs indicate deeper compression. *This reliable clinical pearl will help you estimate not only the degree of threat to a nerve, but also the prognosis for the patient and how much treatment they may need.*

- **Grade 1:** Back mildly painful with intermittent paresthesia in buttock, hip and/or leg. No sensory, motor or reflex impairment in the lower extremity. (Sensory fibers minimally compressed. No compression of motor fibers). *Immediate referral not necessary. Patient should be treated, re-evaluated consistently and referred if condition progresses.*
- **Grade 2:** Back moderately painful with constant paresthesia and objectively verifiable sensory loss in buttock, hip, leg and/or foot. (Sensory fibers significantly compressed. No significant compression of motor fibers). *These patients should be treated aggressively and referred for evaluation and possible co-treatment to the patient's PCP on a timely basis.*
- **Grade 3:** Back very painful with paresthesia, constant numbness, weakness, and loss of reflex in leg, and/or foot, but no atrophy evident. (Sensory fibers extremely

compressed, motor fibers mildly compressed). *These patients should be treated aggressively and referred on a semi-urgent basis to their PCP, spine specialist or neurosurgeon if a PCP is not available.*

- **Grade 4:** Back severely painful and/or numbness and/or paresthesia with inability to move some muscles and muscle atrophy in buttock, hip, leg and/or foot. (Major compression of sensory and motor fibers). *Acupuncture treatment should not delay a semi-urgent referral to the patient's PCP or neurosurgeon if no PCP is available.*

Relevance to acupuncturists: When low back pain is accompanied by symptoms of compression neuropathy (radiculopathy in the case of nerve roots), it is especially important for the acupuncturist to know when referral should be made. *A surgical referral will not necessarily mean that surgery will be performed, since many neuropathies will respond to non-surgical treatments over time.* The importance of proper referral is that, if surgery does become necessary, a surgeon will be available and prepared.

ACTUAL CASE

- **History:** Bill was a physically active 43-year-old who had been lifting boxes at home when he felt a "catch" in his low back. Later that day he couldn't find a comfortable position for sitting, lying down or standing. After two days he began feeling "shocks" and tingling sensations traveling down his right leg to the ball of his foot.
- **Physical findings:** The patient walked into the exam room in obvious pain with his trunk bending to the left. He could forward flex at the lumbar spine only a few degrees. Further motion caused a "jolt" down the back of the right leg to his foot. When standing on his heels, his right foot dropped to the floor. Right plantar reflex was diminished compared to the left. No muscle atrophy or loss of tone was visible in the right leg. In preparation to needle UB 62 and UB 64, he couldn't feel the cotton ball or the cool, wet sensation of the alcohol.
- **Impression:** Severe/grade 3, acute lumbar disc herniation with radiculopathy
- **Plans:** Lacking a PCP, the patient was referred on a semiurgent basis to a physiatrist (physical medicine specialist) specializing in spine disorders. The physiatrist ordered an MRI and advised the patient that aggressive treatment and a neurosurgical consultation were both indicated. The patient deferred the neurosurgical consultation but was treated with electro-acupuncture for six visits over three weeks and was prescribed home exercises.
- **Follow up:** The patient's leg weakness, sensory deficits, pain, and paresthesias were resolved at the end of three weeks of treatment, although he continued to suffer residual back pain. At one month follow-up, the back pain had improved to self-management levels.

DISCUSSION

History and Symptoms

Surprisingly, some cases of disc rupture seem to occur with minimal or even no history of trauma. I distinctly remember several cases in which patients had reached to scratch a foot while in bed and traumatized a disc. More typically, however, disc injury and accompanying nerve root compression occurs as the result of a lifting injury, especially lifting and twisting. However it occurs, it is generally followed by lower back pain and possibly tingling and numbness which the patient may describe as sciatica, buttock, hip, groin, knee, or leg pain. The leg pain can be worse than the back pain, and symptoms may even appear only in the legs. In unusual cases the leg symptoms are bilateral, but unilaterality is the norm.

Physical Exam Findings

The patient may walk or sit in obvious pain, generally leaning away from the affected side. Decreased range of motion (ROM) on forward flexion and backwards bending and increased paraspinal muscle tension is present in almost all cases because the paraspinal muscle stand "on guard" trying to prevent further injury. Diminished sensory function may be evident in foot dermatomes corresponding to particular nerve roots (see standard anatomical texts for these patterns).

Patellar or Achilles tendon reflexes may be diminished on the affected side. Decreased strength in dorsiflexion of the foot leads to possible "foot slap" (dorsiflexion weakness) if the L5 root is involved or decreased toe plantar flexion strength if S1 is involved. In some cases the weakness is so profound that the patient will not be able to walk on their heels or on their toes. Visible/palpable muscular atrophy in distal muscles is a late and serious sign which increases the urgency of referral.

The straight leg raise test is a key physical exam maneuver that acupuncturists who commonly treat low back pain must become proficient with. A positive straight leg raise test indicates compression radiculopathy.

Incidence and/or Prevalence

Multiple studies were reviewed to determine the prevalence of lumbar radiculopathy in the U.S. The estimates range from 2.2–8%. If we take a mean figure of 5% of the population and multiply it by 305 million (U.S. population in 2009) we get approximately 15,250,000 citizens with lumbar radiculopathy in the U.S. at any given sample time.

Risk Factors

Personal and family medical history/co-morbidities

- Significant personal history of acute, recurrent or chronic back pain
- History of trauma involving lumbosacral-pelvic regions (including slips/falls, motor vehicle accidents or other impacts, surgery, labor and delivery)
- Family history of significant chronic back pain
- Muscular deconditioning, especially abdominals and core trunk muscles
- Obesity
- Chronic gait abnormalities (such as leg length discrepancies, altered gait secondary to lower extremity injury, osteoarthrosis, etc.)
- Tobacco use (acidifies pH of nucleus pulposus causing chemical inflammation)

Demographics

- Peak incidence in fifth decade of life. May occur at any age (rare in preadolescents).
- Male>female predominance

Lifestyle & Social History

- Recent heavy/repetitive lifting activity
- Frequent/prolonged/ongoing sitting (including driving)
- Workplace stress and dissatisfaction
- Sedentary lifestyle

Mechanism Producing the Red Flag

Direct pressure on nerve roots as they exit the neuroforamina of the lumbosacral area causes painful ischemic necrosis of the nerve. Nerve root pressure can occur from several causes, more than one of which is sometimes present. These include, from most to least common: disc herniation, bony impingement and tumor.

Other Important Considerations

- The most common nerve root involved is L5-S1, forming the sciatic nerve and giving the classical true sciatica symptoms of pain in the buttock radiating down the lateroposterior aspect of the leg. Other causes of pain radiating down the posterior and lateral legs from the back and hip (such as myofascial pain) may also be present, but should not distract the practitioner from assuming the presence of L 5-S 1 radiculopathy if its red flag is present.
- The L 4 nerve root is also frequently affected and produces radiation from the anteromedial thigh to the medial calf and great toe, a highly-diagnostic pain pattern not shared with any other cause.
- Upper lumbar (L 1-3) nerve root injuries comprise <5% of lumbar radiculopathies. They radiate into the inguinal region where they may be mistaken for common groin pain conditions such as hip joint arthritis or hip tendonitis or uncommon causes including clot in the deep femoral vein or an inguinal hernia.
- Radiculopathies can usually be distinguished from myofascial pain by the presence of paresthesias as well as physical exam findings of numbness, loss of reflex, motor weakness, and muscle fasciculation and atrophy. Radicular and associated low back pain is also typically more acute and severe than pain from muscle/tendon/joint pain, but may not be more severe than pain from deep vein thromboses or inguinal hernias.
- The practitioner should not be misled by reductions in pain late in the course of compression neuropathies when such reduction is also accompanied by declining sensory and motor function in the leg. As nerves die, they are progressively less capable of sending any kind of signal, including pain.
- The efficacy of acupuncture for low back pain, the possibility of self-resolving radiculopathy or the higher prevalence of pseudo-radiculopathy (myofascial radiation patterns) may make it tempting to continue treating radicular symptoms without referral. The possible dire consequence of progression of radiculopathy, however, is so serious that referral is recommended if the patient's symptoms and signs are not improving over time according to our recommended grading scale above.

Specific red flags:
Back pain with insidious onset and progressive, unintentional weight loss

Condition assumed present until proven otherwise:
Cancer of the spine

Possible consequences of missing the condition:
Disability and death

Stabilization, referral and management:

1. **Stabilization:** There are no specific stabilizing steps to take.
2. **Consultation and Referral Options, Transportation:** The referral should occur on a timely to semi-urgent basis to the patient's PCP who will then also refer to the right specialist, perhaps a neurologist or neurosurgeon if neurological features are most prominent. A cancer specialist (oncologist) may also be involved early. The cancer may or may not be operable depending on its staging and other factors. Transport can be by patient and/or family members.

ACTUAL CASE

- **History:** A previously healthy 23-year-old male college student came to the office complaining of mild, vague back pain. His only other concern was that, despite lifting weights and drinking protein supplements to gain weight, he had lost eight pounds over the prior two months. He had never tried to lose weight in the past and had never lost any weight before. He was most concerned about his weight loss.
- **Physical findings:** The patient was a muscular young man, 6'1" and 180 pounds. His back motion was normal and there was no tenderness to palpation of the paraspinal muscles. Reflexes and strength in the lower extremities were normal.
- **Impression:** Suspected carcinoma of the spine.
- **Plan:** Patient was referred for MRI of his LS spine
- **Follow up:** The MRI showed a mass – possible malignant meningioma of the spine with mild extension into spinal cord. Subsequent surgery removed most of the meningioma. The patient was lost to further follow up.

DISCUSSION

History and Symptoms

Cancer pain is usually insidious and gradual in onset. There is generally no history of trauma, although trivial injury can act as a red herring to derail us from considering cancer if it happens to occur before symptoms appear. In multidisciplinary spine centers, patients with spinal cancer average 65.3 years of age and reported night pain, aching, spontaneous onset of symptoms, history of cancer, and unexplained weight loss. Compressive pain from tumor eventually tends to be dull and constant and is usually less responsive to palliative and provocative factors such as sitting, walking, rest, sleep, or change in position than is pain from "mechanical" causes.

Physical Exam Findings

If there are radicular symptoms, the straight leg raising test, reflexes, motor strength, and sensation in the leg and feet may be abnormal (see also radiculopathy section). Weight loss is objectively measurable. Generally, a significant weight loss of > 8-10 lbs over several months is an ominous sign because it means the tumor mass is large enough to be consuming calories (catabolic).

Incidence and/or Prevalence

The incidence of spinal tumors is 1.2/1000 in private practice spine centers. Cancer of the spine is *most commonly* metastatic from other primary sources, the most common being: breast 31%, lung 24%, GI 9%, prostate 8%, lymphoma 6%, melanoma 4%, thyroid 2–6%, kidney 1%, others (including myeloma) 13%, for a total of 100% of the metastatic types. The remainder of spinal cancer is primary from spinal structures themselves (primary spinal tumors) including bone, meninges, etc. The vertebral body itself is the most common site of metastatic involvement.

Risk Factors

- General cancer risk factors including: family history, smoking, alcoholism, carcinogenic diet, toxic exposures.

Mechanism Producing the Red Flag

The back pain is caused by direct tumor compression on bone and/or compression on nerves.

Other important considerations

- "Cancer of the spine" is a general phrase. Treatment will vary according to tissue type and staging (the extent of the cancer and possible spread).

Specific red flags:
Back pain, progressive bilateral leg weakness and erectile dysfunction in a man > 40

Condition assumed present until proven otherwise:

Cauda equina syndrome – lower spinal canal narrowing (spinal stenosis) that puts pressure on sacral nerves causeing neurological symptoms

Possible consequences of missing the condition:

Permanent weakness in lower extremities, anal incontinence, impotence

Stabilization, referral and management:

1. **Stabilization:** There are no particular stabilizing strategies except for the patient to avoid trauma and standing for long periods of time until consult can be obtained.
2. **Consultation and Referral Options, Transportation:** The referral should be made in a timely manner, within a few weeks if cauda equina syndrome has developed. Referral can first be made to the patient's allopathic PCP if one is available. The final consultant will be an orthopedic surgeon.

Relevance to acupuncturists:

Acupuncturists who treat back pain will undoubtedly see many patients with spinal stenosis and some patients with overt couda equina syndrome.

ACTUAL CASE

- **History:** A 48-year-old construction worker came to the office complaining of the gradual onset of "weakness in my legs" and vague low back pain. He had some trouble standing up after being seated in a chair. He'd hurt his back several times in the last 20 years on the job, but there was no particular trauma that precipitated this problem. His other complaint was of erectile dysfunction over the last year.
- **Physical exam:** Patient was 5' 8" and 210 pounds, and had bilaterally slightly decreased muscle strength in his quadriceps muscles.
- **Impression:** Possible spinal stenosis with cauda equina syndrome
- **Plan:** Patient was referred to his family physician. A neurological exam was positive for a "saddle anesthesia" pattern and decreased anal sphincter tone on digital rectal exam.
- **Follow up:** The patient was referred to an orthopedic surgeon and had an MRI showing bony encroachment of the spinal cord due to extensive degenerative disease and bony spurring in the LS area. The patient opted for a trial of physical therapy and rest. Unfortunately, he did not improve significantly and eventually underwent surgery to enlarge the spinal canal. He gradually regained full neurological function over the next year but remained impotent.

DISCUSSION

History and Symptoms

The classic presentation of spinal stenosis (narrowing of the spinal canal) is radiating bilateral leg pain worsened by standing and walking and relieved by rest. This is called "neurogenic claudication" (Vascular claudication from peripheral artery disease gives calf pain on walking from ischemia). This history is almost invariably present in people whose spinal narrowing advances to the stage of neurological involvement, which is cauda equina syndrome. Bowel and bladder dysfunction with impotence occur in advanced cases. There is often, but not always, a history of hard labor or trauma to the low back.

Physical Exam Findings

The patient generally has decreased LS spine ROM due to degenerative process (osteoarthritis) in the LS spine. There will be bilateral leg weakness on strength testing, but some men who start out being very strong may not seem extraordinarily weak. Saddle anesthesia may be detected in the sacral dermatomes and the anal exam performed by an allopathic physician will show weak anal tone in full blown cauda equina syndrome.

Incidence and/or Prevalence

Incidence of spinal stenosis is 5/1000. There are two types, primary and secondary spinal stenosis. Primary stenosis is congenital and relatively uncommon. Affected patients are younger. Acquired stenosis, the one considered in this section, is much more common. It is a degenerative condition. Patients generally become symptomatic at age 45 or older.

Risk Factors

- Male sex, age >40

- Occupations that cause repetitive trauma to the low back
- Arthritis in other areas of the body
- Prior history of low back pain

Mechanism Producing the Red Flag

Direct compression on the spinal canal (and less commonly bilateral compression of nerve roots) causes the symptoms and signs of cauda equina syndrome. Degenerative changes of the spine can include bony spur (osteophyte) formation, bony swelling of the vertebral facet joints (facet hypertrophy), bulging disks, and hypertrophy of the ligamentum flavum. Any of these processes can result in canal or foraminal narrowing. Degenerative slippage of vertebra on one another (spondylolisthesis) can further compromise the canal. Less frequently, acute central disc herniation (disc rupturing inward causing narrowing of the spinal canal) can compromise the cord. There are other less common causes, including tumor.

Other Important Considerations

- Spinal stenosis often has a very gradual onset, sometimes with minimal back pain. Leg weakness may be noted first when getting up from chairs, etc. Also, since the nerves distributed through the sacral region (pudendal nerves) are injured, a typical "saddle anesthesia" pattern can also develop as a late symptom, along with impotence. There is often quite a bit of narrowing before cauda equina syndrome manifests as a late symptom of spinal stenosis.
- We can use the same basic grading scale that we used for unilateral neuropathy (see radiculopathy in low back pain) to grade the neuropathic progression of spinal stenosis. The progression is: sensory symptoms and signs followed by motor symptoms and signs and finally muscle atrophy as muscle fibers die from lack of neuronal stimulation.

Specific red flags:
Severe, localized midline back pain with spinal process tenderness to percussion

Condition assumed present until proven otherwise:

Vertebral compression fracture with possible underlying osteoporosis or tumor

Possible consequences of missing the condition:

Extreme pain and disability with possible death from lethal complications from prolonged bedrest such as pneumonia and blood clots (DVT)

Stabilization, referral and management:

1. **Stabilization:** The patient should be put at bed rest until referral can be accomplished.
2. **Consultation and Referral Options, Transportation:** Patients can be referred to their primary care physician, but hospitalization is sometimes necessary for pain control so sending a patient to the ED is sometimes appropriate. The patient will often need assistance to help them transfer their weight while getting in and out of the car from family members or others who can provide it. Emergency transport is generally not needed.

Relevance to acupuncturists: Spinal compression fractures are common in the elderly and acupuncturists will undoubtedly see some of these patients.

ACTUAL CASE

- **History:** A 66-year-old Caucasian female was brought to the office by her son for acupuncture for "mid back pain." This started when she slipped on a rug the day before and landed on her buttock. Her pain got progressively worse throughout the day. She had to call her son so he could help her get into her car to make her appointment. She denied radiation of the pain, numbness or tingling to either leg. Past medical history included many missed menses as a young girl and early menopause at age 40, with no vitamins or mineral inges- tion to support bone health. She was sedentary.
- **Physical findings:** The patient appeared to be in severe pain, wincing during the exam. She hesitated to bend to the floor or perform other range-of-motion maneuvers. There was highly localized and severe pain with percussion over her T 12 spinous process. The strength, sensation and reflexes in her legs were normal bilaterally.
- **Impression:** Vertebral compression fracture
- **Plan:** The patient's primary care physician was called and the situation was discussed. She recommended that

we send the patient directly to the ED of a local hospital for workup of her back pain.

- **Follow up:** The patient did indeed have a compression fracture of T 12, as suspected. Her X-rays also showed generalized bone demineralization in her vertebral bodies compatible with osteoporosis. There was no evidence of bone cancer on the X-ray or labs (another reason for compression fracture). She was placed at bed rest on a foam mattress and antiembolic stockings were applied to her legs to keep her from developing DVT for what would turn out to be a two week period of bed rest.

She was eventually discharged home in stable condition with recommendations for a careful exercise program, vitamins and minerals for bone health, and a carefully tailored bio-identical hormone replacement therapy regimen.

DISCUSSION

History and Symptoms

Vertebral compression fractures that result from trauma most commonly occur in post-menopausal women, often at the thoraco-lumbar junction (T12 or L 1). The typical injury is a fall on the buttocks causing a compressive vertical force transmitted up the vertebral column and causing a "wedging" of one of the vertebral bodies. Younger vertebral fracture patients have a history of other kinds of trauma, like auto accidents, and have slightly different types of vertebral body fractures. Compression fractures are usually very painful. Regardless of cause, these patients are much better with rest and worse with activity. There is seldom neurological radiation of pain to indicate radiculopathy, but radiculopathy is possible.

Physical Exam Findings

In the case of a compression fracture in an elderly person, the finding of percussion tenderness over the spinous process (performed by gently striking the spinous processes one by one with the back of your fist until you find the fracture) is highly reliable (pathognomonic) as a sign for vertebral compression fracture. As is all cases of back pain, the examiner should perform muscle testing and sensory exam with reflex testing if there is any doubt about radiculopathy.

Incidence and/or Prevalence

The incidence of traumatic compression fractures of the elderly is high. Older patients, especially postmenopausal Caucasian women, are at greatest risk. About 30% of patients with compression fractures have an identifiable trauma. The percentage is so low because spontaneous fractures as a result of bending over, lifting, or even getting out of bed, can occur with minimal activity if bone mass is low enough.

Risk Factors

- Advanced age
- Female sex
- Caucasians have higher incidence rates than African-Americans
- Activities with high risk of blunt impact physical trauma
- Factors known to decrease bone density such as lifelong hypoestrogenemia in women, smoking, sedentary life style, etc.
- Known personal or family history of osteoporosis

Mechanism Producing the Red Flag

The pain of vertebral compression fracture comes from nerve pain from the periosteum and other supporting structure around the bone. Secondary pain may come from inflammation and involuntary muscle spasm to guard the fracture site.

Other Important Considerations

- Other important factors for bone health in addition to adequate sex hormones include: calcium, boron, weight bearing activity, Vitamin D-3 and vitamin K-2.
- Men can also suffer from osteoporosis associated stress fractures after andropause from inadequate testosterone.
- Compression fractures can occur in bones affected by cancer, in which case they are called "pathological fractures."

Rarely, vertebral fractures may go unnoticed by patients and are picked up incidentally on imaging studies. In these cases the pain probably was blamed on something else.

Specific red flags:
Chest pressure coming on reliably with physical exertion

Condition assumed present until proven otherwise:

Angina pectoris – ischemic myocardial pain secondary to coronary artery disease

Possible consequences of missing the condition:

Disability to sudden death from myocardial infarction (MI)

Stabilization, referral and management:

1. **Stabilization:** The patient should not engage in exercise, nor should the clinician evoke a fear response in the patient. A calm attitude is important.
2. **Consultation and Referral Options, Transportation:** Urgency is proportionate to severity, but angina is at least semi-urgent in all cases because emboli can abruptly form in the area of plaque producing a fatal myocardial infarction.
   - With stable angina (chest pain only with extreme physical exertion, for example), timely consultation with the patient's PCP, or cardiologist if the patient has no PCP, is warranted for an appointment that same day or within days. The transport can be by private vehicle.
   - With history of unstable angina (chest pain brought on by minimal exertion), but no current pain, the patient should be sent to the ED. The transport can be by private vehicle, but the patient should not drive.
   - With an unstable patient (current chest pain, SOB, falling BP, etc.) a 911 call should be made.

ACTUAL CASE

- **History:** Phillip was a 52-year-old sedentary male accountant, smoker, with a positive family history of myocardial infarction in his mother at age 70. He had no personal or family history of diabetes, high blood pressure, or lipid abnormalities. He presented to the office with the complaint of fatigue. He denied shortness of breath or chest pain at first, but upon reflection admitted that on a recent vacation in Europe he had chest pressure when climbing up a large hill to visit a monument, which went away when he stopped climbing. He had another less severe episode since returning from his trip that also occurred with extreme intercourse.
- **Physical findings:** Other than smelling like nicotine, the physical exam was entirely normal.
- **Impression:** Probable angina, fairly stable
- **Plan:** The patient's family physician was contacted and the patient was seen the next day.
- **Follow up:** A physical exam by the patient's PCP was normal, but an ECG showed an old (age indeterminate) inferior MI. The patient was sent to a cardiologist who performed a nuclear medicine treadmill study and found a large myocardial perfusion deficit in the area of the heart supplied by the left anterior descending artery (LAD) and an area of poor movement (hypokinesis) at the base of the heart compatible with an old MI. A subsequent angiogram revealed a 95% blockage of the LAD and milder blockages in several other coronary arteries. The patient underwent a triple bypass heart surgery and did well for the next 10 years. He did quit cigarette smoking but developed lung cancer on his eleventh year post MI which proved fatal.

DISCUSSION

History and Symptoms

The typical patient with angina is a male, usually over 45 years of age, reporting regular onset of chest pain or pressure with physical exertion. The level of exertion required to trigger chest pain varies. The patient often has risk factors (see below), but CAD is so prevalent that few risk factors may be present. There may be radiation of the pain to the left shoulder and/or jaw with angina, although this type of radiation is more common with MI.

Occasionally, the pain of angina may be described as "fullness" or even mistaken for heartburn (just as reflux esophagitis can masquerade as angina). CAD may present with chief complaints other than chest pain. For example, in women, CAD is more likely to present with crescendo malaise, anxiety, fatigue, insomnia, and feelings of impending doom. Because we are organizing our red flags by symptoms rather than disease, however, we are only considering angina from exertion in this section.

Physical Exam Findings

The *resting* physical exam is often, if not usually, entirely normal (the resting electrocardiogram done in the physician's office is often normal as well, but serum tests may show risk factors (see below). There may be abnormalities of the pulse, or the pulse may be perfectly normal.

Incidence and/or Prevalence

CAD is the leading cause of death in men and women in the U.S. It accounts for more than 25% of all fatalities each year. The incidence is 1.26 million new CAD diagnoses per year and the prevalence is 17.6 million angina, heart attack and other forms of coronary heart disease (9.2 million males and 8.4 million females).

Risk Factors for angina and CAD (National Cholesterol Education Program - NCEP)

Demographic

- Advancing age
- Male gender

Lifestyle and Diet

- Tobacco smoking
- Sedentary lifestyle
- High-stress
- Diet high in animal fats, trans-fats, and refined carbohydrates, and low in essential free fatty acids
- Coronary-prone (Type A) behavior or personality

Disease Risk Factors

- Postmenopausal status
- Diabetes mellitus
- Hypertension
- Obesity
- Personal history of atherosclerotic disease
- Low and/or pro-inflammatory type HDL cholesterol
- C-reactive protein elevation
- Homocysteine elevation
- Lipoprotein (a) elevation
- Apolipoprotein B elevation
- Low Apolipoprotein A-1 level
- Lp-PLA2 elevation (an enzyme that causes deposition of LDL into arterial walls)
- Small, dense LDL particle size elevation
- High fibrinogen levels

Family/inherited

- Positive family history of coronary artery disease, peripheral artery disease, or stroke
- Family history of lipid disorder

Mechanism Producing the Red Flag

The heart muscle cells (myocytes or myocardial cells) need much more oxygen with exercise than when at rest. In symptomatic CAD, the blood flow cannot be increased enough to meet the increased demand of these cells during exertion because plaque or emboli blocks the lumen of coronary arteries. Angina results from hypoxic injury to the myocardial muscles.

Other Important Considerations

- Chest pain or pressure that reliably occurs with a certain threshold level of exertion is a highly reliable (highly pathognomonic) symptom for significant CAD. The threshold level of exertion is important to ascertain. If it comes on with little exertion, like carrying garbage out to the trash container, it indicates a more ominous situation than if it comes on with maximal exertion. Pain that is infrequent, irregular, sharp, and not proportionate to degree of physical exertion is more likely to be musculoskeletal.
- Despite the fact that exertional chest pain, angina, is so pathognomonic for CAD, 50% of MI occurs with no preceding history of angina, so the absence of chest pain does not clear a patient of possible CAD.
- "Referred pain" from organs like the heart that radiate to somatic regions like the chest, jaw or left arm validates that organs can communicate with somatic segments and suggests one probable therapeutic mechanism of acupuncture, *i.e.*, communication through spinal cord pathways.

Specific red flags:
Sharp chest pain and SOB with unilateral or bilateral asymmetric ankle swelling

Condition assumed present until proven otherwise:

Pulmonary embolus (PE) – blood clot lodged in the lung

Possible consequences of missing the condition:

Sudden death

Stabilization, referral and management:

1. **Stabilization:** There are no stabilizing steps to take.
2. **Consultation and Referral Options, Transportation:** This is an urgent situation that requires a call to 911 and emergency vehicle transport.

ACTUAL CASE

- **History:** A 45-year-old Caucasian female patient reported chest pain on deep inspiration and mild shortness of breath (SOB) for two days prior to coming to the office. She had a history of bilateral ankle swelling for years and mild heart failure.
- **Physical findings:** The patient was 5' 2" and 170 pounds. Her pulse was 90bpm and regular. Blood pressure was 140/85mmHg and respirations were 15/minute. She appeared slightly short of breath. As was usual for her, she had large ankles bilaterally. Her right ankle had a trace of pitting edema, but her left ankle had 2+ pitting edema and was 4cm larger in diameter than her right.
- **Impression:** Probable small pulmonary embolus (PE) with pre-existing DVT.
- **Plan:** A call was placed to 911 and the patient was transported to the ED of a nearby hospital.
- **Follow up:** The patient was found to have a DVT in the left ankle and a small PE of the lung. The patient was treated and released from the hospital after two weeks. She did well at home, but unfortunately had a massive myocardial infarction and died in her home two weeks later.

DISCUSSION

History and Symptoms

Although a massive PE can strike suddenly and be fatal within minutes, the "classic" presentation with abrupt onset of pleuritic chest pain, shortness of breath and hypoxia isn't always seen according to many authoritative sources. In fact, studies of patients who die unexpectedly of PE reveal they often complained of nagging symptoms for weeks before death. Forty percent had been seen and missed by physicians prior to death. Additionally, as in the ACTUAL CASE presented, ankle swelling may occur in obese individuals who tend not to notice a change in ankle circumference or who may have other reasons for ankle swelling like heart problems that they tend to blame the edema on.

Physical Exam Findings

Patients with moderate to severe PE are not a diagnostic challenge. They appear acutely ill with fast breathing (tachypnea), fast heartbeat (tachycardia), and signs of poor oxygenation, like cyanosis. The signs with small PEs may be quite subtle. Either way, the examiner will always want to look for signs of a preceding DVT. As mentioned in the ankle swelling section of this book, it's important to measure the circumferences of the two ankles to see if there is a significant difference (>3cm) between the two because asymmetric ankle edema has the same significance as unilateral ankle edema. Allopathic physicians will find many other signs compatible with PE on imaging and blood gas studies.

Incidence and/or Prevalence

The average annual incidence of PE is estimated at between 650,000 to 900,000 fatal and nonfatal cases annually.

Risk Factors

Thrombosis is triggered by three factors: venostasis, hypercoagulability, and vessel wall inflammation. These three factors are known as the Virchow triad. All known clinical risk factors for DVT and subsequent PE have their basis in one or more elements of the triad.

- Recent surgery or trauma involving the affected leg
- Smoking
- Leg immobilization or lack of physical activity (including postfracture casting, recent airplane travel, prolonged bed rest, and/or generally sedentary occupation and lifestyle)
- Obesity
- Recent or current chemotherapy
- History of prior blood clots, coagulopathy (thick blood)
- Oral contraceptives, non-bioidentical estrogen replacement, any estrogen replacement given orally (causes inflammation in the liver)

Mechanism Producing the Red Flag

Thrombi to the lungs almost always arise from calf veins deep venous thrombosis in sites of venous stasis. Calf vein thrombosis usually propagates proximally to the popliteal vessels and embolizes from there. To reach the lungs, thromboemboli must travel to and through the right side of the heart to the lung, the path being: (1) right atrium, (2) right ventricle, (3) lung.

Specific red flags:
Sudden, spontaneous, sharp unilateral chest pain, and shortness of breath

Serious condition assumed present until proven otherwise:

Pneumothorax – a collection of air escaping from a lung that gets trapped between the lung and the inner chest wall (in the pleural space) and collapses the lung on the affected side (see figure 4).

Possible consequences of missing the condition:

A small pneumothorax may pass without much trouble. A *tension* pneumothorax, the most severe type, is a life-threatening condition caused when the air within the pleural space is under so much pressure that it pushes the midline (mediastinal) structures within the chest (heart, blood vessels, etc.) to the opposite side, thereby compromises cardiopulmonary function. Respiratory distress and possible death can occur.

Stabilization, referral and management:

1. **Stabilization:** There are no stabilizing steps except to reassure the patient (to prevent hyperventilation) and keep the patient at rest.
2. **Consultation and Referral Options, Transportation:** If there is little pain and respiratory distress (a small pneumothorax) the referral can be made on a semi-urgent basis to the patient's PCP or an urgent care facility if no PCP is available. Transportation can be by private vehicle. Many patients with pneumothorax will be anxious. For this reason, even small pneumothoraces will probably require at least semi-urgent referral so that patients can be reassured of healing by serial chest x-rays that will show the resolving pneumothorax as a shrinking dark (lucent) area on repeated chest films.

If the presentation is severe and unstable, emergency medical services should be activated with a call to 911. The most symptomatic cases should go directly to the ED because they will probably need placement of a chest tube (through an incision between the ribs) to draw out the air until the hole in the lung can heal itself. These patients will also need oxygen, blood pressure monitoring, etc.

Relevance to acupuncturists: Pneumothorax occupies a special place for acupuncturist practice because it is a possible though infrequent complication of acupuncture.

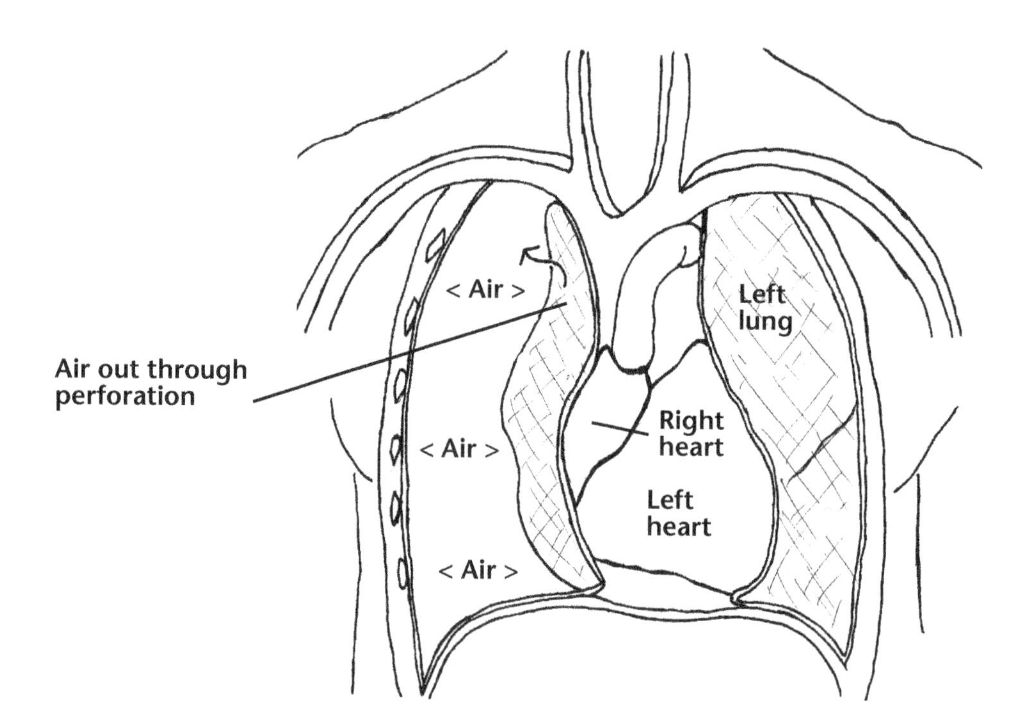

Figure 4. Air within the lung is under pressure because of lung elasticity. The air can escape through a small puncture wound in the lung and build up within the chest between the lung and the inner chest wall causing compression of the lung tissue.

ACTUAL CASE

- **History:** A 38-year-old, thin Caucasian female came into the office for acupuncture and trigger point therapy for back pain. Some of the points used were bladder channel points. One hour after she got home after the treatment, she called to say that she had some shortness of breath and sharp pain on the right side of her chest and wanted to know if it could have had anything to do with the treatment, which helped her back pain a great deal. She denied cough, fever, or symptoms of respiratory tract infection. She was not a smoker and was previously in very good health.
- **Physical findings:** The patient came back to the office. Her lung sounds were unremarkable, but her complaints persisted. Her blood pressure, pulse, and respirations were in the normal range.
- **Impression:** Probable small pneumothorax
- **Plan:** The situation was thoroughly explained to the patient and she was informed about the small incidence of pneumothorax with needling therapy and the possible diagnosis. She was also informed that it would likely resolve spontaneously in a healthy non-smoker, but that it was advisable to have her PCP follow her recuperation to ascertain the exact size of the pneumo- thorax and follow its resolution. The patient understood and agreed. Her PCP was notified about the situation.
- **Follow up:** Plain film of the chest revealed a 10% right pneumothorax seen at the apex of the lung. The midline structures (mediastinal and heart) were in normal position – no tension pneumothorax. Two further serial chest films showed a gradual resolution of the pneumothorax over the next seven days.

DISCUSSION

History and Symptoms

Patients who develop pneumothoraces from needling may not have pain right away because it generally takes some time for the air to accumulate in the pleural space (see mechanism of red flag). Young, healthy, non-mokers with resilient lung tissue tend to have milder symptoms, but the sharp chest pain may be fairly sharp even in some mild cases (10% or less). SOB may be fairly mild, but some overlying anxiety, which is common with shortness of breath, can make the situation seem much worse in anxious patients.

In smokers, the situation can be very much different. Soft, thin, non-elastic areas of the lung (emphysematous blebs) rupture easily and allow more air into the pleural space. The backward pressure of this air against the non-resilient lung tissue of a smoker causes greater deformation of the lung. A larger pneumothorax is possible, even a tension pneumothorax. These patients will have a great deal of air hunger, sharp chest pain and possibly cardiopulmonary symptoms. Patients with tension pneumothoraces may also have them as a result of major trauma, like stab wound and rib fracture that lacerates lung tissue.

Typical Physical Exam Findings

The patient will almost always appear anxious because the combination of shortness of breath and chest pain is frightening for most people, especially if unexplained. They may have reduced breath sounds to auscultation on the affected side of the thorax if the pneumothorax because the air trapped between the lung and the chest wall acts as an insulator of sound transmission. The patient may look urgently ill, pale, sweaty (diaphoretic) and tachycardic if the pneumothorax is large.

Incidence and/or Prevalence

The incidence of pneumothorax from needling in acupuncture has already been given, approximately 1 in 5,000. The incidence of pneumothorax from other forms of trauma is approximately one out of 14,000 men and one out of 50,000 women in the U.S. The worse the injury and more fragile the lungs, the more likely it is that there will be the complication of tension pneumothorax.

The incidence of *spontaneous* pneumothorax (no trauma) is 7.4 cases per 100,000 persons per year for men and 1.2 cases per 100,000 persons per year for women—approximately 8,600 individuals developing spontaneous pneumothorax in the U.S. per year. Tension pneumothorax is a complication in approximately 1-2% of these cases. Spontaneous pneumothorax male to female ratio is 6:1 with the male risk 102 times higher in heavy smokers than in non-smokers.

Risk Factors

- Smoking (because of emphysematous blebs of the lung)
- Frail or thin chest wall
- Combining a thin chest wall in a smoker puts that patient even more at risk.
- Tall and thin body type in a male

Mechanism Producing the Red Flag

It takes time for the air in the lung to leak out of the lung, and the bigger the hole, the more air can leak out with each inspiration because the air in the lung is under pressure from lung elasticity. The air accumulates in the space between the lung and the inner chest wall (pleural space) and eventually starts pushing against the lung tissue, collapsing it (figure 6). This decreases the functional absorptive area of the lung causing shortness of breath, which is increasingly severe as the amount of air progresses. In fact, in the case of tension pneumothorax, so much air is present that it can push the heart and mediastinal structures toward the opposite side of the chest. The pleural surfaces are sensitive to pain which produces the sharp chest pain.

Another Important Consideration

Spontaneous pneumothorax is caused by congenital blebs that ruptured, often with vigorous exercise.

Specific red flags:
Earache, ear drainage, fever, severe tenderness of mastoid process

Condition assumed present until proven otherwise:

Acute Mastoiditis – a serious bacterial infection of the mastoid process of the temporal bone and the most common complication of *otitis media* (middle ear infection). This condition is sometimes also called "acute surgical mastoiditis" (ASM) to emphasis the probability that surgical debridement of the bone will be necessary.

Possible consequences of missing the condition:

Extension of the infection of the middle ear (otitis media, OM) can cause osteomyelitis of the mastoid bone. Infection into other contiguous tissues besides bone can cause thrombosis, abscess, meningitis, and/or facial nerve and/or labyrinth destruction resulting in permanent, partial or complete hearing loss and balance problems.

Stabilization, referral and management:

1. **Stabilization:** There are no particular stabilizing steps to take.
2. **Consultation and Referral Options, Transportation:** The referral should be on a semi-urgent basis to the PCP or urgent care center if no PCP is available or directly to an Ear, Nose and Throat (ENT) physician if neither is available. Deep local acupuncture (*e.g.*, acupoints GB 12, 20, TW 17, An Mian, etc.) is contraindicated because of the risk of spreading infection.

Relevance to acupuncturists: The fact that otitis media can resolve spontaneously in most cases may cause some practitioners to underestimate the potential danger of this condition. Pain severity may be deceptively mild in some cases of acute mastoiditis also, so other features of the red flag, like ear drainage, should signal this possible complication to the alert acupuncturist.

ACTUAL CASE

- **History:** The patient was a 30-year-old computer engineer with a history of otitis media as a child and a recent ear infection, for which he had been taking an antibiotic. He was still having ear pain, fever and had three days of purulent drainage from his right ear. He was seeking acupuncture and herbs to help since he assumed there was nothing more his "conventional doctor" could do beside prescribe the antibiotic.
- **Physical findings:** The patient appeared very uncomfortable. His temperature was 101.2°. The right ear canal had some yellowish fluid in it. The patient's mastoid bone behind the affected ear was exquisitely tender to palpation.
- **Impression:** Probable mastoiditis
- **Plan:** The patient's family physician was called and the patient was directed to an ENT specialist for a same day visit.
- **Follow up:** The consultant agreed with the diagnosis of AM. A CT scan confirmed the diagnosis. Surgery was performed to remove an island of infected bone in the mastoid process. The infecting bacterium was *S. pneumoniae.* The patient made a full recovery other than a 10% hearing loss in the affected ear.

DISCUSSION

History and Symptoms

The patient will always have a recent history of OM. Mastoid pain severity is variable and may be difficult to evaluate in very young patients, but the stronger the pain, the greater the likelihood of AM. Persistent purulent ear drainage (otorrhea) beyond three weeks is a consistent predecessor for AM, but we must assume that that any patient with **earache, ear drainage, fever, and severe tenderness of the mastoid process** has *acute mastoiditis* regardless of the number of days of otorrhea. Pain is localized deep in or behind the ear and is typically worse at night.

Physical Exam Findings

Tenderness and inflammation over the mastoid process is the most consistent sign of AM. High and persistent fever, despite antimicrobial agents, is common due to either a resistant organism or lack of penetration of the antibiotic into the infected tissues. Hearing loss is common in mastoiditis and may already be present to a significant degree when the patient presents to you.

Incidence and/or Prevalence

The exact incidence of AM is unknown. It can occur at any age, but is more common in the very young (median age of 12 months).

Risk Factors

- Recent otitis media is a risk factor.
- As in almost all infectious disease, patients with depressed immunity are at higher risk for mastoiditis (see General Risk Factors: Infectious Disease).
- Low socioeconomic level and inadequate access to primary care medicine.
- People with known severe eustachian tube dysfunction.

Mechanism Producing the Red Flag

Review of an anatomy text is recommended for familiarity with the many structures contiguous with the middle ear. The infection can spread beyond the mucosa of the middle ear to the mastoid bone either directly by bone erosion indirectly via the emissary vein of the mastoid. The dreaded consequence of bone infection (osteomyelitis) covered elsewhere in this book, is one of the most treacherous complications, but the destruction of the hearing and balance mechanisms of the ear is also a dreaded consequence.

▶ Specific red flags:
Persistent elbow pain and stiffness after a fall on an outstretched hand

Condition assumed present until proven otherwise:

Fracture of the radial head of the elbow

Possible consequences of missing the condition:

Permanent stiffness, deformity, posttraumatic arthritis, or nerve damage

Stabilization, referral and management:

1. **Stabilization:** An arm sling can be purchased at a pharmacy and can ease the pain until referral can be achieved.
2. **Consultation and Referral Options, Transportation:** The patient should be referred to their PCP on a semi-urgent (same day or next day) basis. The PCP may be able to handle the fracture or may refer to an orthopedic surgeon. Referral directly to the orthopedist may be necessary if the patient has no PCP.

Relevance to acupuncturists: Radial head fractures of the elbow are fairly common and often underestimated by patient and practitioners. Missing them within the window wherein something can be done risks permanent elbow joint stiffness for the patient. The red flag for this condition is therefore important for acupuncturists to recognize especially if the acupuncturist's practice deals with active and athletic patients.

ACTUAL CASE

- **History:** The patient was an 18-year-old male with elbow pain. He was shoved by a friend during horseplay a week earlier and fell forward, breaking his fall with his outstretched right hand. He did not have a doctor and didn't seek care after the injury because he said it "didn't hurt that much and I can still move my arm."
- **Physical findings:** The patient had mild tenderness to palpation in the lateral right elbow region. He had full flexion, but lacked the last 15 degrees of elbow extension (did not have his full "carrying angle" at the elbow).
- **Impression:** Probable nondisplaced radial head fracture of elbow
- **Plan:** The patient's family physician was contacted that same day and the patient was seen the next day in his office.
- **Follow up:** X-rays revealed a nondisplaced (type I) fracture of the radial head of the right elbow. Because it was nondisplaced and there were no other complications like elbow dislocation or neurological or vascular compression symptoms (tingling in the hand or diminished

pulse on the affected side), a trial of conservative care using an elbow sling and early exercises to restore range of motion was successful in reducing pain and restoring elbow range of motion.

DISCUSSION

History and Symptoms

Patients can have three degrees of radial head fracture. The ACTUAL CASE covers the most common and least dangerous type, the nondisplaced. The severity of symptoms and signs escalate as the type worsens.

Patient with radial head fractures usually presents with the history of a fall on the outstretched hand. If you see the patient several days to a week after the injury, they will almost invariably complain of some stiffness that can be objectively graded as a specific amount of loss of normal ROM. If they also complain of pain in the wrist, a concomitant wrist fracture should be ruled out.

A fracture of the wrist should always be considered when faced with the possibility of an elbow fracture that occurs when patients catch themselves on an outstretched hand. This is because the damaging force is transmitted though the wrist on its way up to the elbow and coexisting fractures of the wrist are always possible.

Neurovascular symptoms of numbness, tingling, or loss of sensation in the distal arm or hand may indicate nerve or vascular injury at the elbow and are ominous additional symptoms not specifically covered by this red flag, but symptoms you should be aware of. They occur more often with Type II and Type III radial head fractures. The tricky thing about type I fractures of the radial head is that the initial pain may not be very severe. Patients will often minimize it. Also, as with some other fractures, like fractures of the scaphoid bone of the wrist, the patient may report having had an initial x-ray that was negative. Subsequent x-rays a week or two later will usually show the fracture.

Physical Exam Findings

Patients with radial head fractures present with localized swelling and tenderness in the elbow region and decreased ROM of the elbow, especially extension. The radial head should be palpated to confirm these findings. The wrist should be examined for stability of the distal radioulnar joint and assessed for pain over the anatomic snuff box (see wrist pain). All three major nerves of the forearm are in danger with elbow fractures, so neurovascular function for the median, radial and ulnar nerves should be routinely assessed. As in all fractures, the presence of bleeding should alert for the possibility of open injury and the possibility of joint infection.

Incidence and/or Prevalence

Radial head fractures are common injuries. They account for 5.4% of all fractures and 33% of all acute elbow fractures. They are more frequent in women than in men and occur most often between 30-40 years of age. Approximately 10% of all elbow dislocations involve a fracture of the radial head.

Risk Factors

- Athletic activities that can cause falls.
- Activities on slippery and irregular surfaces.
- Osteoporosis and osteopenia.

Mechanism Producing the Red Flag

The elbow, like the shoulder, has a propensity to develop permanent stiffness if allowed to remain in a contracted position for too long. This is at least partially due to constriction of the connective tissue around the joint in response to intraarticular swelling and dysfunction. Also because the radial head is intraarticular, bone fragments that do not heal can produce trauma within the joint and posttraumatic arthritis can occur from mechanical grinding. Fractured fragments can lose their blood supply resulting in avascular necrosis and potential nonunion. Finally, displaced and comminuted fractures bring the same kinds of risk seen in more severe elbow fractures (see red flags for supracondylar fractures of the elbow).

Other Important Considerations

- Radial head fracture of the elbow can have a very satisfactory outcome if either conservatively or surgically managed, but the earlier it is managed correctly, the better the outcome will be.
- The reason for false negative initial X-rays in this fracture and in many others is because a bone must be turned at just the right angle to detect a small fracture in its early stages. Also, since the beginning of fracture repair starts with reabsorption of fractured bone before new bone is laid down, the fracture is actually easier to see on film a few days to a week after the fracture than when it is acute. This should be kept in mind for all small fractures.

Specific red flags:
Elbow swelling and pain with diminished radial pulse and/or hand numbness after fall

Condition assumed present until proven otherwise:
Supracondylar fracture of the humerus

Possible consequences of missing the condition:
Ischemic necrosis and/or permanent neurological impairment of the forearm and/or hand

Stabilization, referral and management:

1. **Stabilization:** The patient should ice the area of swelling, but not use a compression dressing because this might further compress nerves and arteries in the antecubital fossa.
2. **Consultation and Referral Options, Transportation:** This is an urgent situation that requires transport as soon as possible to an ED of a hospital (no 911 call, unless there is cardiopulmonary compromise). A call to the triage person at the hospital to alert them to the diminished pulse on the affected side is warranted.

Relevance to acupuncturists: Supracondylar fractures of the humerus are unlikely to present to the acupuncturist as a first resort because they are quite painful. They can be underestimated by the stoical patient as in our ACTUAL CASE history. I have actually seen one of these present in an acupuncture clinic. The main reason we include this red flag is because of the tragic consequences of missing it and the lesson it teaches us generally about being on the alert for *distal* neurological and vascular compromise whenever we see proximal fractures, which can be easily and quickly tested for by the acupuncturist (see physical findings).

ACTUAL CASE

- **History:** A mother brought in her 16-year-old son, a football player, for a sore and "bruised" left elbow after being tackled at football practice several hours earlier. He had intense elbow pain at the time, but decided to "suck it up." The pain had diminished somewhat with icing, but he was having some pain *in his left hand* by the time he arrived at the office, as well as the elbow.
- **Physical findings:** On exam, we noticed that he had swelling and severe tenderness above the left elbow and a weaker radial pulse on the left side compared to the right. Sensation in his left hand was normal.
- **Impression:** Probable supracondylar fracture of the left distal humerus with possible early vascular complications
- **Plan:** Patient was sent directly to the ED of a local hospital after calling and leaving a message with the ED physician about the possibility of vascular embarrassment of the left arm due to possible left supracondylar fracture.
- **Follow up:** The patient had a supracondylar fracture of his left lower humerus on X-ray. By the time he was back from the radiology department he had increased pain and tingling of the left hand and an absent radial pulse. He was taken directly to surgery where his fracture was reduced and the antecubital fossa was explored, revealing an intact brachial artery. Postoperatively his radial pulse returned to normal and he had complete recovery. He is again playing football with no residual problems.

DISCUSSION

Typical History and Symptoms

The red flag captures the essentials of the typical kind of history with these kinds of fractures. Young adults with supracondylar fracture generally sustain them secondary to high-energy trauma such as that sustained in sports like football or in motor vehicle accidents, falls from heights and gunshot wounds. Older individuals and children with weaker bones require far less trauma.

Physical Exam Findings

The key sign for this fracture is the *severe tenderness and swelling directly over the fracture.* The invariable presence of tenderness to palpation in fractures is the reason that careful palpation should *always* be done whenever a supracondylar fracture, or any other type of fracture, is suspected. It only takes a few seconds to palpate every part of a bone to make this determination (starting with gentle palpation to avoid inducing unnecessary pain).

In fact, point tenderness, determined by careful and thorough palpation, is more sensitive test for fracture than an X-ray. Nature has given us a clue: **fractures are always tender** in the conscious patient. The next step is to determine if there are complications from the fracture, specifically injuries to nerves and/or vessels in the area of the fracture site.

To help us determine this, we get another diagnostic clue: If there is pressure on nerves and/or vessels from bony fragments, excessive bleeding or generalized swelling in the antecubital fossa, the downstream (distal) nerves and vessels will be affected. There will be a diminished radial pulse with pressure on the brachial artery, or diminished or abnormal sensation in the case of compression on nerves serving the hand. Thus, a quick check of sensation and pulse distally can tell us if potentially disastrous neurovascular complications are possible.

Incidence and/or Prevalence

Fortunately, fractures of the distal humerus, some of which are supracondylar fractures, are relatively uncommon, representing only three percent of all fractures in adults. Complications with supracondylar fractures are not unusual, however. Radial nerve injury, for example, occurs in 11.8% of such fractures.

Risk Factors

Risk factors for supracondylar fractures are the same as risk fractures for many other fractures.

- Young age (from accidents)
- Old age (from falls and osteoporosis)
- Osteoporosis
- Risky sports and severe trauma in young adults
- History of malignancy, particularly metastatic (causing "pathological fractures")
- Paget's disease of bone

Mechanism Producing the Red Flag

Supracondylar fractures may be associated with injuries to nerves or blood vessels which are much more serious than the fracture itself.

Other Important Considerations

- Early and adequate treatment of vascular and neurological complications may require surgical exploration and decompression of the antecubital fossa space and repair of an injured segment of the brachial artery. Adequate and early treatment of acute vascular injuries usually ensures a good prognosis. Delay may lead to permanent disability.
- Palsies of nerves should be observed for a few weeks after adequate reduction of the fracture. If no improvement in function is observed, surgical exploration is advisable. The acupuncturist may see the patient during this interval; so you should know this.

Specific red flags:
Facial pain over sinuses, fever, purulent drainage from nose continuously for > 3 months or recurrently for > 6 months

Condition assumed present until proven otherwise:

Chronic bacterial sinusitis – infection of air-filled spaces behind the forehead (frontal sinuses), cheeks (maxillary sinuses), and eyes (ethmoidal sinuses)

Possible consequences of missing the condition:

Abscess formation leading to possible damaged vision, osteomyelitis of facial bones, meningitis and infection of the brain (encephalitis) and/or possible death

Stabilization, referral and management:

1. **Stabilization:** Measures to promote sinus drainage may be helpful, such as saline nasal rinses.
2. **Consultation and Referral Options, Transportation:** The urgency of consultation should be proportional to the severity of the patient's signs and symptoms, which may vary widely. In most cases, if the fever is not high and the patient is not too uncomfortable, patients can be referred in a timely fashion to their PCP or an urgent care center. ENT consultation is probably not necessary in these cases. Patients presenting with abnormal high fever, visual disturbances, and/or neurologic signs/deficits should be referred on a same day basis to their PCP for referral to an ENT, or even sent to the ED if they are extremely ill. Transport may generally be by private vehicle but emergency transportation should be called for patients presenting with shock.

Relevance to acupuncturists: Because chronic sinusitis can present much less dramatically than acute sinusitis, it's easy to underestimate the *potential* harm of chronic sinusitis. The key is for the acupuncturist to distinguish whether or not the sinusitis is improving, regardless of what therapies are being used, and refer those cases that are becoming chronic before infection spreads beyond the sinuses. Always remember that different patients have different degrees of immune competence and some patient, with low immune function (chronic prednisone use, AIDS, etc.), can have high risk with ordinary infections.

ACTUAL CASE

- **History:** A 45-year-old Caucasian female presented to the office with a three week history of sinus congestion with yellowish nasal drainage and mild facial pain over her eyes, her third such episode in the last six months. She had taken antibiotics for the first two episodes but was using sinus rinses, herbs, and antihistamines for this episode. She claimed to feel feverish at times but said her temperature was "not high." Her only other problem was severe rheumatoid arthritis which was under control with 15 mg of prednisone daily.
- **Physical findings:** The patient was mildly obese with a slightly moon-faced appearance. Her temperature was 100.8° F. There was tenderness to percussion over her maxillary and frontal sinuses. The nasal mucosa was hyperemic.
- **Impression:** Recurrent (chronic) sinusitis in an immune suppressed patient (from the prednisone).
- **Plan:** The patient's primary care physician was contacted and the patient made an appointment for two days later.
- **Follow up:** We later learned the patient had to reschedule her appointment with her PCP for two weeks and a prescription for an antibiotic was called in for her during the intervening time, but she was unable to pick it up because of expense. The patient did not make her rescheduled visit with the consultant, however. She passed away in her bed the night before her appointment. An autopsy revealed that the infection in one of her ethmoidal sinuses had eroded through the bone separating it from the brain (cribriform plate), causing fatal encephalitis.

DISCUSSION

History and Symptoms

Chronic sinusitis may begin with symptoms of "a cold" that doesn't go away. Some patients mistake the chronicity of chronic sinusitis for allergy. The report of persistent purulent (yellow or yellow-green colored drainage) marks the sinusitis as bacterial rather than allergic, which has clear discharge. Mixed cases of viral/allergic/bacterial sinusitis are common, however, and patients who initially report eye itching, sneezing, and clear drainage consistent with allergy may later present with chronic bacterial sinusitis. Other typical symptoms include facial pain or headache around the eyes, forehead, or cheeks, in the roof of the mouth or teeth, chronic fatigue, and sometimes cough (from backward drainage of purulence from the sinuses).

Chronic sinusitis will usually present with milder and vaguer symptoms than will acute sinusitis (although patients with chronic sinusitis may well have passed through a stage of acute symptoms). A sinus infection is generally considered chronic after 3 months of continuous symptoms or > 6 months of recurrent symptom. As our ACTUAL CASE makes clear, a history of immune suppression should be sought out to help determine the urgency of the consult.

Physical Exam Finding

The practitioner may witness purulent nasal discharge. Temperature may be low to high. Facial tenderness with percussion over the sinuses is a common finding. Otoscopic observation of the tympanic membrane is important to identify whether infection has travelled retrograde up the eustachian tube to also cause otitis media.

Incidence and/or Prevalence

Chronic sinusitis is the most commonly reported chronic disease. The prevalence of chronic sinusitis is approximately one in seven or 12.6% or 34.3 million people in the U.S. (1996 statistics).

Risk Factors

- Blockage from allergies, nasal polyps, nasal tumors, or a deviated nasal septum
- Dental infections such as tooth abscess
- Allergy to the *aspergillus* species of fungus
- Aspirin sensitivity that causes respiratory symptoms
- Cystic fibrosis and gastroesophageal reflux (GERD)
- Immune compromise from disease (HIV/AIDS, leukopenia) or chronic immunosuppressive drug use (prednisone, chemotherapy, etc.)
- Asthma — about one in five people with chronic sinusitis have asthma.
- Regular exposure to air pollutants such as cigarette smoke

Mechanism Producing the Red Flag

Infection can become trapped in the sinuses by polyps or by swelling from allergy or the infection itself. Abnormal anatomy can also block the openings (ostea) of the sinuses. Sequestration of the purulent puts the infected mass under pressure and promotes its penetration into other contiguous structures, including nearby bone. Bone infection (osteomyelitis) is a dreaded complication, but some of the bones housing the sinuses are relatively thin and the infection can erode them into the brain with catastrophic consequences.

Specific red flags:
Bunion deformity (hallux valgus) of great toe displacing adjacent toes

Condition assumed present until proven otherwise:

Serious hallux valgus deformity with subluxation of adjacent joints

Possible consequences of missing the condition:

Chronic pain, disability and irreversible cartilage, bony, and soft-tissue degeneration of metacarpophalangeal (MP) joints of great and adjacent toes

Stabilization, referral and management:

1. **Stabilization:** There are no stabilizing steps to take except to discourage use of shoes that cause the great toe to deviate laterally.
2. **Consultation and Referral Options, Transportation:** The patient should be referred on a timely basis (within a week or two) to their PCP who will probably refer to a podiatrist (or an orthopedic surgeon who subspecializes in the foot).

Relevance to acupuncturists: Acupuncturists will see many bunion deformities when searching for acupoints on the feet and ankles, but they may be somewhat surprised find that such a "garden variety" problem would show up in a red flags book about serious conditions. It does because not all bunions follow a benign course. This red flag helps us identify those that don't.

ACTUAL CASE

History: A 35-year-old Caucasian female complained of bony swelling pain on the medial aspect of the 1st MP joint of the right foot that had been gradually increasing over several months prior to her office visit.

Physical findings: A typical bunion (hallux valgus deformity) was observed in the area of complaint. The lateral (valgus) displacement of the great toe was severe enough to displace the second and third toe of the same foot at their respective MP joints

Impression: Hallux valgus with probable dislocation of adjacent toes

Plan: The patient was referred to a podiatrist.

Follow up: Radiographs by the podiatrist revealed the beginning of significant displacement of the MP joints of the second and third toes on the right foot. The patient had surgery to correct the valgus deformity of the right great toe and has done well since then.

DISCUSSION

History and Symptoms

The pain or discomfort that people experience with bunion deformity varies widely with different patients. Some patients with small deformities are very uncomfortable and others with significant deformities seem to have less pain and maintain normal activities. Although podiatrists often use the amount of discomfort to help decide which patient needs surgical intervention and which do not, the signs we review below give you additional information that can help you decide what cases need referral.

Physical Exam Findings

The key physical finding in this red flag is the observation that the lateral deviation of the great toe is enough to displace the proximal phalanges of the second and third toes from their articulation with their respective distal metatarsals (figure 5).

Incidence and/or Prevalence

Hallux valgus deformity affects one percent of adults in the United States. The incidence increases with age: 3% in 15-30 year-olds, 9% in 31-60-year-olds and 16% in > 60-year-old people with females to male ratio of 2:1 to 4:1. A much smaller number of these are severe enough to displace adjacent phalanges.

Risk Factors

A common cause of bunion deformity is wearing shoes (especially high heels) with a narrow and pointed toe-box that forces the great toe laterally. The condition can also occur or be worsened by other factors, including those listed below.

Arthritic/metabolic conditions

- Gouty arthritis
- Rheumatoid arthritis
- Psoriatic arthritis
- Connective tissue disorders such as Ehlers-Danlos syndrome, Marfan syndrome, Down syndrome, and ligamentous laxity

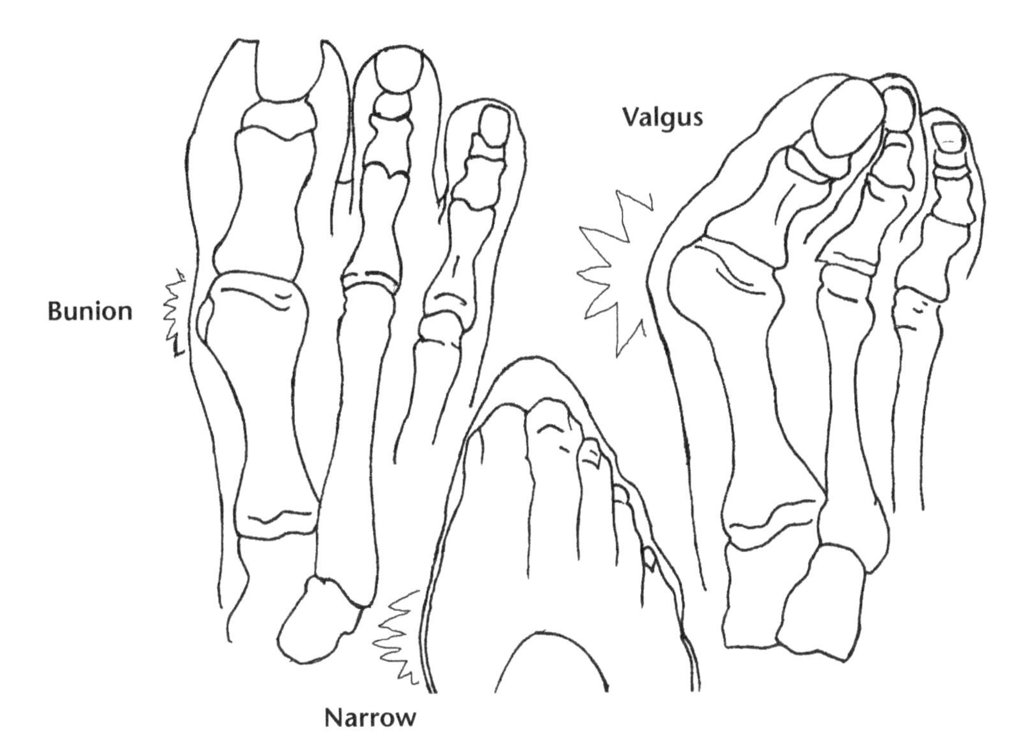

Figure 5. Mild to moderately severe bunions are ignored by many patients. This is not the case when the valgus displacement of the great toe begins to dislocate nearby toe joints as shown in this figure.

Neuromuscular disease

- Multiple sclerosis
- Charcot-Marie-Tooth disease
- Cerebral palsy

Traumatic conditions and structural deformities (a partial list)

- Malunions
- Dislocations
- Malalignment of articular surface or metatarsal shaft
- Abnormal metatarsal length

Mechanism Producing the Red Flag

The big toe of the foot is called the hallux. When it deviates laterally toward the small toe of the same foot, the condition is called hallux valgus. As the hallux drifts into valgus, a bump develops on the medial aspect of the big toe over the first metatarsal (MT) bone. This bony prominence on the inner edge of the metatarsal is referred to as a bunion. As further deviation occurs, the lateral pressure from the great toe can dislocate adjacent joints. The discomfort is caused by pressure against bones, ligaments and tendons of the toes.

Other Important Considerations

- The treatment of a bunion depends mostly on how uncomfortable it is, which often corresponds to how much damage it is doing to the foot. Symptoms will often depend on the type and size of shoes worn.
- In the elderly, padding and strapping may be the best options if surgical correction is medically contraindicated.
- Some clinicians use the "L is vaLgus" as a memory device to recall that vaLgus refers to Lateral deviation of a distal bone in relation to a proximal bone.

Specific red flags:
Headache, eye pain, blurry or haloed vision, nausea, vomiting

Condition assumed present until proven otherwise:

Acute closed-angle glaucoma – one of a group of eye diseases that progressively damage the optic nerve

Possible consequences of missing the condition:

Acute closed-angle glaucoma can yield total loss of vision in affected eyes if not treated within hours.

Stabilization, referral and management:

1. **Stabilization:** There are no stabilizing steps to take.
2. **Consultation and Referral Options, Transportation:** The patient with signs and symptoms of mild glaucoma may be sent on a semi-urgent basis to the patient's PCP or to urgent care if no PCP is available. Referral may also be made directly to an ophthalmologist if the patient lacks a PCP. Transportation may be by private vehicle, but the patient should not drive. If the patient has severe symptoms, they should be sent directly to the ED.

Relevance to Acupuncturists: The symptoms of acute closes-angle glaucoma noted below resemble classical migraine headache symptoms and may easily be diagnosed as such. Differences are addressed below. The acupuncturist should keep a high index of suspicion for this disorder and early stages of all types of glaucoma because the condition is easily treated if caught early.

ACTUAL CASE

- **History:** A 35-year-old African-American female presented to the office for right shoulder pain, but also mentioned having headaches recently, accompanied by eye pain. She attributed these to her migraines. Her only other complaint was seeing blind spots in her peripheral vision, but, unlike the spots that appeared with her migraines, these did not come and go.
- **Physical findings:** There were no specific physical findings.
- **Impression:** Possible early angle closure glaucoma
- **Plan:** The patient was sent to her family doctor who sent her to an ophthalmologist.
- **Follow up:** The eye exam at the ophthalmologist's office demonstrated increased intraocular pressure and visual field defects in the patient's peripheral vision. She was placed on eye drops and her intraocular pressure has returned to normal.

DISCUSSION

History and Symptoms

This red flag necessitates that we understand the symptoms of all types of glaucoma, because all can progress to eventual vision loss, though none as rapidly as acute, closed-angle glaucoma. There are basically four types of glaucoma. We are primarily interested in the first two, closed-angle and open-angle glaucoma.

1. Closed-angle glaucoma may progress gradually without manifesting symptoms until long after it starts, but it can also present acutely when intraocular pressure builds as it does in our red flag. In this case, the rapid progression produces severe eye pain, headaches, blurred vision, halos, nausea, and often vomiting. Increased light sensitivity (photophobia) is another symptom.
2. Open-angle glaucoma, the most common type, produces no initial symptoms, but the patient will eventually begin to experience loss of peripheral vision, which can be irreversible and lead to total blindness if untreated. Open-angle glaucoma is generally bilateral. Patients can have 20/20 vision when looking straight ahead but note blind spots in their peripheral vision.
3. Normal-tension glaucoma (low-tension glaucoma) is a condition in which optic nerve damage and vision loss occurs despite normal intraocular pressure. Normal-tension glaucoma may result in loss of peripheral vision like we see in open angle glaucoma.
4. Symptoms of congenital glaucoma in infants or young children are infrequent due to the inability to communicate at that age. The clinician must rely upon signs noted below.

Physical Exam Findings

Patients with acute glaucoma are in obvious pain. There is often excessive blinking and excessive tearing. Children with congenital glaucoma have cloudy corneas, white, hazy, enlarged, or protruding eye, sensitivity to light, excessive tearing, and eyelid spasm. Defects in peripheral vision and increased extraocular pressure will be found by the ophthalmologist in all patients except in those with normal tension glaucoma.

Incidence and/or Prevalence

Prevalence estimates for all types of glaucoma in the U.S. range from approx 0.74%–1.10%. Two million people are thought to be visually impaired by glaucoma in the U.S.

Risk Factors

- Elevated internal eye pressure (intraocular pressure)
- Age > 60 years old
- Ethnicity: African-Americans are 6-8 times more likely to get glaucoma than Caucasians.
- Family history of glaucoma
- Diabetes, high blood pressure, heart disease, and hypothyroidism increase risk.
- Severe eye injuries can increased eye pressure by dislocating the lens and closing the drainage angle. Other eye conditions that can increase risk include retinal detachment, eye tumors, and eye inflammations, such as chronic uveitis and iritis or eye surgery.
- Prolonged corticosteroid use, including corticosteroids eye drops
- Nearsightedness

Mechanism Producing the Red Flag

The symptoms and signs of acute closed-angle glaucoma, as well as some other types, are caused by a blockage of the outflow of aqueous humor from the eye causing increased intraocular pressure that damages the optic nerve. Open-angle glaucoma begins by damaging the nerve fibers that are necessary for peripheral vision, but fibers for central vision are eventually lost as well, causing total blindness if the condition is not treated.

Specific red flags: *Sudden, cataclysmic headache in a middle-aged hypertensive patient*

Condition assumed present until proven otherwise:

Nontraumatic subarachnoid hemorrhage (NTSAH): A type of intracranial bleed between the arachnoid membrane and the pia mater surrounding the brain (see figure 1).

Possible consequences of missing the condition:

Paralysis and/or sudden death

Stabilization, referral and management:

1. **Stabilization:** Efforts to stabilize the patient will only waste precious time. Herbs which decrease blood coagulability (mostly herbs with "Move Blood" functions) are contraindicated until the condition is stabilized due to risk of increased bleeding.
2. **Consultation and Referral Options, Transportation:** If the patient appears stable, a phone call should be made to the patient's PCP for advice and possible direct admission to the hospital. If the PCP cannot be reached immediately the patient should be sent directly to the ED. The unstable patient will require a call to 911 and urgent medical transport. A phone call should be made to the ED physician or triage nurse to tell them about the situation so they can prepare to call in a neurosurgeon.

Relevance to acupuncturists: Although it is unlikely that a person with a massive intracranial bleed will go to an acupuncturist's office, we have seen cases of early intracranial bleed when symptoms are not overwhelming and are underestimated by patients, family members, and practitioners. NTSAH symptoms can also be dismissed as a flare-up or variant of the usual symptoms of a patient who already experiences severe headaches or facial pain from previously-diagnosed conditions such as trigeminal neuralgia, migraines or cluster headaches. A patient who describes their current headache as "new" or "different" and more severe than their typical headaches should be re-evaluated and screened for the presence of NTSAH.

ACTUAL CASE

- **History:** A 45-year-old Caucasian female patient with history of severe migraines and poorly-controlled high blood pressure arrived late for an acupuncture appointment because she earlier had "the worst headache of my life," which she reported as due to "stress."
- **Physical findings:** The patient's blood pressure was 145/90mmHg. She appeared anxious but also somewhat sleepy. She spoke and moved slowly. Her neurological exam was normal.
- **Impression:** Possible subarachnoid hemorrhage
- **Plan:** The patient had no PCP. She was discharged from her last physician due to non-compliance with her blood pressure medications. She was sent to the ED of a local hospital.

- **Follow up:** The patient was found to have a subarachnoid hemorrhage on a CT scan at the hospital resulting from a saccular aneurysm. The aneurysm was repaired and the patient survived the incident. She was discharged home and given the name of a new PCP.

DISCUSSION

History and Symptoms

Symptoms of a large NTSAH include a severe headache with a rapid onset ("thunderclap headache"). There can also be vomiting, confusion, and decreased level of consciousness reported as feeling fatigued or having difficulty concentrating. Seizure may occur. Lesser bleeding may result in less rapid deterioration, but the "worse headache of my life" complaint is highly characteristic.

Physical Exam Findings

Decreasing level of consciousness is often found. In extreme cases, meningeal signs appear, a very stiff neck with extensor muscle spasm being the most common.

Incidence and/or Prevalence

Nontraumatic subarachnoid hemorrhage (NTSAH) has an estimated annual incidence of six cases per 100,000 persons in the U.S. Patients with NTSAH have 35% mortality in the first six month and 15% additional mortality in the next six months. Intracranial saccular aneurysms represent the most common etiology for NTSAH, with about 80% resulting from ruptured aneurysms. NTSAH is responsible for the death and/or disability of 18,000 persons each year in the U.S. alone.

Risk Factors for NTSAH

- Smoking
- Hypertension
- Drinking 150g or more of alcohol per week
- Use of oral contraceptives
- Certain types of hormone replacement therap

Diseases associated with higher incidence of aneurysms (a partial list):

- Hypertension, idiopathic or from fibromuscular dysplasia or polycystic kidneys
- Increased blood flow from cerebral arteriovenous malformation (AVM)
- Blood vessel disorders like SLE and granulomatous angiitis
- Genetic disorders like Marfan syndrome
- Congenital – Persistent fetal circulation
- Metastatic tumors to cerebral arteries
- Infectious – Bacterial and fungal

Mechanism Producing the Red Flag

Whether the SAH occurs as the result of head trauma, or spontaneously (NTSAH), blood in the CNS acts is an irritant to the meninges. This blood irritates nerves going to the peripheral areas of the body producing signs of meningeal irritation like a stiff neck and headache.

Other Important Considerations

- NTSAH is one type of intracranial bleeding. It is bleeding inside the skull, but outside of the brain (extraxial), as contrasted to bleeding within the brain itself (intraaxial). Extra-axial bleeding falls into three subtypes:

1. Epidural (extradural) hemorrhage – between the dura mater (the outermost meningeal layer) and the skull. This type is caused by trauma that usually lacerates an artery and is very dangerous because the bleed is from arteries.
2. Subdural hemorrhage results from tearing of the bridging veins (lower pressure system) in the subdural space between the dura and arachnoid mater and is covered elsewhere (see confusion).
3. Subarachnoid hemorrhage, the type of extraxial bleeding we consider in this red flag, occurs between the arachnoid and pia meningeal layers and can result from trauma or from ruptures of aneurysms or arteriovenous malformations, as noted earlier.

Specific red flags:
Atraumatic, progressive, intermittent hip pain on movement and decreased hip ROM

Condition assumed present until proven otherwise:
Avascular necrosis of the hip (also called "Legg–Calvé–Perthes syndrome," "Perthes disease" or "aseptic necrosis of hip")—Death of a portion of the ball of the femur due to inadequate blood supply.

Possible consequences of missing the condition:
Severe and disabling osteoarthritis of the hip

Stabilization, referral and management:

1. **Stabilization:** There are no stabilizing measures except to tell the patient to avoid activities that cause pain until seen by a consultant who can rule the condition in or out.
2. **Consultation and Referral Options, Transportation:** Timely to semiurgent referral should be made to the patient's PCP. The ultimate consultant will be an orthopedic surgeon. Transportation can be by the patient or family member.

Relevance to acupuncturists: Acupuncturists will see many cases of hip pain as well as back pain so it is important to be able to recognize instances of hip pain that represent serious conditions like this. Although fairly rare, recognition of this red flag is important to keep patients from avoiding irreversible damage to the hip joint.

ACTUAL CASE

- **History:** The patient was an 8-year-old Caucasian male brought in for acupuncture for left hip pain. The boy said he had been having pain for about one month after running with his friends on the playground at lunchtime. He described it as a dull ache behind the left knee.
- **Physical findings:** The child had a slight limp when he entered the office. He said he had a little pain in the left knee because he ran "extra hard" that day. His left hip range of motion was slightly limited in flexion and the ROM exam caused him mild discomfort. His right hip exam and his left knee exam were normal.
- **Impression:** Possible early Perthes disease of left hip.
- **Plan:** Patient's PCP was called, but they PCP wanted the child referred directly to the orthopedist and gave us the orthopedist's telephone number, which we used to refer the patient.
- **Follow up:** The patient had an X-ray of the left hip, which was normal, but an MRI showed an early aseptic necrosis of the femoral head. The child was placed on limited weight bearing for two years and carefully followed until his symptoms resolved. He had no permanent damage to the hip and is doing well as of last check.

DISCUSSION

History and Symptoms

Pain is the primary complaint in Perthes disease, but it may be intermittent over a period of weeks, or even months, leading the parent or clinician to think it is "growing pain." The pain usually starts hours after activity and lasts for an hour or two afterwards. Rest pain is present in 75% of cases and night pain in 45%. When pain is present, it is worsened by prolonged standing, walking, running or kneeling, and relieved by rest, only to return at night. Pain may be felt in other parts of the leg, such as the groin, thigh, or knee. The pain in the knee (referred pain) is usually in the back of the knee and can feel like a "charley horse." Pain is sometimes felt in the unaffected hip because the patient uses that side to spare the injured side, placing the majority of the weight on the "good leg."

Physical Exam Findings

When patients complain of moderate to severe pain, a painful (antalgic) gait on ambulation can be present. They also have decreased ROM in all directions of the hip on ROM testing. There may be atrophy of thigh muscles from disuse and an inequality of leg length (with the affected leg being shorter) in more severe cases.

Incidence and/or Prevalence

Perthes is fortunately rare, occurring in approximately 5.5 of 100,000 children. Caucasians are affected more frequently than other races. The condition is very rare in African-Americans. The male to female ratio is 4:1. The peak incidence is in children aged 4-10 years old, with a median age of 6 years old. *Perthes disease has another peak incidence again at between 25-45-year-olds.* Perthes was originally described a century ago as a type of "childhood arthritis."

Risk Factors

- Systemic steroids
- Alcoholism

- Sickle cell disease
- Underground or undersea work
- Genetics do not appear to be a determining factor.
- Possible (unproven) deficiency of anticoagulating blood factors

Mechanism Producing the Red Flag

Perthes disease occurs because of reduction in blood flow to the capital epiphysis of the femur (the ball of the femur that articulates with the acetabulum). This is possibly the result of lack of development of one of the arteries that supplies it. It leads to weakness and flattening and/or fracture of the femoral head. The bony areas and surrounding tissue can become intensely inflamed and irritated, causing the pain. Muscle spasms may also occur, adding to the pain.

Other Important Considerations

- Perthes is generally diagnosed between 4-10 years of age (preadolescence). Remember this age range to help distinguish this disorder from the next hip disorder we'll examine in children, slipped capital femoral epiphysis (SCFE), which generally starts at adolescence.
- Typically, Perthes is unilateral, but bilaterality is seen in up to 10% of children.
- Avascular necrosis of the hip is a process of gradual deterioration that occurs in stages. Early treatment in the course of any particular case yields optimal results. Treatment before 6 years of age is recommended because regenerative capacity is better before 6.
- Treatment of Perthes may require periods of immobilization or limitations of usual activities. The long-term prognosis is good with proper treatment. Most children return to normal activities without major limitations after 1.5-2 years of treatment. Surgery is required in a minority of cases.

Specific red flags:
Hip, knee, groin pain with limp in obese adolescent with or without trauma with decreased hip ROM on exam

Condition assumed present until proven otherwise:
Slipped capital femoral epiphysis (SCFE) – Slippage in a backward direction of the capital epiphysis due to weakness of the growth plate (see figure 6).

Possible consequences of missing the condition:
Severe hip arthritis and loss of hip function

Stabilization, referral and management:

1. **Stabilization:** As with Perthes disease, the patient should avoid prolonged standing or other activities that cause hip pain until consultation has occurred.
2. **Consultation and Referral Options, Transportation:** For patients with stable SCFE (see history and physical section), referrals should be made on a timely basis to the patient's PCP or directly to an orthopedist if a PCP is not available. Patients with unstable SCFE will need to be hospitalized under the care of an orthopedic surgeon for possible hip surgery. This can also be expedited by the patient's PCP or may require an admission through the ED. Family transport is usually appropriate.

Relevance to acupuncturists: Like the previous hip problem of Perthes disease, SCFE represents a real threat to the future function of the hip, and since it is a painful condition, may show up at the acupuncturist's office. As in many red flags, early and possibly mild cases can be spotted for optimal healing outcome.

ACTUAL CASE

- **History:** A 14-year-old high school student was brought for acupuncture for complaints of "off-and-on" hip pain by his mother that had started a few weeks earlier at basketball practice.
- **Physical findings:** A young African-American man walked into the office with a slight limp. He was 5'6" and 190 pounds. He had decreased range of motion (ROM) of hip flexion and internal rotation and complained of pain at the extremes of motion.
- **Impression:** Probable SCFE – stable
- **Plan:** The patient was referred to his family doctor, who referred the patient to an orthopedist. X-rays of the hip revealed a slipped capital femoral epiphysis. The patient was placed on limited weight bearing and told to avoid basketball for at least one season. He was followed periodically.
- **Follow up:** The patient couldn't resist a "pick-up" game

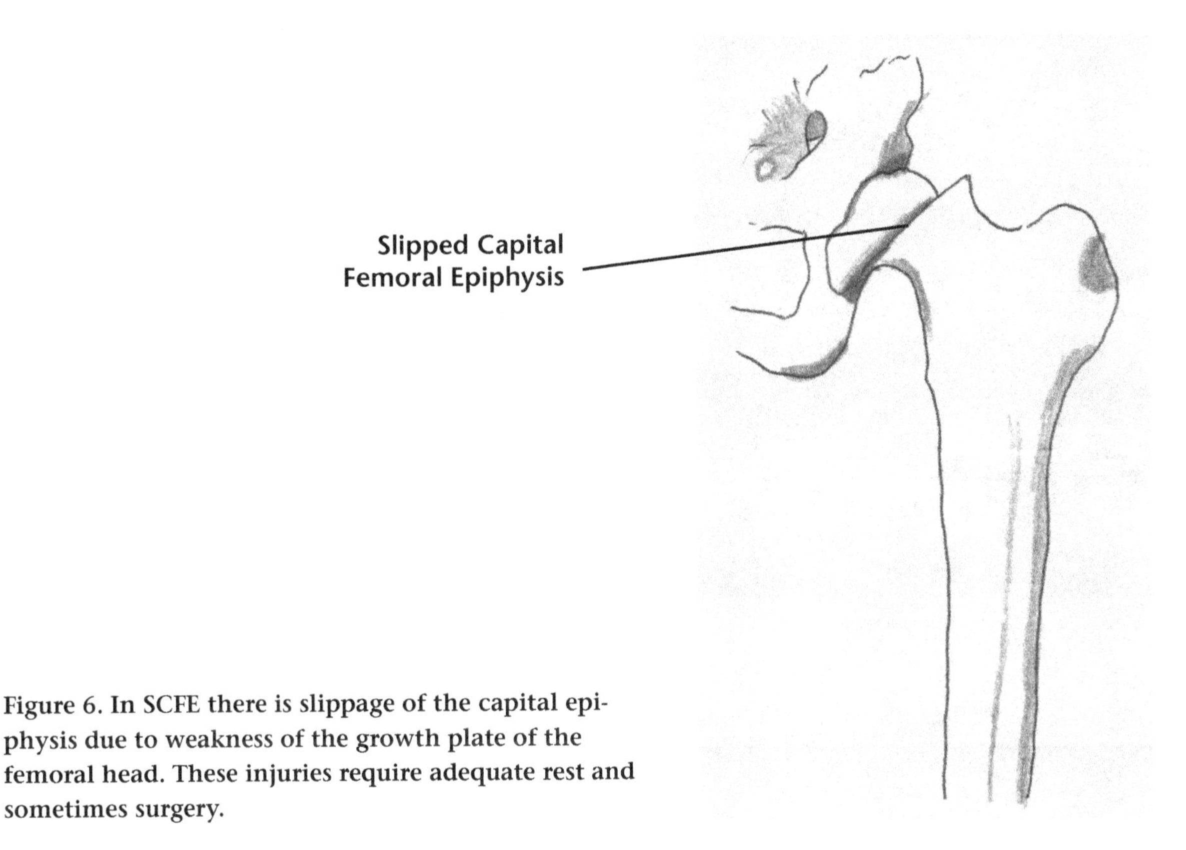

Figure 6. In SCFE there is slippage of the capital epiphysis due to weakness of the growth plate of the femoral head. These injuries require adequate rest and sometimes surgery.

of basketball one day after school. After vying for a rebound, he landed on the foot of his affected side and felt exquisite pain in the hip. He proved to have a displaced femoral epiphysis on X-ray and was taken to surgery for an internal fixation procedure. The patient healed well and played basketball the next season.

DISCUSSION

History and Symptoms

An adolescent who has *stable* SCFE may present with stiffness in the hip rather than pain. The pain may get better with rest or may evolve into a limp. It may come and go. The pain is not necessarily in the hip, but may be referred to the groin, thigh, or knee. In the later stages, the adolescent may lose some ability to move the involved hip. He or she may not be able to do simple tasks such as bending over to tie shoes, etc. *Unstable* SCFE produces extreme pain and an inability to move the injured leg.

Physical Exam Findings

The appearance of the adolescent is often characteristic. There is often a limp (antalgic gait). In severe cases, the adolescent will be unable to bear any weight on the affected leg. The affected leg may be externally rotated in this case and may also appear to be shorter. The hip will have some limitations of normal range of motion with sometimes a complete loss of hip flexion and inability to fully rotate the hip inward. Pain at the extremes of motion and involuntary muscle guarding and spasm is noted.

Decreased ROM of the hip on exam, is the common sign for any kind of hip pathology that interferes with the normal movement of the ball of the femur. It is common to Perthes, SCFE, and even osteoarthritis of the hip joint in adults. The take home message is this. If there is hip pain, but the ROM of the hip is normal, we are in a better position to think we might really be dealing with a "growing pain" in a child or adolescent, rather than a destructive process like SCFE.

Incidence and/or Prevalence

SCFE usually develops during periods of accelerated growth, shortly after the onset of puberty. The overall incidence in the U.S. is 10.8 cases per 100,000 children (boys 13.35/100,000 and girls 8.07/100,000). African-American children and Hispanic children have higher incidence rates than Caucasians (3.94 and 2.54 times higher incidence respectively).

A recent Scottish study showed a two and a half times increase in incidence of SCFE over the last two decades and a fall in the mean age at diagnosis from 13.4-12.6 years for boys ($p = 0.007$) and 12.2-11.6 for girls ($p = 0.047$). This was closely correlated with the rising incidence of childhood obesity over the last 20 years in Scotland.

Risk Factors

- Overweight in relation to height
- African-American ethnicity
- Male sex (3:1 male to female ratio)
- Hypothyroidism, low growth hormone, pituitary tumors, Down's syndrome, and several other rare medical conditions.

Mechanism Producing the Red Flag

The pain is from inflammation and bony displacement of the ball of the hip joint through the growth zone of the femoral head, the epiphysis.

Other Important Considerations

- SCFE and Perthes disease covered previously are often confused. Perthes disease is never traumatic, however, whereas SCFE can be. Also, Perthes often occurs in preadolescents (4-10 years old), whereas SCFE occurs with the onset of adolescence (11-16 years old). Finally, Perthes is rare in African-Americans, whereas SCFE is more common.
- A child is considered to have "stable" SCFE if he or she can walk with or without crutches. More than 90% of cases of SCFE are stable. Unstable SCFE often occurs after trauma. Trauma can also cause a stable SCFE to become unstable.
- An orthopedic surgeon should ideally follow SCFE cases to follow progression and because surgery may be necessary. If surgery is necessary, a single central screw keeps the epiphysis from slipping further.
- The most serious complications of SCFE are avascular necrosis and chondrolysis (degeneration of the cartilage of the joint). Avascular necrosis is more common in patients who have unstable SCFE. Chondrolysis, or loss of articular cartilage of the hip joint, is a major complication of SCFE and may cause permanent loss of motion, flexion contracture and pain.

Specific red flags:
Knee trauma with pain and immediate and severe swelling of the knee

Condition assumed present until proven otherwise:
"Internal derangement of knee"—a general term indicating tearing of one or more of the major ligaments and/or menisci of the knee: the anterior cruciate ligament (ACL), posterior cruciate ligament (PCL), and/or medial or lateral menisci

Possible consequences of missing the condition:
Permanent pain and disability of the knee

Stabilization, referral and management:

1. **Stabilization:** Ice and elevation are useful as long as there is swelling, and use of crutches should be advised.
2. **Consultation and Referral Options, Transportation:** In the acute phase, this timely to semiurgent situation referable to the patient's PCP or an orthopedist if a PCP is not available. The orthopedist will be the ultimate consultant because this can be a surgical problem in many cases. The patient should be driven by a friend or family member because the knee is often painful and unstable. In chronic cases, the referral depends on symptoms of pain and swelling. Many patients who pass through a period of acute internal derangement learn to live with recurrent swelling, pain and dysfunction, but others have enough discomfort to require referral.

Relevance to acupuncturists: Because patients with internal derangement of the knee may present for treatment weeks to even months after the injury, this red flag will often be picked up by history as a "swollen knee," or patients may come to you for cotreatment after surgery. Many things can make a knee swell, including inflammation from crystal deposition, inflammatory arthritis or infection. The swelling will generally be of slower onset in other conditions, however. Only a major tear of an internal structure of the knee compatible with an internal derangement can cause the kind of immediate swelling presented in this red flag because blood vessels attached to the internal contents of the knee are also torn with the injury.

ACTUAL CASE

- **History:** The patient was a 27-year-old athletic male who worked as a window washer. He gave the history of stepping down off a ladder, missing a rung and landing "hard" on his left foot 3 weeks earlier. The left knee twisted and he heard a "pop." It felt "wobbly" to stand on afterwards. By the time he hobbled over to a curb and rolled up his pant leg, the knee had swollen "to the size of a grapefruit." He didn't see a health care practitioner right after the accident because he didn't have insurance and thought he would get better on his own.
- **Physical findings:** The patient walked in with an antalgic limp. On exam, his affected knee was swollen almost one and a half times larger than the opposite knee. The swelling was soft. A fluid wave was induced in the swollen knee by tapping on one side of the swelling and watching the impulse cross to the other side. There was a positive anterior drawer sign of one-half inch (the proximal tibia could be displaced forward one-half inch from the femur with the patient seated and the examiner's hands behind the proximal calf pulling forward). There was medial joint space tenderness (tenderness to palpation of the space between the distal femur and the proximal tibia medial to the patellar tendon) and there was an equivocal McMurray's test.
- **Impression:** Internal derangement of the left knee: probable complete ACL tear and also possible tear of the medial meniscus
- **Plan:** The patient had no PCP to consult and was referred to an orthopedic surgeon.
- **Follow up:** An MRI showed complete rupture of the ACL and partial tears of the medial and lateral menisci. Because the patient was active and athletic, the surgeon and patient agreed to reconstructive surgery of the knee (ACL repair and removal of torn fragments of the medial and lateral menisci). The patient is back to his usual athletics, including surfing.

DISCUSSION

History and Symptoms

The exact structures torn in an internal derangement cannot be diagnosed by history alone, though a loud pop at the time of injury suggests a tear of the anterior cruciate ligament (ACL) and/or meniscus. Immediate swelling appearing over minutes is the usual case. The knee can feel unstable to the patient. Despite the dramatic presentation of this injury, a sizable number of patients may not present soon after the injury, but may come in for evaluation weeks, months, or even years after the initial tear. Patients with older cases will often describe knee instability, episodes of the knee buckling or shifting and recurrent swelling. If a meniscal tear is involved, a torn piece of cartilage can get stuck in the joint and cause the knee to "lock."

Physical Exam Findings

In acute cases, there will invariably be a large amount of bloody effusion within the knee, which feels fluctuant to touch. The examiner can induce a fluid wave that can be seen to travel to one side of the effusion to the other side by tapping one side of the effusion. The swelling tells you that a major structure has been torn. Further exam is needed to tell if the ACL or the menisci are torn, or both. These will be briefly discussed below, but you should consult a standard orthopedic test for the details of these special tests.

To see if the ACL is torn, the tibia can be pulled (displaced) anteriorly in relationship to the femur. An intact ACL would prevent such displacement. This can be done with either the anterior drawer test or the Lachman's test. To be accurate, these tests must be done either before muscle guarding has set in or after it has resolved, otherwise muscle spasm of the thigh muscle may prevent accurate testing. Due to normal differences in ligamentous tightness between different individuals, the degree of laxity in the injured knee must be compared to that of the normal knee before determining if any displacement indicates ACL tear.

To see if a meniscus is torn, we must perform a test that puts pressure on the meniscus like the McMurray test, which involves compressing the joint line while stressing the meniscus. Joint space tenderness is also characteristic of meniscal damage, especially of the medial meniscus. The lateral meniscus is more difficult to assess on physical exam than the medial.

Incidence and/or Prevalence

Injury to the ACL is common, especially in athletic individuals. The overall incidence of ACL tear is about 1 in 3,000. An estimated 200,000 ACL injuries occur annually in the U.S., with approximately 95,000 complete ruptures. Approximately 100,000 ACL reconstructions are performed each year. Adjusted for sports participation, a higher prevalence of injury is observed in females than males (2.4–9.7 times greater). Meniscal tears alone are more prevalent than ACL tears, but approximately 50% of patients with ACL injuries will also have meniscal tears.

Risk Factors

The incidence of ACL injury is higher in people who participate in high-risk sports such as basketball, football, skiing, and soccer.

Mechanism Producing the Red Flag

The disruptions in the knee are caused by mechanical forces and the knee laxity by tears of supporting ligaments and cartilage. The extreme swelling is caused by breakage of arterial vessels and the pain by neuronal injury and subsequent inflammation.

Another Important Consideration

- A completely torn ACL will never grow back on its own. Surgery is required if the patient wants the former level of stability to be restored. Yet, many people do opt to have a loose and dysfunctional joint rather than go through reconstruction of the ACL which is not always successful.

Specific red flags:
Posterior calf pain reliably occurring after walking a specific distance

Condition assumed present until proven otherwise:

Intermittent claudication from peripheral artery disease (PAD)–an analogue of angina that comes on after a specific amount of exercise.

Possible consequences of missing the condition:

Loss of limb (15% of those with intermittent claudication lose a limb). Also, claudication pain is a marker for severe arteriosclerotic disease possibly present in coronary or carotid arteries that could cause sudden disability or death from (MI) or stroke (20% of people with intermittent claudication have MI or stroke within five years).

Stabilization, referral and management:

1. **Stabilization:** There are no specific stabilizing steps to take except to advise against maximal exercise until the patient can be evaluated for widespread arteriosclerotic disease.
2. **Consultation and Referral Options, Transportation:** Patients with intermittent claudication from PAD can have a timely consult with their PCP or an urgent care center if no PCP is available if there are no signs and symptoms of coronary and carotid insufficiency. Patient transport, in these cases, is appropriate. If these additional signs are present, follow recommendations under chest pain to assess referral options.

ACTUAL CASE

- **History:** The patient was a 38-year-old male, a national labor union leader, a one-pack-per-day smoker for 25 years. He complained of right sided posterior calf pain that came on reliably at mile one of his two mile biweekly walk. He would typically slow down or stop, at which time the pain would go away, and he could then resume his walk at a slower pace without the pain. He incidentally described some erectile dysfunction, but denied chest pain on exertion. His father died from an MI at age 42 and his paternal grandfather having had an MI at 55 and died of stroke at 61. Several relatives in his maternal lineage had history of adult-onset diabetes mellitus.
- **Physical findings:** The patient appeared to be a "take charge" kind of individual. He had a normal physical exam except for a diminished dorsalis pedis pulse in the right foot compared to the left.
- **Impression:** Intermittent claudication from PAD and probable high risk for MI and stroke with possible partial occlusion of the dorsal penile artery.
- **Plan:** The patient had no PCP and was sent to a cardiologist.
- **Follow up:** The patient proved to have significant right iliac artery stenosis, coronary artery disease and carotid stenosis. He had a stent placed in the left anterior descending artery of his heart due to a 98% occlusion and he eventually underwent bypass grafting of the blocked portion of his right iliac artery. His carotid plaque was not occlusive enough to need surgery. He stopped smoking and was placed on an aggressive lipid lowering and anti-atherogenic protocol. He initially did well, but one year after his last procedure was smoking again, blaming it on the stress of his job. He had developed diabetes as well. On last check he was also impotent.

DISCUSSION

History and Symptoms

Half of the people who have PAD have no symptoms at all. Those who do have symptoms most commonly complain of pain, cramping, weakness or heaviness in the hip, thigh, or lower leg (depending on the artery affected). Claudication pain in the posterior calf is most common and it is more often unilateral than bilateral. Usually, the discomfort goes away in a few minutes when ceasing the exercise. The patient often, but not always, has a history compatible with atherosclerotic risk (see CAD risk factors in chest pain).

Physical Exam Findings

PAD diagnosis begins with a physical examination by checking for weak pulses in the feet and legs. Typically, the popliteal pulse behind the knees, posterior tibial pulse behind the medial malleolus and the dorsalis pedis on the dorsum of the feet are checked and compared to the opposite side. All acupuncturists should be adept at quickly checking these pulses and can become so with little practice and by consulting standard texts on physical exam. Suspicious cases identified by history and/or exam can get a noninvasive screening test called ankle/brachial index test. This inexpensive test compares the blood pressure in the ankles with the blood pressure in the arms. The ankle pressure is usually at least 90% of the arm pressure. With severe narrowing of leg arteries, it may be less than 50%.

Incidence and/of Prevalence

Peripheral arterial disease is more common in people > 50 years old and in men than women. The prevalence of PAD, as assessed by noninvasive tests, is about 14-17% in men and 11-17% in women over 55. The overall annual incidence of intermittent claudication is 4.1-12.9 per 1,000 men and 3.3-8.2 per 1,000 women yearly.

Risk Factors

- Advanced age
- Male gender
- Factors and processes that injure the inner lining (endothelium) of arteries like cigarette smoking, diabetes mellitus, hypertension (see also CAD risk factors).
- Other factors like hyperlipidemia, obesity, and physical inactivity
- The strongest associations are with smoking (relative risk 2.0–4.0 x normal) and diabetes mellitus.

Mechanism Producing the Red Flag

The mechanisms producing the vascular injury and occlusion are listed above and in the chapter on chest pain and CAD. The cause of the pain in the muscles is ischemic pain from poorly oxygenated muscle cells.

▶ Specific red flags:
Late teen to early adult with focal, persistent shin pain after increasing running distance

Condition assumed present until proven otherwise:

Stress fracture of tibia–a crack in the bone caused by the stress of exercise (The tibia is one of many places where stress fractures can appear–see incidence)

Possible consequences of missing the condition:

Complete fracture of the tibia

Stabilization, referral and management:

1. **Stabilization:** The patient should be strictly cautioned to avoid exercise that brings on pain until the condition is evaluated by a consultant.
2. **Consultation and Referral Options, Transportation:** The referral can be in a timely fashion to the patient's PCP or a sports medicine orthopedist if a PCP is not available. Some PCPs have extra training in sports medicine (certificate of added qualification) and may be able to handle the condition themselves, or some may refer to an orthopedist. Transportation can be by private vehicle.

Relevance to acupuncturists: This is another common problem that the acupuncturist can encounter and it can easily be underestimated. The possible or probable need for imaging studies and strict supervision to ensure complete healing can be tricky enough that consultation for comanagement is often advisable.

ACTUAL CASE

- **History:** A 20-year-old 800-meter college track star presented to the office with tenderness of the right shin bone that came on toward the end of his long run.
- **Physical findings:** The patient was lean, muscular and appeared quite healthy. He had a normal examination except for an area of specific tenderness of the medial

aspect of the distal right tibia. There was no significant tenderness in the corresponding area of the left tibia.

- **Impression:** Probable stress fracture of the distal right tibia
- **Plan:** The patient had an important track meet coming up in a week. He was cautioned to train only on an exercise bike until his injury could be better assessed. He was referred to his PCP who, confirmed that he had experience dealing with stress fractures.
- **Follow up:** The PCP saw the patient the next day and obtained an X-ray, which was negative, and a nuclear medicine bone scan, which showed the suspected stress fracture. The patient was issued an airpadded type tibial splint to wear and advised to be on strict nonweight-bearing aerobic exercise for at least two weeks to maintain conditioning. Unfortunately, the patient did not comply and competed in the track meet he considered too important to miss, during which he shattered his tibia.

DISCUSSION

History and Symptoms

The patient with a stress fracture is usually an adolescent or adult with a history of long-distance running who has increased training intensity or distance fairly quickly. It is also seen in other sports and occasionally in workers who have excessive weight bearing and walking as part of their job. The pain usually occurs gradually during exercise and generally gets better when slowing down or stopping.

A tip-off that a stress fracture may be present in the tibia, rather than the more common condition of "shin splints" (posterior tibialis periostitis) is that stress fractures tend to be unilateral, wheras shin splints are often bilateral. The patient may, however, have shin splints *and* a stress fracture or bilateral stress fractures, although these are less common presentations.

Physical Exam Findings

The general rule about fractures presented in other areas of this book was that *fractures are always tender to careful and sufficient palpation.* Stress fractures are no exception to this general rule. Patients with stress fractures have focal bony tenderness and poorly resolving soft tissue tenderness near the fracture site. This point tenderness is somewhat different from the more generalized tenderness found in shin splints. Knowing the likely locations of stress fractures (see below) helps direct your palpation.

Although the bone edges have not become displaced from one another, the X-ray will generally show a small discontinuity of the periosteum over the site of the fracture. In early stages of stress fracture, however, as in our ACTUAL CASE study, the X-ray might be negative and a "bone scan" may be required for the definitive diagnosis (the radionucleide is avidly "taken up" by inflammatory tissue at the fracture site and shows up as a "hot spot" on the bone scan).

Incidence and/or Prevalence

Stress fracture frequency in various locations: tibia 34%, fibula 34%, metatarsal 20%, femur 14%, pelvis 6%.

Risk Factors

- Amenorrhea and oligomenorrhea (infrequent, light menses), low body fat, dieting ("female athletic triad" with osteopenia risk in female athlete)
- Long-distance running events–especially competitive
- Occupations requiring repetitive weight-bearing activity

Mechanism Producing the Red Flag

Stress fractures are caused when the strength of bone is exceeded by demands of exercise, making both factors equally important in the equation of who will develop a stress fracture and who will not. Disruption of pain fibers in the periosteum is responsible for the pain.

Other Important Considerations

- Most stress fractures take about 4–6 weeks to heal with "conservative management."
- Rest is needed, but the concept of "training around the injury" in sports medicine tells us that the patient can maintain conditioning and strength levels while the stress fracture heals by shifting to exercises that do not cause pain.
- In the case of tibial stress fractures, more challenging activities can sometimes be restarted somewhat earlier (after two weeks or so) with the use of a splint that redistributes the forces on the tibia away from the fracture site. This must be carefully supervised, however, by someone familiar with stress fracture management.
- Factors that encourage bone strength like adequate calcium, vitamin D3, vitamin K, boron, and other nutrients should be given during healing and sometimes beyond.

Specific red flags:
Neck pain with tingling, numbness or pain radiating down one arm

Condition assumed present until proven otherwise:
Cervical nerve root radiculopathy – compression of major spinal nerve as it exits through the neuroforamina of the spine

Possible consequences of missing the condition:
Permanent neuromuscular deficit in arm or hand

Stabilization, referral and management:

1. **Stabilization:** There are no stabilizing steps except to have the patient avoid unnecessary bending of the neck or weight loading on the head.
2. **Consultation and Referral Options, Transportation:** Even with some neurological deficits, if the patient has adequate movement of the arm and strength to perform everyday duties, the consult can be on a timely basis to their PCP or orthopedic surgeon if a PCP is not available. The urgency of referral is similar to that described for compression of nerve roots in the lumbosacral (LS) region and will be reiterated here in reference to the neck. A major difference between the two is that cervical radiculopathy tends to resolve spontaneously more often than LS radiculopathy.

Grade 1: Neck mildly painful with intermittent paresthesia in shoulder, forearm, and/or hand. No sensory, motor, or reflex impairment. (Sensory fibers minimally compressed. No compression of motor fibers.) *Immediate referral not necessary. Patient should be treated and reevaluated consistently and referred if condition progresses to stages noted below.*

Grade 2: Neck moderately painful with constant paresthesia and objectively verifiable sensory loss in shoulder, arm, and/or hand. (Sensory fibers significantly compressed. No significant compression of motor fibers.) *These patients should be treated aggressively and referred for evaluation and possible cotreatment to the patient's PCP on a timely basis.*

Grade 3: Neck very painful with paresthesia, constant numbness, weakness, and loss of reflex in arm and/or hand. No atrophy present. (Sensory fibers extremely compressed. Motor fibers mildly compressed.) *These patients should be treated aggressively and referred on a semi-urgent basis to their PCP, spine specialist or neurosurgeon if a PCP is not available.*

Grade 4: Neck severely painful and numbness or paresthesia with muscle weakness and muscle atrophy in shoulder, arm and/or hand. (Major compression of sensory and motor fibers). *Acupuncture treatment should not delay a semi-urgent referral to the patient's PCP or neurosurgeon if no PCP is available.*

Relevance to acupuncturists: Acupuncturists see a great deal of neck pain as well as low back pain, most of it self-resolving. That is why it is particularly important to be able to identify the few cases that pose a greater danger to the patient and be able to refer these patients for timely comanagement or further diagnosis and/or treatment when appropriate.

ACTUAL CASE

- **History:** The patient was a 35-year-old right- handed ironworker who felt a "twinge" in his neck and a tingling in his right shoulder, arm and hand while pulling on the end of a crescent wrench at work. The neck pain had gotten a little better in the several days before his appointment, but he still had some tingling and numbness in his arm and hand. The pain was worsened by sleeping on his stomach, which he tried to avoid. He did not notice weakness in his hand.
- **Physical findings:** The patient seemed in mild discomfort. His grip strength was slightly weaker in his right hand than his left. There was slightly decreased sensation on the ulnar aspects of the right hand to light touch and pinprick when compared to the left. Reflexes in the right arm (bicep and triceps) were normal and matched those in his left arm.
- **Impression:** Grade 2 cervical radiculopathy
- **Plan:** The acupuncturist contacted the patient's PCP. The PCP, who knew the acupuncturist well, advised that the patient need not be referred or have an MRI of the neck unless he got worse or his symptoms did not resolve in two weeks. This was discussed with the patient. The patient agreed with this plan and continued acupuncture treatment with the PCP "waiting in the wings" in case his symptoms did not resolve.
- **Follow up:** The patient's neck pain and right arm tingling gradually resolved over the next month. He regained full strength in this right hand and went back to work

DISCUSSION

History and Symptoms

The most common symptom of cervical radiculopathy is neck pain with radiation down into the shoulders, arms, and hands. The quality and type of pain can vary from dull, aching, and difficult to localize to sharp, burning, and focal, or there can be some hypersensitivity to touch as well as numbness in the area of skin supplied by the nerve root. Sensory symptoms are more common than motor symptoms. If we understand the typical composition of nerves that contain both sensory and motor fibers, we can easily understand why this is so. Specifically, sensory fibers tend to be arranged around the periphery of major nerves that contain both sensory and motor fibers, whereas motor fibers are more centrally located. Thus, compression from outside the nerve tends to produce sensory symptoms first, then motor symptoms as the pressure pushes further into the nerve. This is the reason that the presence of motor involvement always indicates greater threat to the nerve than sensory symptoms alone.

This is a reliable clinical pearl that will help you determine not only the degree of threat to a nerve, but also give you an idea of prognosis for the patient and how much treatment they may need to get well. Well established compression neuropathies with motor symptoms have a significantly worse prognosis and will require more treatment than compression neuropathies with sensory symptoms only. Practitioners should prepare their patients for this.

Physical Exam Findings

As the above discussion of radiculopathy suggests, testing of increasingly severe radiculopathy will first reveal areas of abnormal sensation in the shoulder, arm, and/or hand and progress to muscle weakness (testable by grip strength, for example) and decreased reflexes in the service of the affected nerve root, and eventually to atrophy of muscles. The reader is directed to charts of dermatome and specific muscles served by specific nerve roots to be able to perform the correct sensory and motor exam (C-7 is the most common nerve root compressed).

Incidence and/or Prevalence

According to a large epidemiological survey of cervical radiculopathy at the Mayo clinic, the average incidence for cervical radiculopathy per 100,000 people was 83.2 with an age-specific annual incidence per 100, 000 peaking at 202.9 for the 50-54-year-old age group.

Surprisingly, a history of physical exertion or trauma preceding the onset of symptoms could only be identified in 14.8% of cases. A past history of lumbar radiculopathy was present in 41%. A unilateral C-7 nerve root compression was most frequent. Disc protrusion was responsible in 21.9% of patients and 68.4% were related to spondylosis, disc or both. 26% had surgery.

Risk Factors

- Activities that place excessive or repetitive load on the spine
- Heavy labor or contact sports
- Family history of radiculopathy or other spine disorders

Mechanism Producing the Red Flag

Cervical radiculopathy is caused by compression of major spinal nerves as they exit the spine through the neuroforamina. This can be caused by mechanical compression of the nerve by a disc herniation and/or bone spur. Less often, a tumor or infection can do the compressing. Scoliosis, though not causative by itself, can contribute to the pressure by the abnormal curvature of the spine (pressure on the concave side of the curve).

Specific red flags:
Neck pain and progressive sensory changes and weakness in both arms and legs

Condition assumed present until proven otherwise:

Spinal cord injury (SCI) – many stages and degrees of injury are possible

Possible consequences of missing the condition:

Possible loss of function of limbs, bowels and bladder and paralysis

Stabilization, referral and management:

1. **Stabilization:** The patient should be cautioned to avoid situations in which a fall or other significant trauma could occur until consultation is accomplished.
2. **Consultation and Referral Options, Transportation:** As long as the patient is not worsening, the consult can be

on a timely basis to the patient's PCP if one is available. If the patient is worsening, the consult should be semiurgent, or even urgent it they are worsening rapidly. The ultimate consultant will probably be a neurosurgeon.

Relevance to acupuncturists: Acupuncturists could well see cases of spinal cord injury, including those from spinal cord contusion and compression, and should be able to recognize those that pose a great risk to the patient.

ACTUAL CASE

- **History:** The patient presenting for acupuncture (with her husband) was a 50-year-old Caucasian female with the main complaint of mild neck pain and weakness in both legs and vague paresthesia in both arms and hands, thighs and feet for approximately three weeks. She initially denied a history of trauma, but her husband reminded her that she had fallen about one month earlier after becoming inebriated at a New Year's dinner. She tripped on a rug and almost landed on her face.
- **Physical findings:** The patient had a normal physical exam except for mild weakness in both quadriceps and questionable decreased sensation to light touch and pinprick in both feet and lower legs. There were no areas of patchy numbness throughout the body (which could possibly have been present with demyelinating diseases like multiple sclerosis (MS).
- **Impression:** Possible spinal cord compression
- **Plan:** Lacking a PCP, the patient was sent directly to a neurosurgeon. The patient's MRI confirmed spinal cord compression secondary to a spinal cord contusion.
- **Follow up:** The patient was followed conservatively over six months and repeat MRI showed a fortunate spontaneous resolution of her spinal cord contusion. One year later, she was stronger and much improved. Unfortunately, she continued to drink alcohol excessively and five years later developed Wernicke's encephalopathy (alcoholic brain damage).

DISCUSSION

History and Symptoms

Spinal cord injury, regardless of the cause, generally causes bilateral symptoms. The higher the compression, the more pervasive the neurological symptoms, because more nerve fibers are compressed before they leave the spinal cord to become peripheral nerves. Since motor, sensory and autonomic fibers are injured, symptoms can manifest as all three types of symptomatic dysfunction. For all practical purposes, however, sensory symptoms (paresthesias and numbness) and motor symptoms (weakness) predominate.

Physical Exam Findings

The signs of spinal cord injury, like the symptoms, are generally bilateral. Symptoms of sensory disturbances can be objectively validated by noting decreased sensation to pin prick or light touch in the dermatomes distal to the spinal cord lesion. Muscle weakness can also be noted in distal muscles. Additionally, signs specific to spinal cord injuries can be elicited. These include abnormal position sense in the toes and deficient vibration sense at the ankle, measured by a tuning fork. Neurological signs such as clonus, muscle spasticity, or bladder involvement also indicate spinal cord (or lower brain) lesions.

Finally the Babinski reflex can be positive. The Babinski reflex is an involuntary upward movement of the big toe with fanning out motion of the other toes when the sole of the foot is firmly stroked along its lateral aspect (see a standard neurological text for the particulars).

Incidence and/or Prevalence

The incidence of traumatic SCI in the U.S. is 30-60 new cases per million. Prevalence estimates vary from 183,000-230,000 cases in the U.S. at any given time. The male-to-female ratio of patients with SCI is 4:1. More than 50% of all cases occur in those between 16-30 years old. The median age is 26.4 years.

Risk Factors

The most common causes of SCI include:

- Motor vehicle accidents, approximately 44%
- Falls, approximately 18%; most common in patients >45 years old
- Older females with osteoporosis have a greater incidence of SCI due to vertebral fractures from falls with associated spinal cord injury.
- Violence accounts for approximately 17%
- Sports injuries cause approximately 13%; diving injuries most commonly
- To give perspective, cancer may cause more SCI than does trauma.

Mechanism Producing the Red Flag

All neurological dysfunctions in SCI are due to compression effects on the spinal cord, causing ischemia.

Specific red flags:
Shoulder pain and progressive inability to abduct the arm due to shoulder stiffness

Condition assumed present until proven otherwise:
Adhesive capsulitis of the shoulder "frozen shoulder"

Possible consequences of missing the condition:
Longtime disability and pain, possibly lifetime

Stabilization, referral and management:

1. **Stabilization:** There are no specific stabilizing steps except to encourage the patient to perform mild ROM exercises of the stiff shoulder pending consultation.
2. **Consultation and Referral Options, Transportation:** The consultation should be obtained in a timely fashion to the patient's PCP, who will refer to a physiatrist (physical medicine specialist) or orthopedic surgeon. If the patient has no PCP, the referral should be to a free standing clinic or urgent care center to start further consultations.

Relevance to acupuncturists: Adhesive capsulitis is very common and always painful as it evolves from minor shoulder pain and stiffness to complete shoulder immobility (frozen shoulder). Because it is so common, it's virtually certain that acupuncturists will see many cases. If detected early in its course, the development of a totally frozen shoulder can often be prevented. Those skilled in treating shoulder problems will tell you that preventing this problem is much easier than treating it. The alert acupuncturist can be in the position to spot incipient cases and intervene and/or refer to a consultant skilled for co-management or referral, if necessary.

ACTUAL CASE

- **History:** The patient was a 40-year-old female who injured her right shoulder six months earlier when she slipped in a shower and tried to stop her fall by hanging on to a towel rack. She had a history of mild diabetes. She began having increasing pain in her right shoulder several days after the injury. The pain become progressively worse and her shoulder became stiff. She said her shoulder was now "stuck" and painful. She had the most trouble trying to reach behind her to put her coat on and when trying to lift her arm over her head.
- **Physical findings:** The patient was obviously frustrated with her condition and seemed somewhat angry that "nobody seems to know what to do for me." Her neck exam was normal. Her left shoulder ROM was normal, but the right shoulder motion was limited to 20 degrees of abduction and very little internal rotation. There was mild atrophy of the right deltoid compared to the left. There was mild swelling of the right hand. Neurovascular function of the right hand was grossly normal.
- **Impression:** Traumatic and inflammatory adhesive capsulitis of the right shoulder
- **Plan:** The patient was referred to physical therapy and an orthopedic surgeon. Acupuncture therapy was continued.
- **Follow up:** The orthopedic surgeon ordered an MRI which showed an attenuated area of the supraspinatus tendon and "beaking" of bone under the acromion. He gave the patient a shot of cortisone in her right shoulder, which gave the patient 30% relief of her pain and slightly increased ROM. Physical therapy to ROM was begun, but the patient had a lot of pain and made little further progress. The patient was eventually taken to surgery. The shoulder adhesions were broken (mobilized) and the subacromial beak was removed. The supraspinatus tendon was repaired. She began a long course of physical therapy and acupuncture following the surgery. She was much improved 1 ½ years after the original injury, but still lacks some abduction and internal rotation.

DISCUSSION

History and Symptoms

Adhesive capsulitis (AC) can be divided into two types, primary and secondary. In primary AC there is no history of trauma preceding the condition. In secondary AC there is preceding trauma. The two types can coexist. The main symptoms of both types are decreased motion of the shoulder, pain, and stiffness. The pain comes first and makes the patient hesitant to move his or her arm, which leads to stiffness and decreased motion. Eventually, the patient may regain most or even all of their lost ROM.

This typical progression of primary AC is sometimes divided into three phases: a painful phase, a stiffening phase and a thawing phase. The first phase lasts from weeks to months and features diffuse shoulder pain. The second phase consists of progressive loss of global motion, especially internal rotation and abduction and lasts up to one year. The thawing phase, during which there can be gradual improvement in ROM, lasts for months. The patient may require an additional nine months to regain a full ROM and continued therapy is often needed.

Return of full ROM is not guaranteed, however. If the progress of this illness starts after significant trauma to the shoulder, the prognosis is not as good. Conditions that may delay or even prevent full recovery of the shoulder include: underlying degenerative condition of the glenohumeral joint, abnormal anatomy (a subacromial beak, for example), or significant degeneration of the rotator cuff tendons and/or weakness of the muscle that moves the tendons. Ongoing inflammation from autoimmune disease may also interfere with healing.

Physical Exam Findings

There may be scattered trigger points in the muscles around the affected shoulder. The ROM, especially in internal rotation and abduction of the shoulder decreases steadily and eventually, in its worst manifestation, causes a completely frozen shoulder with little motion in any direction. Patients invariably have painful motion with the exam and, in early stages, have a "painful arc of motion" as they abduct their shoulder. At this point, due to disuse, there is invariably some atrophy of the muscles of the shoulder. Swelling and mild discoloration of the hand can exist in serious cases, so called "shoulder hand syndrome," which resembles a mild CRPS, but is not as severe as CRPS. Neurovascular function of the right hand remains normal.

Incidence and/or Prevalence

Patients between 40-70 years old are most affected. Estimates are that 3% of people will develop adhesive capsulitis sometime in their lifetime. Females are affected more than males and the nondominant shoulder more often than the dominant one. Patients with diabetes are approximately five times more likely to get the disease and those on insulin are 10 times more likely to get it. They also have an increased incidence of bilateral shoulder involvement.

Risk Factors

Although inflammation and trauma are both implicated in the development of AC and may both contribute to it independently or as cofactors, in many cases the reason for the inflammation remains obscure.

- History of autoimmune disease, like rheumatoid arthritis
- Cervical disk disease
- Diabetes
- Shoulder trauma
- Shoulder surgery
- Shoulder immobilization (from immobilization)
- Open heart surgery (possibly from immobility during the recovery)
- Hyperthyroidism

Mechanism Producing the Red Flag

Both the acuteness of primary AC, its strong association with inflammatory diseases like rheumatoid arthritis and its symptoms and signs strongly suggest that the cause of AC has to do with inflammation, along with dysfunction and/or disruption of:

1. The capsule of the glenohumeral joints and probably its attendant ligaments (superior, middle and inferior glenohumeral ligaments)
2. The subacromial and subdeltoid bursa
3. The rotator cuff muscles and tendons

Inflammation, dysfunction and/or disruption of one or more of these structures sets the stage for stiffness and progressively decreasing ROM because the patient strongly avoids moving the shoulder due to pain. This becomes a catch-22 for the patient because the only way to avoid a frozen shoulder is to move it. Therapy must be done to avoid permanent stiffness. This is why this condition must be handled by someone who has dealt with this problem often enough to know the pitfalls of too aggressive therapy versus therapy that is not aggressive enough.

The shoulder, like the elbow (see red flags for radial head fracture of the elbow), is very unforgiving. It will stiffen permanently if not put through its normal range of motion because the articular capsule and ligaments will contract to freeze the joint if interventions are not made and sometimes even when they are.

Other Important Considerations

- Therapy for AC or to prevent AC is usually conservative, *i.e.*, acupuncture, physical therapy, exercise therapy, heat and cold therapy, etc. Occasionally, anti-inflammatory medications, and shoulder injections are helpful adjuncts to physical types of therapy, especially if bursitis is a strong contributor to the pain.
- Sometimes, AC patients will require surgery, not always because of the contracture of the joint, but because disrupted joint structures need to be repaired. *Even if surgery restores motion, however, physical therapy and/or acupuncture must be continued for months afterward to prevent the joint from refreezing.*

Specific red flags:
Severe sore throat, high fever, drooling and difficulty swallowing in an adult

Condition assumed present until proven otherwise:

Peritonsillar abscess

Possible consequences of missing the condition:

Extreme illness, possible sepsis and death

Stabilization, referral and management:

1. **Stabilization:** There are no particular stabilizing steps
2. **Consultation and Referral Options, Transportation:** The consult should be to the patient's PCP if one is available or directly to an ENT physician if no PCP is available. The ultimate consultant would be an ENT physician because incision and drainage of the abscess is likely, which can be done as an outpatient.

Relevance to acupuncturists: Patients with peritonsillar abscesses are usually quite ill appearing, but some stoical patients can walk into your office for care, or you may well see patients in early stages of this illness and can recognize that it is coming.

ACTUAL CASE

- **History:** The patient was a 20-year-old male, previously in good health, with history of an increasingly severe sore throat over the preceding four days. On his way to his acupuncture visit for an unrelated complaint, he began to have shaking chills and his sore throat worsened. He found himself unable to eat or drink anything due to the pain and said, "I have to spit a lot."
- **Physical findings:** The patient was spitting into some tissues when we walked into the room and was in obvious discomfort. He was reluctant to open his mouth. One of his tonsils was red and had whitish, cotton candy appearing patches on its surface. It was almost twice the size of his other tonsil and extended almost to the midline of the oropharynx. There was no thermometer in the room, but the patient's skin felt hot and flushed.
- **Impression:** Peritonsillar abscess
- **Plan:** The patient's PCP was called and saw the patient within one hour.
- **Follow up:** The patient's PCP sent the patient to an ENT physician who confirmed the diagnosis of peritonsillar abscess. He did an incision and drainage of the abcess under local anesthesia, which released a large amount of pus. The patient later told his acupuncturist that the procedure hurt a great deal but was followed by a great deal of pain relief.

DISCUSSION

History and Symptoms

Fever and throat pain are invariably complaints, sometimes with shaking chills. Patients complain of sore throat in general but usually say it is much worse on the abscessed side. They complain of reluctance to swallow and find it difficult and painful when they do so. Severe malaise, headache, and neck pain (from swollen lymph nodes) are also common complaints, as is ear pain on the affected side.

Physical Exam Findings

Although patients with mild or early cases of peritonsillar abscess can appear only mildly to moderately ill, those with advanced cases look quite ill, even prostrated. They can have tachycardia from fever, which can be > 103.5° F and dehydration from reluctance to swallow. Sunken eyes and poor tissue turgor (skin tenting after being pinched) from dehydration can even be seen. Drooling and salivation are often evident.

The voice is often muffled—a "hot potato" voice—and the breath is often rancid. An exam of the throat reveals a red and enlarged tonsil on one side, sometimes with exudates on one or both tonsils. The other tonsil is often swollen and red as well, but much less so. The affected tonsil can be so large that it extends medially into the oropharynx and pushes the uvula over toward the opposite side of the throat. Anterior cervical lymphadenopathy is usually palpable.

Incidence and/or Prevalence

Although peritonsillar abscess can occur at any age from 10-60, it is most common between the ages of 20 to 40 years old. The incidence in the U.S. is estimated at 30 cases per 100,000 persons/year or 45,000 cases annually, which translates to at least $150 million a year in health care costs. The peak incidence is during November-December and April-May.

Risk Factors

- Age: 20-40 years
- Gender: male
- Recent throat infection or dental infection
- Periodontal disease
- Smoking
- Tongue piercing (possible)

Mechanism Producing the Red Flag

The two palatine tonsils lie on the lateral walls of the oropharynx in the depression between the anterior and posterior tonsillar pillars. Each tonsil is surrounded by a capsule. Purulent exudates get trapped between the tonsillar tissue and the capsule wall. The capsular wall does not allow easy drainage and an abscess forms. The pain and other manifestations of peritonsillar abscess result from the stretching and inflammation of affected tissues.

Specific red flags: *Pain on urination (dysuria) with high fever, chills, frequent urination, pain in back and malaise*

Condition assumed present until proven otherwise:

Kidney infection (Acute pyelonephritis)

Possible consequences of missing the condition:

Kidney scarring, kidney failure, abscess, sepsis, possible death

Stabilization, referral and management:

1. **Stabilization:** The patient should be encouraged to drink water until the referral is made.
2. **Consultation and Referral Options, Transportation:** Acute pyelonephritis is a semi-urgent to urgent problem depending on the stage of the disease and the stability of the patient. In patients with mild fever, dysuria, and stable vital signs, the consult can be a same day consultation, preferably to their PCP or failing that, to a free-standing medical clinic or urgent care center. If the patient is having high fevers, shaking chills, and appears septic, the patient should be sent direct to the ED with the fastest possible transport available (not necessarily through a 911 call unless they are having cardiopulmonary complaints). Admission to the hospital for fluids and IV antibiotics will probably be needed.

Relevance to acupuncturists: Discomfort with urination (dysuria) is such a common complaint and so often due to simple bladder infection that patients and clinicians can easily be lulled into a false sense of complacency when it appears. That is all the more reason that acupuncturists must know those instances wherein dysuria is indicative of possibly life-threatening illness.

ACTUAL CASE

- **History:** The patient was a recently married 19-year-old Caucasian female with an aching and burning sensation in her suprapubic region every time she urinated for two days prior to coming in for acupuncture. She came in at the recommendation of her mother who said that antibiotics for her bladder infections (the mother's) always gave her a yeast infection later, so she advised her daughter to try cranberry extract and Chinese herbs instead. The patient noted that she had been having chills and thought she had a fever as well. She now complained of pain in her right flank and nausea as well.
- **Physical findings:** The patient appeared moderately ill. She appeared to be having chills, in fact, her teeth were chattering. Her temperature was 102.5° F. She had tenderness to percussion at the right costovertebral angle (CVA) and mild suprapubic tenderness.
- **Impression:** Acute pyelonephritis
- **Plan:** The patient's PCP was notified and the situation was discussed. She was seen within one hour by the PCP and had white blood cells (WBCs) in the urine at her office. A portion of the urine sample was sent to the lab for culture and sensitivity (C&S).
- **Follow up:** The patient was given a shot of an antibiotic in the PCPs office and medication orally with instructions that she should go to the ED if she got worse or couldn't take the medicine orally. The patient unfortunately vomited when she took the first capsule of the antibiotic and her fever spiked to 104.5° F at home. She was taken to the ER by her husband and received IV antibiotics and fluids. She was discharged with precautions to try to avoid further urinary tract infections (UTIs) in the future and taught about how to determine the difference between a simple bladder infection (cystitis) and pyelonephritis (the presence of fever).

DISCUSSION

History and Symptoms

This red flag contains many of the important symptoms of kidney infection. Dysuria (stinging or sharp urination pain or possibly aching, burning, pressure or vague discomfort), symptoms shared by patients with simple cystitis. That's because patients with kidney infection usually also have bladder infection so they share the "lower urinary tract" symptoms of dysuria and frequency. Patients with pyelonephritis, however, have important additional symptoms not found in simple cystitis. Although bladder infection patients may have some vague low back pain, pyelonephritis patients often have pain in the flank or over the kidney. They can also have high fever, whereas *patients with simple cystitis do not have significant fever*. Additional symptom of chills, nausea and vomiting make it virtually certain that the patient is having acute pyelonephritis.

Physical Exam Findings

Although patients with early or mild pyelonephritis may not appear very uncomfortable, in the full-blown case they will look quite ill with high spiking fevers, sometimes to 105° F and shaking chills. They will often have CVA tenderness on the affected side.

Incidence and/or Prevalence

About 1 out of 7,000 people develop pyelonephritis each year in the U.S. Of the 250,000 cases in 1995, approximately 200,000 required hospitalization. Pyelonephritis is more common in females. It can become potentially fatal when secondary complications develop: tissue destruction (20-80% mortality), abscess (20-50% mortality) or sepsis (>25% mortality).

Risk Factors

- Pregnancy
- Bladder procedures and bladder catheterization
- History of bladder and kidney problems
- Immune deficiency status
- Immunosuppressant drugs
- High dose corticosteroids use
- Poor hygiene habits

Mechanism Producing the Red Flag

Organs like the kidney have a duct component (the collecting tubules) and a solid, cellular component (the parenchyma). Infection of the parenchyma is associated with greater morbidity and mortality than infection within the tubules. This makes sense because there is an "escape route" for infection in tubules due to the natural egress of fluids that does not occur in parenchyma. This is the reason that bladder infections are less serious than pyelonephritis, for example, since the bladder is like a dilated tubule, whereas kidney infections are infections of kidney parenchyma as well as tubules.

Specific red flags:
Chronic tenderness in anatomic snuff box; pain of wrist after fall on outstretched hand

Condition assumed present until proven otherwise:
Occult fracture of the scaphoid (navicular) bone of the wrist

Possible consequences of missing the condition:
There is high risk of malunion, delayed union, non-union, or avascular necrosis of the scaphoid bone with permanent dysfunction and pain.

Stabilization, referral and management:

1. **Stabilization:** Patients with this red flag should be advised to avoid situations that could produce wrist trauma and to wear a wrist splint pending consultation.
2. **Consultation and Referral Options, Transportation:** A timely consultation to the patient's PCP or a free-standing medical clinic or urgent care is warranted. The ultimate consultant will be an orthopedic surgeon, because careful assessment and care will be necessary to prevent non-union and avascular necrosis from occurring. Referral may also be made directly to an orthopedist if the patient lacks a PCP. Transportation may be by private vehicle.

Relevance to acupuncturists: Scaphoid fracture of the wrist is common and can present with subtle symptoms. Acupuncturists will see some of these cases and can be in a position to avert a poor outcome for the patient if the red flag is picked up and the patient is referred.

ACTUAL CASE

- **History:** An 18-year-old male came in to the office complaining of wrist pain. Three weeks earlier, he fell while roller skating and broke his fall on an outstretched hand. He had some pain in the right wrist initially, but didn't think much of it at the time. His parents insisted he get an x-ray the day after the injury in the ED, which was negative. He was told he had a sprain and went home. Despite this reassurance, the pain persisted. His parent wanted to see if acupuncture would help the pain since he did not have a fracture.

- **Physical findings:** The patient had point tenderness in the anatomic snuff box (on the radial aspect of the wrist in the indentation between the abductor and extensor tendons of the thumb). He had full range of motion of his hand and wrist.
- **Impression:** Possible undiagnosed fracture of the scaphoid bone of the wrist
- **Plan:** The patient did not have a PCP and was sent to an orthopedic surgeon.
- **Follow up:** Wrist films were obtained eight days after the injury that clearly showed a nonhealing fracture of the scaphoid bone at its waist. The scaphoid is just under the base of the thumb and is shaped like a bean or boat – thus the alternate name "navicular" for this bone of the wrist. A trial of casting for three months was instituted to attempt healing. Unfortunately, the bone did not heal. Finally, an internal fixation with a screw was accomplished with a bone graft from the pelvis. The patient is doing well one year after the accident.

DISCUSSION

Typical History and Symptoms

Typical symptoms of a scaphoid fracture are pain and swelling on the thumb side of the wrist. Patients suffer the fracture by falling on an outstretched hand or as the result of direct wrist trauma. Many patients are self-diagnosed or misdiagnosed as having a wrist sprain, so you may see patients who are convinced they have only a sprain. This misapprehension can be augmented because the initial X-ray is often negative. Although the pain may initially diminish somewhat, the dull pain from a poorly healing or scaphoid fracture goes on alerting us to the fact that there is still a problem.

Typical Physical Exam Findings

Patients with acute scaphoid fractures have tenderness in the area of the previously described anatomic snuff box. The tenderness in this region never goes away if there is non-union or avascular necrosis of the scaphoid so that this sign is reliable for all stages of scaphoid fracture.

Incidence and/or Prevalence

The incidence of scaphoid fractures of the wrist is 345,000 yearly in the U.S. It is the most frequently fractured wrist bone, accounting for 71% of all carpal fractures. The peak occurrence is in those 15-60 years old, but the fracture can occur in children and is often missed in this younger age group. About 5-12% of scaphoid fractures are associated with other fractures. 90% of acute scaphoid fractures heal if treated early. 30% of cases with negative X-rays turn out to have fractures on later X-rays. Avascular necrosis of a segment of the scaphoid occurs in 15-30% of all scaphoid fractures.

Risk Factors

The risk of developing a non-union of the scaphoid depends most importantly on the location of the fracture in the bone. Other factors that can contribute to nonunion are smoking, certain medications, and infections.

Mechanism Producing the Red Flag

The scaphoid bone (also called the navicular bone) is one of eight carpal bones. It is prone to slow healing or non-union due to the way the fracture site is related to the unique arrangement for blood supply to the bone. The scaphoid has a retrograde blood supply. The arterial vessels that feed the bone enter the distal part of the bone, rather than the proximal, and flows back through the bone to nourish the bone cells. A scaphoid fracture can sever the arteries and stop blood flow to proximal bone segments, which may cause non-union of the proximal segment of the bone. This can lead to a dead piece of bone and arthritis of the articulation with the thumb metatarsal bone and cause chronic pain, difficulty gripping objects, and other dysfunction.

Other Important Considerations

- Scaphoid fractures of the wrist are commonly mishandled by all types of practitioners. Understanding the clinical pearl that all fractures are tender to careful and adequate palpation helps.
- If the red flag is present, we should assume the fracture is present until proven otherwise by a repeat radiograph two weeks after the injury. Until the situation is determined, the patient should be kept in a wrist splint.
- Often, orthopedists will initially treat scaphoid fractures with casting if the fracture is not displaced. If it does not heal, surgery can be considered. If the scaphoid fracture is displaced, surgery may be an early option to reposition the bones and fix them in place with a screw or pins. A bone graft may also be used for healing the fracture site. After surgery, a cast is used to immobilize the scaphoid bone.

- Recent studies have shown that the chance of developing chronic regional pain syndrome (CRPS) in patients with wrist fractures is lower in patients who take high doses of vitamin C after wrist fracture.

Review What You Have Learned
Chapter 16 Pain

Chapter 16—Pain, General

1. The timing of pain – when it comes on, how long it lasts, etc., is important from a red flag point of view because

a. Pain from non-serious causes generally diminishes over time

b. Pain that has an increasing slope after approximately two weeks can indicate that the patient is developing a chronic pain condition

c. Increasing rather than decreasing pain after two weeks could indicate ongoing tissue damage

d. All of the above

2. Persistently inflamed and painful joints are red flags because

a. There is the possibility of permanent joint destruction in such cases

b. They indicate wear-and-tear arthritis

c. They indicate possible serious autoimmune (connective tissue) disease

d. All of the above

e. A and C

3. Progressive and unrelenting bone pain is a red flag for

a. Infection

b. Tumor

c. Myalgia

d. Multiple sclerosis

4. Conscious patients with fractures will always exhibit

a. An inability to move the affected limb

b. Positive x-rays in the site of fracture

c. Decreased sensation in the joints distal to the fracture

d. Tenderness to sufficient palpation over the fracture site

5. Complex regional pain syndrome (CRPS)

a. Can be a complication of severe injury to a limb

b. Causes pain, but not dysfunction

c. Has also been called reflex sympathetic dystrophy

d. All of the above

e. A and C

6. Abdominal pain and rigidity can be

a. A sign of peritonitis

b. A sign of blood or pus in the abdominal cavity

c. A sign that surgery may be necessary

d. All of the above

e. A and C

Chapter 16—Pain, Abdominal

1. Hematemesis (vomiting blood) is a red flag for

a. Lower gastrointestinal bleeding

b. Upper gastrointestinal bleeding

c. *Helicobacter pylori* infection

d. Lung cancer

2. What is true regarding chronic heartburn?

a. It can be aggravated by cigarette smoking, alcohol ingestion and fatty foods

b. It can lead to Barrett's esophagus

c. It can lead to esophageal cancer

d. All of the above

3. Pancreatitis pain

a. Is made better by lying flat on the back

b. Is accompanied by nausea and vomiting

c. Is colicky in nature

d. Never recurs more than once in any individual's life

4. The classical progression of appendicitis symptoms and signs is

a. High fever, right lower abdominal pain, vomiting and a rigid abdomen with rebound tenderness

b. Midepigastric pain, vomiting, pain moves to the right lower quadrant, rebound tenderness

c. Vomiting and pain in the left lower quadrant, high fever

d. Generalized abdominal tenderness, unaffected appetite, pain moves to the right lower quadrant

5. Sudden lessening of appendicitis pain indicates

a. The body's immune response has beaten back the infection

b. The patient has adapted to the pain

c. The patient has entered a "honeymoon period" ushered in by appendiceal rupture

d. The danger point has been passed

6. Severe pain, vomiting and abdominal distention herald the possibility of

a. Acute appendicitis

b. Acute gastroenteritis

c. Bowel obstruction

d. Acute pancreatitis

Chapter 16—Pain, Back

1. What percentage of the U.S. population will have significant back pain sometime in life?

a. 50%

b. 20%

c. 80%

d. 5%

2. In a patient with back pain and paresthesia (pins and needles) we should be concerned about the possibility of a

a. Herniated disc

b. Tumor

c. Sensory compressive neuropathy of some kind

d. All of the above

3. The straight leg raising test is positive for compression of a lumbosacral nerve root when

a. Performing the test properly elicits pain in the back of the calf and low back

b. Performing the test properly elicits pain, paresthesia or numbness in the area served by the compressed nerve

c. The test properly results in back pain and calf pain

d. All of the above

4. Back pain with unexplained weight loss is a red flag for

a. A spinal tumor

b. A disc compression

c. A back sprain and poor diet

d. None of the above

5. In what type of patient would cauda equina syndrome most likely occur in?

a. An obese woman in her seventh decade in life

b. A 50-year-old male construction worker

c. A 60-year-old female accountant who sits all day long

d. A 25-year-old male cyclist

6. An elderly women with severe central back pain might have

a. A spinal tumor

b. A "pathological fracture" of a vertebral body

c. Osteoporosis

d. All of the above

MATCHING

A. Compression neuropathy

B. Radiculopathy

C. Compression fracture

D. Peripheral nerve compression neuropathy

7. ____ Localized spinous process tenderness to percussion

8. ____ Carpal tunnel syndrome

9. ____ Compression of a spinal nerve at a neuroforamina

10. ____ General term for pressure on any neural tissue

11. Nutrients and other substances especially helpful for bone strength include

a. Calcium, boron, potassium

b. Calcium, estrogen, vitamin B12

c. Calcium, boron, vitamin K2

d. Calcium, vitamin D3, cortisol

Chapter 16—Pain, Chest

1. Independent risk factors (other than lipid abnormalities and smoking) strongly associated with an increased incidence of coronary artery disease include

a. Increased serum homocysteine level

b. Increase serum C-reactive protein

c. Increase lipoprotein A elevation

d. All of the above

2. In which of the following clinical scenarios is it most likely that a patient has significant coronary artery disease?

a. A patient with severe, sharp chest pain

b. A patient with shortness of breath (SOB) and left arm pain at rest

c. A patient with severe chest pain and dizziness

d. A patient with chest pain reliably occurring with exertion

3. Sudden, sharp chest pain and shortness of breath several days to weeks after a patient has been discharged from the hospital following major surgery should alert the clinician to

a. A probable heart attack

b. A possible pulmonary embolus (PE)

c. A possible deep venous thrombosis (DVT)

d. A probable pneumothorax

4. According to the Japanese study cited in this book, the incidence of pneumothorax following acupuncture is approximately

a. 1 in 100,000

b. 1 in 5,000

c. 1 in 20,000

d. 1 in 50,000

5. The direction of air flow into the space between inner chest and outer lung in pneumothorax is

a. Through the puncture in the chest into the space

b. Through the puncture in the lung into the space

c. Through a puncture in the esophagus into the space

d. None of the above

6. Pneumothorax pain is

a. Sharp

b. Dull

c. Colicky

d. Aching

7. Patients at particular risk for developing the dreaded consequence of tension pneumothorax include

a. The frail and the elderly

b. Patients with muscular chest walls

c. Smokers

d. All of the above

e. A and C

Chapter 16—Pain, Ear

1. The significant signs and symptoms that indicate the probable presence of acute mastoiditis (infection of the air cells of the mastoid bone) are

a. Tenderness over the sinuses and high fever

b. Earache, decreased hearing bilaterally and facial pain

c. Earache and drainage, fever, tenderness over the mastoid bone

d. High fever, sore throat and hoarse voice

Chapter 16—Pain, Elbow

1. A fall on an outstretched hand can fracture the head of the radius. What characteristic symptoms and signs might a clinician note two weeks after such a fracture that had not been properly treated?

a. Persistent and severe pain and tenderness in the area of fracture – the "anatomic snuff box"

b. Diminution of the strength of the radial pulse on the affected side

c. The fracture would generally have healed without residual effects by this time

d. Lack of the last 10 degrees of extension at the elbow

2. What is the most dreaded consequence of an untreated supracondylar fracture of the humerus?

a. Permanent loss of the last few degrees of elbow extension

b. Ischemic necrosis of distal structures

c. Arthritis of the elbow

d. All of the above

3. What is the most reliable symptom or sign leading a clinician to suspect a fracture of an extremity in a conscious patient?

a. Tenderness at the fracture site to careful palpation

b. Inability to move the extremity distal to the fracture

c. Swelling and pain

d. All symptoms and signs are unreliable – an x-ray must be taken

Chapter 16—Pain, Facial

1. Chronic purulent (bacterial) sinusitis can lead to disability or death in some cases because

a. Some patients may be immune suppressed

b. Osteomyelitis can be a consequence of chronic purulent sinusitis

c. Infectious material can be trapped in sinuses by polyps or swelling and erode into the brain

d. All of the above

Chapter 16—Pain, Foot and Toe

1. Hallux valgus deformity (bunion) can be a red flag if

a. The laterally deviated great toe is very painful at the MP joint

b. The other toes of the foot have to bear additional weight due to bunion pain

c. The laterally deviated great toe dislocates other MP joints of the foot

d. High heels can no longer be worn

Chapter 16—Pain, Headache

1. Headache can be a component of which of the following illnesses?

a. Subarachnoid hemorrhage

b. Acute closed-angle glaucoma

c. Migraine

d. All of the above

2. Which of the following types of bleeding would be most likely to result in hemorrhage?

a. Epidural

b. Subdural

c. Subarachnoid

d. All of the above

e. A and C

Chapter 16—Pain, Hip

1. Persistent hip pain with significantly decreased range of motion in an adult or adolescent is suspicious for

a. Severe myofascial pain around the hip

b. Significant bursitis of the trochanteric bursa

c. Significant injury of degenerative pathology of the ball and socket joint

d. Significant likelihood of faking illness (malingering)

2. Which statement is true regarding Perthes disease (death of a portion of the ball of the femur—a mashed ball) and slipped capital femoral epiphysis —SCFE—(slippage of the ball portion of the femur at the epiphyseal growth plate)?

a. SCFE occurs more often in adolescents, especially African-Americans, whereas Perthes disease is more common is preadolescents, more commonly Caucasians

b. SCFE results in decreased range of motion of the hip joint whereas Perthes does not

c. Perthes disease occurs more frequently as the result of trauma than does SCFE

d. All of the above

Chapter 16—Pain, Knee

1. The immediate severe swelling that accompanies a severe traumatic internal derangement of the knee is the result of

a. A severe inflammatory reaction

b. A rapid buildup of reactive synovial fluid in the knee

c. Rupture of arteriolar or arterial vessel(s)

Chapter 16—Pain, Calf

1. Calf pain brought on reliably by walking is a red flag for peripheral artery disease (PAD) and can be associated with

a. Coronary artery disease

b. Impotence due to blockage of the dorsal penile artery

c. Diabetes mellitus

d. Smoking cigarettes

e. All of the above

Chapter 16—Pain, Shin

1. Which of the following statements accurately characterize the difference between shin splints and stress fractures of the tibia?

a. Shin splints and stress fractures are usually bilateral

b. Stress fractures are a total fractures of bone whereas shin splints are small cracks in bone

c. Shin splints are more common in women with osteoporosis whereas stress fractures are not

d. Shin splints are more often bilateral than stress fractures

Chapter 16—Pain, Neck

1. Cervical nerve root compression neuropathy (radiculopathy), like LS radiculopathy, generally progresses in the following order of signs and symptoms

a. Neck pain>paresthesia>numbness>weakness> atrophy

b. Neck pain>weakness>areas of numbness>atrophy

c. Neck pain>paresthesia>weakness>numbness

d. None of the above

2. Neck pain and progressive weakness in both arms is most indicative of

a. Cervical radiculopathy

b. Spinal cord injury

c. Polio

d. Multiple sclerosis

Chapter 16—Pain, Shoulder

1. An inability to lift (abduct) the shoulder is most compatible with

a. Partially torn rotator cuff tendons and a normal ligamentous capsule around the shoulder

b. Total adhesion of the capsule of the shoulder and normal rotator cuff muscles and tendons

c. Paralysis of the muscle of the rotator cuff and shoulder

d. All of the above

e. A and C

Chapter 16—Pain, Throat

1. A patient with severe sore throat, fever drooling, and painful swallowing should be sent to an ENT physician for

a. Emergency tonsillectomy

b. Incision and drainage of a peri-tonsillar abscess

c. Removal of an aspirated object in the back of the throat

d. None of the above

Chapter 16—Pain, Urination

1. Major similarities and/or differences between untreated bladder and kidney infections include

a. Both can feature high fever and hematuria (blood in urine) with back pain

b. Both can be the result of yeast infections

c. Both can cause yeast infections

d. Bladder infections do not produce significant fever whereas kidney infections do

Chapter 16—Pain, Wrist

1. Occult fractures of the scaphoid of the wrist are susceptible to

a. Malunion

b. Delayed union

c. Nonunion

d. Avascular necrosis

e. All the above

2. Scaphoid fractures of the wrist are often missed because

a. Initial x-rays of the wrist may be negative

b. They don't hurt when carefully palpated

c. They are often falsely diagnosed as wrist sprains

d. A and C

Chapter 17: PSYCHOLOGICAL PROBLEMS

Because acupuncture clinics see so many cases of mental-emotional pain and dysfunction, with and without other somatic symptoms, it is very important to be able to recognize potentially serious psycho-emotional issues when they are present in our patients.

Recognizing red flags for serious psychiatric illness is an essential skill for acupuncturists because of the high volume of patients with these problems. In many studies, psychological complaints are second only to pain as a motivating reason for patients to seek acupuncture in the U.S. We must always remember, however, that patients who appear to have purely psychological problems can have physical as well as psychological causes.

For example, hyperthyroidism and hypoglycemic reactions cause symptoms often indistinguishable from anxiety and hypothyroidism can make a patient look and feel depressed. Drugs and other intoxicants can make patients delusional. The ways in which hormones influence thinking and mood and the way thinking and mood effect hormones is a fascinating subject beyond the scope of this book. We should always keep in mind, however, that psychological symptoms can have physical causes and vice versa.

The red flags in this section are named according to the *Diagnostic and Statistical Manual of Mental Disorders, Fourth Edition (DSM-4)*. Anxiety and depression are listed in the category of "mood disorders". Delusions are listed as belonging to "thought disorders." Red flags for drug dependence and addiction are listed in "substance abuse disorders." Unlike other chapters in this book, there are no general red flags in this section so we'll go directly to the specific red flags.

Specific red flags:
Sudden severe anxiety, smothering sensation, chest pain with complete recovery

Condition assumed present until proven otherwise:
Panic disorder

Possible consequences of missing the condition:
Possible multiple emergency room visits, development of agoraphobia (fear of going out in public), lifelong psychological disability

Stabilization, referral and management:

1. **Stabilization:** Reading material to help patients with panic disorder is available online. Cognitive distortions (unhelpful things people tell themselves on an unconscious level) are common in panic disorder. A list of them and what to do about them can be found in David Burn's book *Feeling Good*. This can be recommended until consultation.
2. **Consultation and Referral Options, Transportation:** Since Chinese medicine can be effective in panic disorder, the emphasis should be on the recognition that the disorder is present. If Chinese medicine treatments are not effective to the acupuncturist's satisfaction, the patient's PCP can be consulted if one is available because medication is sometimes helpful. The PCP may then refer to a psychologist or counseling center. The referral can be on a timely basis.

Relevance to acupuncturists: Panic attacks will be common in any acupuncturist's practice. The emphasis should be on recognition of panic disorder because it can be so life-disrupting.

ACTUAL CASE

- **History:** Jill was a 33-year-old business woman and community leader. Since so many others looked to her for guidance, she was reluctant to tell us that she had been having sudden attacks of "extreme anxiety" in the daytime and sometimes in the middle of the night. She would wake suddenly with chest heaviness, shortness of breath and a feeling that she was going to die. On one of these occasions she went to the ED where a complete cardiac workup was negative for heart disease. She was particularly concerned that she was increasingly unwilling to go out of her house on errands for fear she'd have an attack and she was making up excuses to her friends to avoid leaving home.

- **Physical findings:** The patient appeared worried, but her exam was otherwise normal. She had a normal pulse rate.
- **Impression:** Panic disorder
- **Plan:** Patient was referred to her PCP for co-treatment with the acupuncturist. A psychologist was consulted by the PCP to help her deal with her stress.
- **Follow up:** The patient made great inroads in dealing with stress and the frequency and severity of panic decreased. She did have another fairly severe attack after two months, however, and was started on a selective serotonin receptor inhibitor (SSRI) by her PCP. She improved. The SSRI was gradually discontinued six months later, and with continued acupuncture and counseling, she has been panic free for six years.

DISCUSSION

History and Symptoms

The patient may have a past history of anxiety or the panic disorder may have come on without prior complaints of anxiety. Often, there is history of a significant psychological trauma. A family history of anxiety and/or depression and/or panic disorder and/or substance abuse is often present suggesting inheritable patterns of neurotransmitter imbalances. The disorder can result from unconscious conflicts.

Physical Exam Findings

Usually the patient will appear somewhat anxious between the panic episodes. The pulse rate will usually be normal at rest (<80 bpm).

Incidence and/or Prevalence

Panic disorder is common. The prevalence is 1.4% of the U.S. population (2009 census is 305M x 0.014 = 4.27 million people in the U.S. with panic disorder). The mean age of presentation is 25 years old with onset generally between 17-30.

Risk Factors

- Family history of panic disorder or manic depressive illness. First degree relatives of those with panic disorder have double the risk of occurrence than control subjects.
- Female/male ratio = 3/1
- High stress situations

Mechanism Producing the Red Flag

The mechanism producing the symptoms is a full throttle stress response similar to what occurs in the face of grave danger. There is a massive release of catecholamines (epinephrine and norepinephrine) and cortisol. This produces the expected responses of increased rate and strength of cardiac contractions, breathing rate, sweating, and feeling that a person is in grave danger ("feeling of doom"). Epinephrine and norepinephrine are *hormones* that act at distant sites in the body and also *neurotransmitters* that work at synapses in the brain. They are excitatory at all locations.

Other Important Considerations

- A panic attack is a terrifying disorder to anyone who has experienced one. It often happens when a patient feels relaxed or is asleep, but can occur anywhere at any time.
- There is often significant anxiety between panic attacks because patients anticipate a future attack. Many patients are treated by medical doctors with benzodiazepines for the anxiety, which is sometimes necessary, but carries a risk of addiction.
- Panic attacks and agoraphobia (literally, fear of the marketplace) are related, but are not the same. A patient with agoraphobia is afraid of leaving their home and venturing into public places for fear of a panic attack. Agoraphobia can be brought on by panic attacks that occur when a patient is out.
- Panic disorder is often associated with depression as well as generalized anxiety and phobias. Phobia (to social situations, animals, storms, heights, illness and death) is actually the most common type of anxiety disorder with an incidence of an astounding 15-20% in the U.S. population (65.27 million people).

Specific red flags:
Non-drug induced auditory hallucination, delusions, tangential thinking

Condition assumed present until proven otherwise:
Schizophrenia

Possible consequences of missing the condition:
Lifetime mental disability, declines in familial and socio-economic functioning, premature death through neglect or suicide

Stabilization, referral and management:

1. **Stabilization:** An attempt should not be made to talk a patient out of their delusions because it can cause a lot of anxiety and resistance. Better to start the referral process and reassure family and patient that help is on the way.
2. **Consultation and Referral Options, Transportation:** Psychiatric consult is always indicated, but the degree of urgency depends upon the practitioner's best estimate of the patient's impairment *and the degree of danger they represent to themselves or others.* Private transport is almost always adequate unless the patient is actively suicidal or violent, in which case county-supported psychiatric emergency services or 911 must be called.

Relevance to acupuncturists: Acupuncturists will see many schizophrenics for several reasons. Firstly, schizophrenia is very common (see below). Secondly, although antipsychotic agents are undeniably extremely helpful in many patients, they also commonly have significant side effects and many patients do not take them reliably because they don't think they need them or don't like the side effects. These patients, or more likely their family members, may seek out gentler treatment for the condition. Many experienced acupuncturists will want patients with severe schizophrenia to also be on an antipsychotic medication as well as receive acupuncture care. Another reasons patients may seek acupuncture is the relatively lower cost of acupuncture treatment versus standard medical treatment. For these reasons, relatively high numbers of schizophrenics may become acupuncture patients.

ACTUAL CASE

- **History:** A mother and father brought their 22-year-old son to the office wanting to know if acupuncture could help her son with a newly acquired problem with "insomnia." Their son, Robert, had not seen a doctor and they could not afford insurance. The mother stated that her son seemed to have "his days and nights mixed up." He wandered around the house at night and would find him fascinated by infomercials on TV in the middle of the night. He would be laughing uproariously as if watching a comedy. Other times, he sat on the roof of the house outside of his room, staring at the moon. He had been scribbling meaningless repetitive phrases and numbers in notebooks he had been using for his college classes until recently. He was not attending classes because he was "sleeping all day" according to his mother.
- **Physical findings:** Robert sat quietly, smiling occasionally to himself, throughout his mother's description of the problem. When asked what he thought was going on, he said he had lost interest in school because it "was the devil's work." He admitted he had been receiving messages from the TV and beamed down from the moon that he was a messenger of God. At this point he looked quite distressed. When asked why his demeanor changed, he admitted that some of the voices that spoke to him were not friendly "God voices" but told him he was evil and worthless. When asked what he was filling his notebooks with, he said that he needed to write the devil's name in as many ways as possible in order to be safe.
- **Impression:** Schizophrenia, hebephrenic type
- **Plan:** The family was informed about the severity of the problem and referred to the county mental health clinic. It was agreed that the patient would be seen for Chinese medicine care after being stabilized on medication. At this point, the father, who had said little up to this point, said "I'm not going to let my son be experimented on like some kind of animal" (in reference to psychiatric care).
- **Follow up:** At last check with the mother, the patient had not been seen for stabilization. She thought the father would agree soon, however, because "my son is completely out of control."

DISCUSSION
History and Symptoms

Schizophrenic patients often do not report their symptoms easily and may even deny them. Some seem not to mind receiving special messages from TV sets or hearing voices. Unfortunately, many schizophrenics are not happy in their separate world because some of their hallucinations may be terrifying. Regardless of how the patient perceives their malady, or whether they perceive it at all, the family is usually profoundly concerned and is much more likely to seek help than the patient.

The symptoms and signs of schizophrenia are divided into positive and negative categories.

Positive symptoms include:

- Hallucinations (usually auditory) – voices in their head
- Delusions of grandeur, persecution, or control
- Disorganized speech and thought processes that may shift rapidly in speed and topic, with tangential thinking, loose associations, and tendency towards unusual symbolism
- Rapid and unpredictable shifts in mood incongruent with the external environment
- Hypersensitivity to stimuli of any sort, feelings of enhanced or extra-sensory awareness
- Unstable and inappropriate laughter, behavior and social boundaries
- Motor function generally reduced but may alternate between frenzy and stupor
- Obsessive thoughts and/or behaviors or compulsions
- Absorption with inner pre-occupations, often involving religion or sex

Negative symptoms or deficits include:

- Flattened affect, lack of enthusiasm or pleasure, catatonia (freezing in posture)
- Difficulty in speech.
- Disorganized and disrupted behavior, confused social roles and work/study routines.
- Decline in overall function.
- Social withdrawal and disruptions, hostility and suspiciousness.
- Deterioration of personal care and hygiene.
- Depressed affect is often present.
- Oversleeping, insomnia, fragmented and disordered sleep – mixing up nights and days
- Depersonalization (feeling like you are an actor on the stage of your life).
- Impaired concentration.
- Dependency on others, low self-esteem.

Schizophrenia represents a large class of thought disorders that can be variable in presentation. Not all, or even a majority, of the signs/symptoms listed above need be present to warrant referral to psychiatry. Also, some types of schizophrenia, like paranoid schizophrenia in a previously well-functioning adult, leave patients considerably more functional than other types, because the delusion(s) may be relatively isolated (CIA plots, etc.) and may not affect thinking in other ways. Some people with psychotic disorders may remain relatively high-functioning in certain areas of life such as work, hobbies, or artistic endeavors while showing significant declines and disruptions in other areas.

Typical Physical Findings

Hebephrenic schizophrenics (usually younger patients) can be observed to laugh at inappropriate times and to have a flat affect, tangential associations, and flights of ideas. They will often be more attentive to their inner dialogue than to any outer dialogue. They may exhibit poverty of movement to the point of catatonia. Paranoid schizophrenics will often look worried and may, with some coaxing, let you in on some or all of their conspiracy theories, which often include the FBI, CIA, KGB, and other such government agencies watching them or trying to trap or catch them.

Incidence and/or Prevalence

Schizophrenia is a common illness and the most common psychotic condition. Our streets are filled with schizophrenics who, by their dysfunction and/or the inability of society to provide for them, are homeless and wander aimlessly. The prevalence rate for schizophrenia is approximately one in 123 or 0.81%, which makes for 2.2 million people in the U.S. This illness can occur at any age, and is particularly severe if it occurs in childhood. It most commonly occurs between the onset of adolescence and young adulthood (15-24 in men and 24-32 in women). Although the incidence of schizophrenia declines with age, there is another peak at about 45 years old and again in the mid 60s, the latter mostly in women. Late-onset schizophrenia (after the teens) is often the paranoid type and carries a somewhat better prognosis.

Risk Factors

Inherited/familial

- Older father
- Family history of schizophrenia and other mental illnesses
- Prenatal maternal bereavement, famine, and malnutrition

Social and personal

- Poor friendships and social support

- Divorced and nonmarried status
- Low socioeconomic status
- Major adverse life event (death, divorce, personal failure, illness)

Iatrogenic & toxic

- Central nervous system damage during obstetrics
- Alcohol and street drug use (hallucinogenic drugs are particularly risky)

Co-morbidities/medical history

- Depression, sadness, anxiety, pessimism
- Left-handedness
- Obsessive compulsive traits
- Epilepsy
- Post-menopausal status in women (suggest a possible neuroprotective effect of estrogen and/or progesterone on the brain)
- Traumatic brain injuries

Mechanism Producing the Red Flag

Although the symptoms and signs of schizophrenia suggest a dysregulation of the neurotransmitters dopamine and serotonin in specific brain regions, the ultimate cause of schizophrenia is unknown. Rather, there is probably not one cause, but multiple interrelated factors including a genetic predisposition and the influence of many factors outlined above.

Another Important Consideration

- Schizophrenia is included as a red flag here because of the hope that early referral might mean an earlier intervention and improved outcome. Schizophrenia generally requires combined interventions including social work, behavioral, psychology, and medication. Chinese medicine can play a beneficial role in multidisciplinary interventions.

Specific red flags:
Patient who feels pessimistic, hopeless, and helpless

Condition assumed present until proven otherwise:
Major depression

Possible consequences of missing the condition:
Brain deterioration and disability, declining/disrupted quality of life, family/friend relationships, and socioeconomic functioning, increased risk for other serious medical conditions and suicide.

Stabilization, referral and management:

1. **Stabilization:** Acupuncturists can offer empathetic listening and supportive counseling as well as continue helpful herbal and acupuncture treatments.
2. **Consultation and Referral Options, Transportation:** Options will depend upon level of risk for suicide and the patient's ability to pay for services, transportation and other factors. Psychological emergency services should immediately be contacted for patients with plans to commit suicide and who refuse to sign a "no self-harm" contract (see sample form, appendix D). Those with strong suicidal ideation, but no plans for suicide, should have semi-urgent consultation with the patient's PCP who may be able to handle the situation or may make a psychological and/or psychiatric consult within days to a week. Patients with fleeting thoughts of suicide, or no thoughts of suicide, should receive timely referral to their PCP. Depression severe enough to disrupt and destabilize the patient's occupational and social functioning is best handled by a multi-disciplinary team including professionals with specialized training in treatment of depression, which may well include the acupuncturist.

Relevance to acupuncturists: Mood disorders (depression and anxiety) represent the second most common reason patients seek acupuncture in the U.S. This may be because of the generally high prevalence of this condition, compounded by the difficulty of treating depression and sometimes a desperate search for alternatives by patients and/or family members. Careful screening for depression severity and possible suicide risk is essential, but sometimes challenging, because depressed patients commonly underreport and/or deny symptoms or blame some other cause for the way they feel. Fortunately, depression may also be discovered by observation and questioning in addition to self-reporting of complaints (see history and physical exam findings sections for full discussion).

ACTUAL CASE

- **History:** A 30-year-old man came to the office complaining of constipation and vague abdominal pain, 2/10 at its worst intensity, generally relieved with bowel movements. It started about one week after his girlfriend moved out because he was having an affair with another woman. When he was asked if he was depressed, he said, "Yes." When asked if he had thought about suicide, he said, "Yes." When asked if he had plans to hurt himself, he says, "I might as well."
- **Physical findings:** The patient appeared depressed. He was sighing and making poor eye contact. His abdominal exam was normal.
- **Impression:** Major situational depression with suicide risk
- **Plan:** The patient was willing to sign a no self-harm contract. He was referred back to his PCP who already knew the patient's situation.
- **Follow up:** The PCP referred the patient to a community health service that agreed to see the patient on a sliding scale fee schedule within one week. The patient was seen by a psychologist over several weeks, but made little significant progress with his depression. He was eventually placed on an antidepressant by his PCP. His depression improved significantly. The patient was lost to further follow up.

DISCUSSION

Typical History and Symptoms

Often, direct questioning will prompt depressed patients to acknowledge depression and its severity, but patients may also deny or under-report depression because they are unaware of it, feel ashamed, or fear stigmatization. Depressed patients may instead complain of decreased interest in people and activities that were formerly interesting, a sense that life is not rewarding or, in more severe cases, hopelessness and helplessness. Often, if asked if they see "light at the end of the tunnel," they will say, "No."

Feelings of low self-esteem, guilt, worthlessness, inappropriate responsibility, dependence, self-criticality or pessimism are common. They may also report poor sleep, early awakening, weight gain or loss, or non-specific or vague symptoms like constipation, fatigue, vague chest or abdominal pain and digestive disturbances, difficulties with concentration and memory, general malaise, headaches, low back pain or loss of appetite. These often present as chief complaints rather than depression itself. The frequency and chronicity of medical visits for such complaints can be indicators of the severity of the depression.

Other clues include symptoms that do not follow recognized anatomically or physiologically based patterns regarding location, onset, triggers, palliative factors, etc. or symptoms that respond adversely to all attempts at care. Depressed patients have sometimes had extensive diagnostic testing that has turned out negative. The presence of risk factors for depression can also help identify its presence (see risk factor section below).

Physical Exam Findings

Depressed patients may look down often, sigh, avoid eye contact, and look like the "weight of the world" is on their shoulders. They may appear lethargic or to have slow thought and movement. They may respond in a monotone voice and be vague or hyporesponsiveness to questions. They may have an unkempt appearance and poor hygiene and appear pessimistic. Even though they come to you for treatment, they may seem to have a negative attitude regarding treatment. They may cry, be anxious, irritable, or show smoldering resentment or excessive guilt. They may have trouble making decisions and concentrate poorly.

Incidence and/or Prevalence

The prevalence of significant depression in the U.S. is estimated at 5.3% of adults, or 17 million people. Of those with major depression, approximately 4% are adolescents, 12% are women and 7% are men. The lifetime risk for an episode of significant depression is highest in women at 20% (the percentage of women that will experience major depression sometime in their life).

Risk Factors

Lifestyle, demographics, family, and social history

- Sedentary lifestyle
- Social isolation, poor family, friendship and community support
- Divorce, bereavement
- Caregiver to loved one with major or chronic medical condition with associated severe pain, discomfort, disability or risk of death
- Women have higher incidence rates than men
- Low socioeconomic status

- Major disruptions in socioeconomic functioning or status: loss of employment, finances, property or home
- Family history of depression or suicide
- Irregular sleep and work habits, particularly, swing or night shift work
- Lifestyle with inadequate daylight exposure or sudden move from equatorial to polar latitudes
- Excessive, non-essential internet use

Co-morbidities and medical history

- Alcohol or drug abuse
- Abuse (physical, sexual, emotional, psychological, spiritual or financial)
- Any major or chronic medical condition with associated severe pain, discomfort. disability or risk of death, in particular, cancer, HIV/AIDS, heart disease, Alzheimer's, stroke, complex regional pain syndrome, trigeminal neuralgia, unremitting tinnitus
- Postpartum state
- Traumatic brain injuries or surgery
- Depressed mood as child or adolescent
- Diet low in omega3 free fatty acids and low vitamin D3 levels

Iatrogenic

- Long-term use of certain medicines like some antihypertensive meds or sleeping pills

Mechanism Producing the Red Flag

Depressed thoughts and feelings or maladaptive responses to major life stressors can lead to a depressed affect and lack of functionality and enthusiasm, as well as an internal retreat from the world. Major depression has a negative physical effect on brain tissue causing a significant decrease in the volume of the hippocampus, a region important in memory and learning. In other words, depression causes physical brain deterioration, which may worsen the ability to cope, leading to more depression, which may then cause more brain deterioration, on and on in a negative cycle of deterioration.

Other Important Considerations

- In addition to the significant decreased quality of life that depressed patients face, there is also the short and long term risk for suicide to consider. The risk is especially high in severe depression. In fact, half of all suicide victims suffer from major depression and suicide occurs in 25% of people with chronic depression.
- Severe anxiety and depression often go hand in hand as "agitated depression." Some patients will tell you that their anxiety is so extreme that it causes their depression.

Specific red flags: *Depression followed by an episode of hyper-excitation and euphoria*

Condition assumed present until proven otherwise:

Manic phase of bipolar disorder—one illness in the family of illnesses known as "bipolar spectrum disorders" (BSD) defined by the presence of cycling, recurrent episodes of abnormally elevated mood interspersed with episodes of depressive mood.

Possible consequences of missing the condition:

Episodes of bipolar illness are often associated with severe distress and disruption of a patient's life and that cause a significantly elevated risk of suicide during depressive episodes and risky behavior during manic phases that can lead to death.

Stabilization, referral and management:

1. **Stabilization:** There are no immediate stabilizing steps to take
2. **Consultation and Referral Options, Transportation:** The referral should be made on a timely to semi-urgent basis depending on symptoms. Patients who are mildly to moderately depressed can be referred in a few days to a week to their PCP. The ultimate allopathic consultant for manic-depressive illness is generally a psychiatrist, although some PCPs have additional expertise in psychiatry and may be able to treat the patient. Patients with severe depression may represent an immediate risk to themselves, or occasionally to others, and should be handled and referred as outlined in the previous red flag on major depression.

Relevance to acupuncturists: Acupuncturists will undoubtedly see many bipolar patients due to the high incidence of the disorder (see below). Also, like other health care providers, acupuncturists will often miss the red flag for this illness because the history of the manic episode (which may be only "hypomania") will often not be obtained. Due to the inherent greater dangers of bipolar illness compared to ordinary depression, however, the red flag for this illness should be recognized.

ACTUAL CASE

- **History:** The patient was a 35-year-old male former gymnast in college who presented to the office with a history of recurrent depression for several years. He denied that he was having suicidal thoughts or plans, but was nonetheless concerned about his condition because he thought he might be in danger of harming himself. When asked what he meant by this, he explained that he was afraid he would hurt himself on the job, where he often had to climb telephone poles to repair equipment. He went on to explain that his episodes of depression were interspersed with intervals during which he felt fine. In fact, he felt "super-fine" like he was "on top of the world." The feeling was so intense that he was convinced he could "jump from the top of the pole and land on my feet like a cat."
- **Physical findings:** The patient was a fit and muscular looking Caucasian man who had a totally normal examination and did not appear especially depressed, although he did look worried.
- **Impression:** Bipolar disorder
- **Plan:** After Chinese medical treatments did not seem to adequately improve his illness (it often does), he was referred to a local psychiatrist because he had no PCP.
- **Follow up:** The patient was diagnosed with bipolar illness and was placed on several medications in an attempt to control his bipolar illness, his mania in particular. They met with little success and some side effects. He was finally placed on Lithium, which worked well and gave him no significant side effects. He has done well since then.

DISCUSSION

History and Symptoms

Bipolar patients cyclically experience abnormally elevated (manic or hypomanic) episodes followed by abnormally depressed episodes that are severe enough to interfere with their normal functioning. Hypomania is higher than a good mood, though not as high as mania. Although the mood swings classically last for at least a week, some individuals have rapidly alternating moods, known as rapid cycling bipolar episodes. Though there can be variation on how high and how low the moods are and how rapidly they cycle, the cycling nature of mood is necessary to make the diagnosis of bipolar disease.

Mania is characterized by feelings of irritability, euphoria or excessive expansiveness. It is common to experience increased energy and a decreased need for sleep. Thoughts may race and speech may be pressured and grandiose. Attention span may be short as the patient races from thought to thought. Judgment in a number of arenas may become impaired. There may be uncharacteristic spending sprees, risky drug taking, and promiscuous sexual behavior.

Patients in mania may be intrusive, aggressive, and intolerant of others. Sometimes, they experience symptoms that overlap with symptoms of thought disorders like schizophrenia. They may have delusions of grandeur and feel they're a "chosen one" with special insight not given to other mortals, or feel they have extraordinary physical and psychic powers. These delusions may become so strong that they experience a psychotic break with reality. They may have auditory hallucinations as well. Some manic patients are consumed with anxiety and irritability, while others are euphoric, grandiose, and convinced of their superiority.

The diagnosis may be difficult if one phase, the manic or the depressed, is dominant in relationship to the other. In patients who primarily experience mania, clinicians and patients may think that simple anxiety is the diagnosis. Conversely, patients with dominant depressive episodes may be diagnosed as having unipolar depression. Additionally, hypomania must not be mistaken for the sense of relief that unipolar depression patients experience when their depression lifts.

Physical Exam Findings

The physical findings depend on the stage that the patient is in when they present to you. Between up and down episodes they may appear perfectly normal. During mania, they will exhibit pressured speech, grandiose and unrealistic self-concept and other findings as outlined in the symptoms section. In the depressed phase they will exhibit the classical physical signs of depression as discussed in detail under the red flag for depression such as downcast eyes, frequent sighing, a look of sadness, slouched shoulders, etc.

Incidence and/or Prevalence

The best estimate we could find is that bipolar disorder

afflicts approximately 5.7 million people in the U.S., one out of every 45 adults. Prevalence is equal in men and women. It is found across all cultures and ethnic groups. The median age of onset for bipolar disorders is 25 years of age.

Risk Factors

- Family history: people with an immediate family member with depression or bipolar disorder are at higher risk, implicating genetic factors.
- Environmental influence – early childhood psychological trauma
- Childhood precursors – hypomania or cyclothymia (milder mood swings than bipolar disease)

Mechanism Producing the Red Flag

Like most psychological disorders, the cause appears to be an imbalance of neurotransmitters in critical areas of the brain, although the specific alterations are unknown. Functional MRI scanning show maldistribution of blood patterns contrasted to what is seen in normal patients.

Other Important Considerations

- Bipolar disorder is frequently under-diagnosed and most often misdiagnosed as anxiety disorder, borderline personality disorder or schizophrenia.
- In some cases bipolar disorder can be devastating, but it has also been associated with creativity and high achievements when patients are in the manic phase. Possibly one of the best known examples of this was the creative genius Vincent van Gogh.

▶ Specific red flags:
Personality change, social withdrawal, unstable relationships, evasiveness and decreased academic performance in an adolescent or adult

Condition assumed present until proven otherwise:
Drug abuse (partial loss of control over drug use) or addiction (loss of control over drug use)

Possible consequences of missing the condition:
Decreased productivity in school and life, possible fatality, societal cost

Stabilization, referral and management:

1. **Stabilization:** There are no immediate stabilizing steps, but the maintenance of a nonjudgmental affect is helpful in dealing with patients and family.
2. **Consultation and Referral Options, Transportation:** Depends on the situation. If substance use is acknowledged, referral to substance abuse treatment facility and/or a family physician or psychiatrist is appropriate. If suicide risk is present and the patient refuses to sign a "no harm contract," psychological emergency services must be activated for safety (see red flag for depression).

Relevance to acupuncturists: Every acupuncturist will have many patients who are abusing or are addicted to drugs, both prescription and recreational. The recreational use of drugs is so common among preteens, teens and college-aged people that it might seem a legitimate "rite of passage" or a non-harmful or even beneficial practice to some users. It is also true that individuals differ widely in their ability to "handle" drugs. Unfortunately, many people do not pass through habitual or even occasional drug use unscathed physically and/or psychologically. This seems to hold true for all recreational drugs, even some of the relatively less harmful ones, like marijuana. The recognition of patients who abuse or are addicted to drugs is important so we can help patients deal with life issues and feelings in a way that sets them free, rather than keeps them enslaved in sometimes dangerous drug routines.

ACTUAL CASE

- **History:** A concerned mother brought her 17-year-old son, Jake, into the office because of what she thought was depression for about one year. She based this on what she saw as Jake's withdrawal from other family members and poor concentration on school work. His grades had dropped from Bs to Ds and Fs. Jake was not concerned about his declining performance. He said school was boring. We agreed that the mother would leave the room so Jake could talk privately. We assured Jake that his private conversation would be confidential unless he agreed to share it. When asked about health issues, worries, possible tensions at home, or problems with friends, he denied any difficulties. When asked about drugs he said, "I blow a little weed every now and then. I think they should be legal anyway."
- **Physical findings:** Jake made poor eye contact through

out the interview and seemed morose and a little angry, glaring at his mother several times before she left the room for our private conversation.

- **Impression:** Possible drug abuse
- **Plan:** The patient and his mother were sent to a psychologist skilled with adolescent problems without mention of drug abuse. The son said he would go "to keep my mom from flipping out."
- **Follow up:** The patient had several individual sessions with his counselor and several family sessions. They made some progress initially with Jake being able to express his feelings better. The counselor finally advised drug treatment for Jake, but Jake refused. Two months later, Jake hit the side of a bridge in his mother's car at top speed while driving drunk. His passenger was killed instantly, but Jake survived. He lost most of his upper teeth, smashed his jaw and cheekbone and lost one eye. He had extensive plastic surgery and is making a slow recovery. At last check, he was no longer doing drugs but was facing charges of involuntary manslaughter.

DISCUSSION

History and Symptoms

Symptoms vary somewhat depending on the age and personality of the patient. In adolescents, families often report withdrawal from family members and often from former friends in favor of new friends. Depressive affect or behavior is often evident. Some degree of hostility and dissatisfaction with their family are common in many "normal" adolescents, but this behavior is often heightened by drug abuse.

In adults, the personality change and problems functioning are generally noticed by employers and coworkers. Hiding of substances, evasion and dishonesty is common among spouses. Drug abusing patients and family members generally deny drug use as an explanation for changes in mood and behavior and offer alternative explanations. Codependency and enabling often occurs with family and sometimes friends until the situation can no longer be ignored.

Physical Exam Findings

The physical signs differ somewhat depending upon the drug of choice, but signs of depression are frequent: poor eye contact, downcast gaze, verbal responses to questions that are slow, evasive, withheld or hostile, a sad expression, or more frequently, apathy, and poor compliance with health advice. If stimulants are preferred there may be some anxious or even manic behavior.

Adolescents and young adults can express paranoid thinking, ideas of victimhood, unrealistic fantasies, grandiosity, and melodramatic language. Morbid themes may be espoused. Ideas about death are not unusual. Although sometimes considered "normal" in some adolescents, they are often carried to an extreme. Declining dental health is evident in long-term methamphetamine users. Users of injectable drugs usually make efforts to hide needle marks. Drugs inhaled nasally may produce increased sniffing or snorting.

Incidence and/or Prevalence

Drug abuse can begin at any age, but lifetime drug habits most often begin during the teens. The *Monitoring the Future* (MTF) study has measured drug, alcohol, and cigarette use and attendant attitudes among adolescent students nationwide since 1975. This survey indicates that drug use is the rule rather than the exception by senior year in high school. Almost 70% of all twelfth graders use alcohol, 3.4 % use cocaine, 3.5% use methamphetamine, 4.7 % use hallucinogens, 32.8 % use marijuana, 10% have used Vicodin® and 5% have used OxyContin® (use is increasing of the latter two).

A small but significant number of experimental, recreational, and habitual adolescent drug users may progress to drug abuse and addiction (dependency and loss of control of drug use). This progression to abuse and addiction causes incalculable heartache for the user and their family, as well as quantifiable adverse consequences on health, educational, occupational functioning and lifespan. Consider these U.S. statistics from the CDC and other authoritative sources, which is limited to alcohol, opioids, and methamphetamines use only.

1. Yearly deaths from alcoholic liver disease – 13,050
2. Yearly alcohol related deaths excluding accidents and homicides – 22,075
3. Yearly deaths from alcohol related MVA – 16,919 (40% of fatalities)
4. Yearly deaths from alcohol poisoning—50,000 (one person a week in the U.S.)
5. Yearly deaths (2006 data) from opioids 13,800 (tripled

from 6 years earlier. Opioid analgesics were involved in almost 40% of all poisoning deaths in 2006.

6. Yearly deaths from methamphetamine (1992 date) 500

- Total average yearly deaths from the substances mentioned above = 116,312 deaths/year.
- Total average yearly deaths from terrorist attack (over 10 year period including peak year that include 9-11 attack = 322.7 deaths/year.
- This makes for a 360/1 ratio of substance abuse deaths versus terrorist attack deaths/year.
- This does *not include* deaths from smoking cigarettes, 440,000 deaths/year (50 deaths/hour).

Additionally we have these costs to consider (U.S. statistics again).

1. Yearly cost of alcohol prevention, treatment, support programs – $26,338 million
2. Yearly lost productivity costs due to alcohol and drug abuse – $134,206 million
3. Yearly cost from MVA damage – $15,744 million
4. Yearly cost from crime due to drugs – $6,328 million
5. Yearly cost from fires set due to drugs – $1,537 million
6. Yearly social welfare costs due to drugs – $448 million
    - Total yearly cost from drug abuse = $184 billion, 601 million.

All clinicians are obliged to consider the importance of substance abuse and addiction when faced with such data.

Risk Factors

It would be reassuring to say that we could predict those who go from experimentation to abuse to overt addiction on the basis of risk factors alone, but that isn't the case. Some drugs seem to have a power to corrupt genetically predisposed people who have few risk factors. We should therefore look at the following risk factors as relative factors.

- Mood disorders including depression, anxiety, ADHD, and bipolar disorder
- Family history of substance use
- 2:1 male to female ratio
- Poor, fragmented, or unstable family support
- Loneliness
- Experimentation with highly addictive drugs such as heroin, methamphetamines, and cocaine

Mechanism Producing the Red Flag

Addiction permanently affects the structure and function of the brain. In genetically predisposed individuals, substances of abuse cause changes in the dopaminergic mesolimbic system that result in loss of control over the use of the addictive substances. These changes are mediated by a number of neurotransmitters. The permanent nature of these changes is the primary reason for relapse in the addicted patient.

To make matters worse, chronic use of drugs like sedatives and alcohol cause a down regulation (decrease) in gamma-aminobutyric acid (GABA [calming]) receptors in the brain. With cessation of the drug, the GABA receptors increase, but there is too little GABA to bind them. The result is extreme stimulation of the sympathetic (fight or flight) nervous system.

Another problem concerns the role of non-neural cells of the CNS and peripheral nervous system called "neuroglia" or simply "glial" cells. These cells were formerly thought to be merely supportive and to help with neuronal transmission along nerve trunks. We now know that they perform a heretofore unappreciated role in neuronal function that bears directly on drug addiction.

When patients use opiates, for example, the effect on the neuron is to dampen down neuronal transmission. This can, of course, relieve pain. Habitual use of substances like opiates cause glial cells to respond by producing inflammatory products that they send to the neuron in an effort to wake it up. When a person stops taking opiates, not only does the normal neuronal activity pick up again, but the neuron is actually hyperexcited because the glial cells continue their stimulatory efforts, sometimes for months.

This previously unknown compensatory role of glial cells, in addition to psychological factors, at least partly explains why heroin and opium addicts crave their substances of choice long after the acute withdrawal phase is over. It helps clinicians understand the power of drug addiction in relation to opiates and is the reason that treatment for these conditions must usually be handled by experts.

Other Important Considerations

- Marijuana is often touted as the least dangerous drug of those we've considered. In fact, the internet seems saturated with sites arguing that it is completely safe. While alcohol does seem to be the most dangerous commonly used drug in terms of morbidity and mortality, there is good evidence that marijuana may not be as benign as is thought by many people.

- There is evidence that marijuana can produce "amotivational syndrome." In one well-controlled study, college-aged research subjects who smoke marijuana spent significantly less time in productive activities and more time recreating than those who didn't. Many clinicians think it unwise to underestimate the significance of a motivational syndrome in young people just beginning to think about their vocation in life.
- In a study that appeared online in the May 2010 issue of the Archives of General Psychiatry, young adults who smoked marijuana regularly starting around 15 years of age were twice as likely to develop psychosis and four times as likely to have delusional thinking in a "dose response" relationship than those who did not.

Review What You Have Learned

Chapter 17 Psychological Problems

Chapter 17—Psychological Problems, Anxiety

1. A true statement about panic disorder is that it can coexist with generalized anxiety in the same patient. What statements are false about panic disorder?

a. Panic disorder and agoraphobia are the same illness
b. Panic disorder can coexist with depression
c. Phobia is more common than panic disorder
d. Patients with panic disorder can have the sense of impending doom during attacks

Chapter 17—Psychological Problems, Delusions

1. What symptoms are most common and diagnostic in schizophrenia from those listed below?

a. Visual hallucinations, tangential thinking, delusions
b. Tangential thinking, auditory hallucinations, delusions
c. Paranoid thinking, delusions, anxiety, visual hallucinations
d. Social withdrawal, visual hallucinations, delusions

2. The prevalence rate of schizophrenia in the U.S. is closest to

a. 10%
b. 5%
c. 20%
d. 1%

Chapter 17—Psychological Problems, Depression

1. Depression is a serious medical disorder because

a. It can lead to suicide
b. It can lead to deterioration (loss of volume) of a portion of the brain called the hippocampus
c. It can lead to a deterioration of memory and learning
d. All of the above

Chapter 17—Psychological Problems, Mood Swings

1. A patient whose mood range between euphoria to depression is likely suffering from

a. A lack of understanding by family members
b. A bipolar spectrum disorder (manic depressive illness)
c. Phobias and obsessive thoughts
d. Depression and anxiety

Chapter 17—Psychological Problems, Substance Abuse

1. Patients who abuse drugs may self-report that they have no problems in controlling their use. What signs are likely to be present in individuals who are having problems with abuse or addiction?

a. Change of personality, hiding and hording addictive substances, dishonesty about substances
b. Tensions at home with relatives or with nonusing friends
c. Decreasing school performance in students and withdrawal from family members
d. All of the above

2. Marijuana may be the least dangerous of commonly abused drugs compared to alcohol, opiates and methamphetamine in terms of mortality. One can find many statements about how safe it is on the internet. Regardless of this "reassurance," concerns about habitual use include

a. Possible lung damage in those who smoke it
b. Possible "amotivational syndrome" that may interfere with achievement in the young
c. A possible quadrupling of the lifetime incidence of psychosis in regular users who start young
d. All of the above

Chapter 18: PULSE ABNORMALITIES IN GENERAL

Since pulse diagnosis is an important part of Chinese medical patient assessment, acupuncturists have the possibility of being the first practitioner to become aware of a serious pulse abnormality. In this chapter, we learn more about which abnormalities are considered serious by Western care professionals, and why.

In this chapter, we examine red flags that have to do with the pulse, the rhythm of the heart beat. Specifically, we examine problems that have to do with *quantitative* or timing abnormalities of the pulse, not *qualitative* aspects (how the pulse feels, for example), from which acupuncturists derive additional valuable clinical information.

A person who lives 70 years with a pulse of 70 bpm will have 2,575,440,000 heartbeats in a lifetime. The great majority of which will be well regulated. Small, infrequent and non-sustained deviations from normal will be well tolerated. Major deviations will not. In general, there are only three things that can go wrong with the heartbeat (or some combination of the three). Not counting asystole, a complete cessation of the heartbeat, we can expect one or more of the following:

1. The rhythm can be regular, but too slow (bradycardia).
2. The rhythm can be regular, but too fast (tachycardia).
3. The rhythm can be irregular (many patterns of irregularity are possible).

To note the quantitative aspects of heart rhythm, we must take the pulse, listening to the heartbeat or watch the electrical timing of the heart on an ECG. When the pulse and/ or heartbeat are monitored by the examining clinician, we call abnormalities of timing "arrhythmias." Although this word literally means "irregular," bradycardia and tachycardia (regular rhythms) are also generally categorized as arrhythmias.

Arrhythmias are *signs* because they are observed by the clinician. When patients complain of what they *sense* as abnormal heartbeats, we call their *symptoms* "palpitations." A distinction between arrhythmias and palpitations is necessary because there can be significant disagreement between what patients feel and what clinicians observe.

For example, a pulse can be normal when timed simultaneously when a patient feels palpitations. Similarly, a 24-hour monitoring of the heartbeat can reveal normal heart rhythm when a patient reports significant palpitations. Conversely, some patients will not feel subtle arrhythmias seen on their 24-hour tracing as palpitations. Why this happens so frequently is unknown, but it does seem that stress, worry, or possibly depression make some patients more aware of their heartbeat than nonstressed patients.

What this means to the clinician is that we must objectively note arrhythmia before we can definitively say that a heartbeat or pulse abnormality is present. A patient's report of palpitations, however, should always be taken seriously and spur the clinician to carefully check the heart rhythm because an arrhythmia may be present. Severe arrhythmias will almost invariably be symptomatic.

Not all arrhythmias are considered in this section because symptoms like dizziness or syncope may occur so quickly with some arrhythmias that they may be presenting complaints, rather than the palpitation itself. Bradycardia, for example, is covered in the dizziness section because dizziness due to inadequate cerebral perfusion is often the first complaint with significant bradycardia.

Neither do we consider very serious and/or lethal arrhythmias here, because these patients won't make it to the acupuncturist. We do cover one instance of tachycardia as a specific red flag following this introduction, as well as one instance of irregular pulse, however. This is by no means an exhaustive look at the fascinating subject of arrhythmias, but it does capture a few important red flags of conditions in which alert intervention can be lifesaving.

Before examining the specific red flags in this section, however, we should take a look at an important general red flag that involves palpitations. As mentioned, palpitations can be caused by anything from worry and over-sensitivity of one's normal heart beat, to potentially life threatening conditions.

It behooves us and our patients to know, therefore, in what instance palpitations could generally indicate serious illness.

Palpitations that are absent with exercise and present at rest are almost always benign, whereas **palpitations that occur reliably with exercise and go away with rest** are a general red flag for ***some type of heart disease*** in the same way that **chest pain that occurs reliably with exercise and goes away with rest**, previously discussed under chest pain, is a red flag for *coronary artery disease*. Please refer to the chest pain red flag for risk factors for "malignant" palpitations that appear with exercise.

Specific red flags:
Resting heart rate > 100/min, hypervigilance, warm skin

Condition assumed present until proven otherwise:
Hyperthyroidism (thyrotoxicosis)

Possible consequences of missing the condition:
Ten percent of untreated hyperthyroid patients can enter a dangerous escalation of hyperthyroidism called "thyroid storm" leading to heart failure and death

Stabilization, referral and management:

1. **Stabilization:** There are no immediate preventative steps to take.
2. **Consultation and Referral Options, Transportation:** Hyperthyroidism without fever warrants a timely or semi-urgent referral to the patient's PCP depending on severity of symptoms. Thyroid storm (fever is present) requires emergency treatment and hospitalization. Patients can be sent by private transportation with someone else driving. As always, 911 should be called for unstable patients.

Relevance to acupuncturists: A rapid pulse rate and anxious affect are so commonly attributed to anxiety in many primary care practices that hyperthyroidism may not be suspected as the actual cause. Additionally, hyperthyroidism often comes on so gradually that patients and clinicians usually don't notice it until symptoms are pronounced. Likewise, the often fatal complication of thyroid storm that requires immediate and aggressive treatment may escalate slowly from hyperthyroidism and may be missed in early stages.

ACTUAL CASE

- **History:** A 27-year-old female presented to the office with her husband with anxiety, a fast heart beat and the feeling of being overheated. She had also lost five pounds without attempting to do so. Her husband accompanied her and stated he was concerned about her "change in personality" and was worried about her mental health.
- **Physical findings:** The patient appeared emotionally labile: anxious, tearful and *hypervigilant*. Her pulse was 105 bpm and her temperature was 101.0° F.
- **Impression:** Hyperthyroidism with possible early thyroid storm
- **Plan:** The patient was sent to the ED of a nearby hospital
- **Follow up:** The patient was found to have very high T4 and T3 concentrations in the blood and was started on aggressive IV fluid management and oxygen in the ICU. She fortunately recovered from her illness, which proved to be Graves disease. She was discharged on medication to suppress the thyroid gland and eventually underwent partial ablation of the thyroid gland as an outpatient to bring the thyroid hormones to normal.

DISCUSSION

History and Symptoms

The symptoms of hyperthyroidism usually increase so gradually that patients may have mild to moderate symptoms for weeks or even months before suspecting a problem. Because the body's metabolism is increased, patients often feel hotter than those around them and are uncomfortable in warm environments (heat intolerance). They may complain of warm, moist skin and easy perspiration, mild diarrhea, and light or skipped menses. They are often fatigued at the end of the day, but may also have trouble falling sleeping.

They complain of trembling hands and a pounding or irregular heartbeat (palpitations). Family members may note they have mood swings and irritability (emotional lability). Their hypervigilance (from fast thinking) is usually interpreted as anxiety. They often complain of weight loss despite eating more. The only exception to these generalizations about the symptoms of hyperthyroidism is in the elderly. In many elderly people, some or even all of the typical symptoms of hyperthyroidism may be missing. These patients may merely complain of weight loss, fatigue, depression, and/or anxiety.

As hyperthyroidism becomes more severe, patients become short of breath and have chest pain and muscle weakness. Symptoms of thyroid storm are the same as in hyperthyroidism, but heightened and with the addition of fever and tremor. The temperature may rise above 105.5° F and be accompanied by nausea, vomiting, diarrhea, dehydration, delirium, and eventually coma. Thyroid crisis can sometimes take a different form called "apathetic storm" in the elderly, which is characterized by extreme weakness, emotional apathy, and confusion rather than delirium and agitation. Fever may also be minimal in this case.

Physical Exam Findings

The most reliable sign of hyperthyroidism is tachycardia of > 100 bpm at rest. Warm, moist skin noted by the patient may also be observed on physical exam, as well as oily hair. The patient almost always appears hypervigilant and somewhat nervous. This increases dramatically with thyroid storm. The hyperthyroid patient may have rapidly cycling emotions and may cry for no apparent reason. Deep tendon reflexes may be hyperactive. A goiter or bulging eyes are not reliable signs of hyperthyroidism.

Incidence and/or Prevalence

Prevalence for hyperthyroidism in the U.S. varies from < 1% to < 2%. We favor the higher estimate, because hyperthyroidism is often undiagnosed in milder cases. Hashimoto's is the most common cause of hypothyroidism, but Grave's disease more commonly causes thyroid storm. Thyroid storm occurs in as high as 10% of patients with untreated hyperthyroidism. The mortality of thyroid storm approached 100% in the early 1900s. The death rate is now slightly less than 20%. Both hyperthyroidism and thyroid storm are more common in women than men.

Risk Factors

- Infections, especially of the lung in patients with hyperthyroidism
- Stopping medications given to suppress hyperthyroidism
- Excessive dose of thyroid hormones
- Pregnancy
- Heart attacks
- Other autoimmune diseases

Mechanism Producing the Red Flag

There are multiple causes of hyperthyroidism. Regardless of cause, the mechanism of this red flag is secondary to an overabundance of T3 and T4. Since these hormones set the overall metabolic rate of the body, their overabundance increases the rate of all activities, including thinking (hypervigilance), heart rate (tachycardia) and nerve conduction (hyperactive reflexes). The increased metabolic rate creates heat (fever). The increase in heart rate can be so severe in thyroid storm that there is inadequate time for the left ventricle to fill before each contraction, leading to greatly diminished cardiac output, heart failure and possible death.

Other Important Considerations

- Hyperthyroidism must always be considered in the anxious, tachycardic patient.
- *Tachycardia is the most reliable sign of hyperthyroidism, the rate >100 bpm. Tachycardia with fever are the most reliable signs of thyroid storm.*
- Thyroid storm is often associated with Graves' disease, but has also been reported with toxic nodular goiter.

Specific red flags: *Irregularly irregular pulse with rate >100 bpm*

Condition assumed present until proven otherwise:
Atrial fibrillation (A-fib) with an uncontrolled ventricular response – A-fib is a fluttering of the heart chamber that contains the natural pacemaker of the heart, the sinoatrial (SA) node. This red flag specifically indicates a specific type of A-fib, A-fib with a rapid ventricular response.

Possible consequences of missing the condition:
Disability, stroke, heart failure, sudden death

Stabilization, referral and management:

1. **Stabilization:** The patient should avoid stimulant herbs and substances like caffeine, etc., until consultation and restoration of normal sinus rhythm is accomplished or, failing that, the ventricular response is controlled.
2. **Consultation and Referral Options, Transportation:** With an uncontrolled V response, the situation is at least semi-urgent. Stable and relatively younger patients with the rapid response who are not otherwise symptomatic can be driven directly to the ED. 911 should be contacted for elderly patients with tachycardia or for patients with severe shortness of breath, chest pain, lightheadedness, weakness, or an even more rapid heartbeat (>120, for example).

Relevance to acupuncturists: Acupuncturists are taught about intermittent or regularly irregular pulses or irregularly irregular pulses in acupuncture school. This red flag is an example of an irregularly irregular pulse, a pulse that is completely unpredictable and has no discernable pattern. A good number of acupuncture patients will be found to be in A-fib because at least 1% of the general population is. Of that number, a small subset, often those not previously diagnosed by a medical doctor or those who have gone off their anti-arrhythmic medicine, will present to the acupuncturist with uncontrolled A-fib and complaints of palpitations.

ACTUAL CASE

- **History:** The patient was a 35-year-old Caucasian male with "flip-flopping" sensations in his chest for the prior 2 weeks. They seemed to start suddenly one day at a picnic after he drank a six-pack of beer and followed that with a strong mug of coffee so he could drive home. They were now continuous. He had periodic dizziness and found it impossible to take his normal nightly walk on the beach due to shortness of breath. He came in for an acupuncture treatment because he "didn't trust doctors." His PMH was unremarkable. He smoked a pack of cigarettes/day and drank two six-packs of beer on weekends.
- **Physical findings:** The patient was thin and anxious appearing, heavily tattooed male who looked a little older than his stated age. He was friendly, open, and seemed fairly intelligent. His pulse was irregularly irregular and the rate was 110 bpm on checking for one full minute. He appeared slightly short of breath.
- **Impression:** Probable atrial fibrillation with an uncontrolled ventricular response
- **Plan:** When impressed with the urgency of his situation, the patient reluctantly agreed to go to the ED of a local hospital and was driven by his girlfriend on their Harley.
- **Follow up:** The patient was found to be in A-fib in the ED. A cardiologist was consulted and the patient was cardioverted back into normal sinus rhythm. Unfortunately, the normal rhythm did not hold and he went back into A-fib with a more rapid ventricular response of 120 bpm. He was given medication to control his ventricular response (to "block down" impulses across the AV node) and left the hospital with a rate of 80-90 bpm. An echocardiogram showed an enlarged heart from presumed alcoholic cardiomyopathy which was thought to be the etiology of his A-fib.

DISCUSSION

History and Symptoms

The situation we face in this red flag is uncontrolled A-fib, but we should first explore symptoms of A-fib in general because A-fib may precede uncontrolled A-fib. Symptoms of A fib vary from person to person. Many patients have no symptoms. Others have a sensation of the heart fluttering in the chest. The most common symptom in people with *intermittent* A-fib is palpitations, the sensation of a rapid or irregular heartbeat. Some patients have lightheadedness and feel faint. Other symptoms include weakness, lack of energy, or shortness of breath with effort. Some have fleeting chest pain as well. In uncontrolled A-fib, all of these symptoms are worsened and patient can become unstable.

Physical Exam Findings

Stable patients may exhibit no signs except irregularly irregular pulse. Patients in uncontrolled A-fib will almost invariably appear anxious and somewhat short of breath. If very unstable, they may look "shocky" with facial pallor, sweating, and low blood pressure.

Incidence and/or Prevalence

Atrial fibrillation is the most common arrhythmia, affecting about 1% of the population, mostly people older than 50. About 5% of people older than 80 have atrial fibrillation. The risk of stroke, a common complication of A-fib, is about 1.5% for people aged 50-59 years old and 30% for those aged 80-89 years old (3-5 times higher than the general population). The rate for all types of complications in people who have an uncontrolled heart rate >100 is much greater than those who have controlled A-fib. The incidence of uncontrolled A-fib is unknown.

Risk Factors

- Advancing age
- Previous heart disease like CAD, valvular heart disease, cardiomyopathy, sinus node disease (see red flag for bilateral ankle swelling in this book for brief explanations of the different kinds of heart disease)
- Pericarditis (inflammation of the pericardium surrounding the heart)
- High blood pressure, especially uncontrolled
- Other chronic problems like thyroid disease and sleep apnea increase risk for A-fib
- Alcohol consumption, especially if excessive or with binge drinking
- Family history of A-fib or other heart problems
- Previous pulmonary emboli, serious pneumonia or lung disease, like emphysema
- Cigarette smoking

Mechanism Producing the Red Flag

A-fib most commonly occurs as the result of some other cardiac condition, but it may occur without evidence of underlying heart disease, especially in younger people, about half of whom have no other heart problems. Atrial contractions in A-fib are disorganized and chaotic. The atria may contract at a rate of 400-600 per minute. Even though the AV node lets only a small number of these impulses through, enough may stimulate the ventricle to produce the uncontrolled response we speak of here. The irregularly irregular rhythm is the result of the fact that the AV node allows a random number and sequence of stimulating electrical signals through and the result is a random rhythm.

The complication of stroke is due to the fact that the blood eddies and churns in the atrium due to its erratic activity and clots can form, slip through the mitral valve into the left ventricle and from there can lodge in small arterioles of the brain, causing stroke. The complication of heart failure is due to incomplete filling of the ventricles due to inadequate filling time. If the ventricular rate is high, decreased stroke volume and decreased cardiac output are the result. Fainting, fatigue, and other signs and symptoms of heart failure are also due to inadequate cardiac output to sensitive tissues.

Other Important Considerations

- Most people with chronic or recurrent A-fib take warfarin (Coumadin) to lower the risk of stroke. Warfarin has its own set of possible side effects from its anticoagulant capacity, however. People at lower risk of stroke and those who cannot take warfarin may use aspirin which can cause bleeding problems and stomach ulcers.
- Despite the risk that A-fib can bring in some cases, clinical trials show that patients who have A-fib *with a controlled heart rate* (using medications plus Coumadin) live just as long as those in normal sinus rhythm (AFFIRM trial).
- People with infrequent and brief episodes of atrial fibrillation may need no further treatment than learning to avoid the triggers of their episodes, such as caffeine, alcohol, smoking, or overeating.

Review What You Have Learned
Chapter 18 Pulse Abnormalities in General

1. Palpitations
a. Are arrhythmias
b. Can be measured in the pulse
c. Can be measured by pulse and an electrocardiogram (ECG)
d. Are symptoms that may or may not be associated with an arrhythmia

2. Potentially lethal arrhythmias are most reliably marked as such by
a. Their reliable occurrence at night in bed
b. Their reliable occurrence with exercise
c. Their report as symptomatic by the patient
d. There is no way to predict which arrhythmias might be lethal and which might not be

3. The most reliable sign (not symptom) of hyperthyroidism is
a. Fever
b. Moist skin and heat intolerance
c. Resting heart rate > 100 bpm
d. Weight loss

4. Patients with "thyroid storm"
a. Have already passed through milder and earlier stages of hyperthyroidism
b. Almost always recover spontaneously after several months and then become hypothyroid
c. Most often have Graves' disease rather than Hashimoto's disease
d. All of the above
e. A and C

5. Atrial fibrillation (A fib) is marked by a pulse that is
a. Regularly irregular
b. Irregularly irregular
c. Irregularly regular
d. Regular with skipped beats

6. Which type of patient with untreated A fib most urgently needs referral?
a. A 35-year-old male with no other medical problems
b. A 65-year-old woman on no medications and with no other medical problems
c. A 55-year-old woman on conjugated equine estrogens
d. A 70-year-old female on blood thinners (Coumadin)

Chapter 19: SENSORY AND MOTOR PROBLEMS

Neurological disorders and neuronal damage with attendant symptoms of numbness, weakness, paralysis, or loss of balance are almost always serious. If we have patients with these symptoms, immediate referral for a thorough neurological examination is often indicated.

Persistent and progressive tingling, numbness, or weakness in any part of the body is a general red flag for *progressive neuronal destruction* that can evolve to total and permanent numbness, weakness, or paralysis. Conditions include compression neuropathies like lumbar and cervical radiculopathy (already considered), ischemic injuries like cerebral stroke, traumatic neuronal injury or injury from demyelinating diseases like multiple sclerosis (MS). There are few non-serious causes for progressive neurological symptoms.

Acute paralysis or loss of strength, balance or coordination is also a general red flag, this time for *acute neuronal damage.* Both of these are general red flags because they don't suggest a specific condition we must rule out, but a number of possible neurological lesions. Even though there are a few instances, like Bell's palsy, in which the neurological problem can heal completely, these signs and symptoms are *suggestive enough* of semi-urgent or urgent neurological conditions so that we must assume a serious condition is present until proven otherwise.

Specific red flags:
Fifteen minute episode of unilateral tingling/numbness that resolves completely

Condition assumed present until proven otherwise:

*Transient ischemic attack (TIA)*A TIA is an acute episode of temporary neurologic dysfunction caused by ischemia (tissue threat without permanent damage) due to vascular occlusion with symptoms lasting less than one hour. (A cerebrovascular accident – CVA – is a "stroke" with permanent neurological damage – tissue infarction.)

Possible consequences of missing the condition:

Up to 20% of patients with new TIA will later have a disabling or fatal stroke later.

Stabilization, referral and management:

1. **Stabilization:** If you see a patient during the symptoms of a TIA, you should have them lie down quietly and follow directions below. If they are between neurological episodes, they should be told about the advantages of taking one baby aspirin/day in preventing a possible stroke until the consult is accomplished.
2. **Consultation and Referral Options, Transportation:** Several scenarios are possible and are outlined below.

- *If the patient is in the midst of neurological symptoms,* they should be managed on an urgent basis because it is impossible to say if the patient will recover or progress to a stroke (CVA). They should therefore be transported by the quickest available means to an ED. The same holds true if they are not currently having an attack, but they have been having attacks that are getting more frequent and severe (crescendo pattern) recently. A call should be placed to the triage person at the ED to inform them about the patient's condition. If they also have cardiopulmonary instability, 911 should be called (see red flags for chest pain).
- *If the patient had a TIA that has resolved,* they can receive a same day, semi-urgent consultation with their PCP or a neurologist if no PCP is available. Because of the small incidence of stroke in two or three days (see below), some of these patients may need to be sent to the ED if no consultant can see them within the same day.

Relevance to acupuncturists: TIAs are not uncommon and patients often underestimate their importance once the symptoms pass, especially if they are mild. It is therefore important to recognize this red flag and emphasize its importance to the patient so that timely consult is obtained to avoid a possible stroke.

ACTUAL CASE

- **History:** A 40-year-old female came to the office with fear that "I may have MS." Her mother and one sister had MS. Several days earlier, she had a five minute episode of numbness, tingling, and weakness in her left arm and left leg that resolved completely. Her only medication was an estrogen and progestin containing oral contraceptive. She denied double vision (sometimes seen with MS) or prior episodes of similar symptoms and was otherwise healthy.
- **Physical findings:** The patient was mildly obese. She was alert and oriented and had a normal neurological exam. Her blood pressure was 130/90 bpm.
- **Impression:** Likely TIA
- **Plan:** The patient was sent to her PCP.
- **Follow up:** The PCP placed the patient on one baby aspirin daily and blood pressure medicine to lower her pressure to the 120/80mmhg range. She was taken off her oral contraceptives. She had an echocardiogram to look for valvular problems of the heart, a twenty four hour holter monitor to rule out an arrhythmia, and a carotid doppler study. She also had an MRI of the brain. All studies were negative. After discussing alternatives, a non-hormone IUD was placed for contraception. She was started on a low sugar and animal fat diet and an exercise program to decrease her percentage of body fat. She has not had a recurrent TIA.

DISCUSSION

History and Symptoms

Most patients with TIAs will present to clinicians days to weeks after the attack has passed. It is not uncommon for them to minimize symptoms by the time they see you. Family members or other witnesses should be sought out to provide more information about the attack because they might have noticed subtle abnormalities the patient didn't notice like changes in speech, gait, memory or movement. When they affect the extremities, which is usual, TIAs are almost always unilateral, which can be quite helpful in the diagnosis. TIAs can also present with transient aphasia, wherein patients have difficulty finding words that are common, such as "pencil" or "chair," for example.

This kind of information can only be obtained by careful and thorough questioning about the onset, duration, and intensity of symptoms. We can see from the consultation section that we must know this kind of information in order to stratify the possible risk for the patient. There is a lot of difference between a brief and mild episode of unilateral tingling in one arm that resolves quickly and two hours of unilateral numbness with weakness of an arm and leg or a crescendo pattern of TIAs. (Some define TIAs as lasting under 24 hours, although it's likely that some of these "long-lasting TIAs" are actually small strokes that leave little damage.)

Physical Exam Findings

The symptoms of TIA more often lead you to suspect a TIA than the signs do because, as mentioned, the TIA is usually over when you see the patient and no signs may remain. There will be no residual physical exam signs unless there has been a stroke. Still, it is a good idea to do a neurological exam on patients you think might have had a TIA because they may have actually had a small stroke. For information on a full neurological exam, please consult a text on the physical exam. Here are a few reminders of some of the most useful parts of the exam.

A handy way to remember to do a quick mental status exam is to remember not to OMIT the mental status exam (O for checking Orientation to person, place and time, M for checking Memory function, I for checking their Intelligence function and T for checking their Talking—language function). A standard check on cranial nerves, sensation, muscle strength, reflexes, balance, and special tests as outlined in the spinal cord injury section should give you the information you need to see if damage was done. The heart and carotids should also be checked because TIAs can emanate from blocked carotid arteries (carotid bruit may be present) or the heart (an arrhythmia or heart murmurs indicating valvular damage may be present).

Incidence and/or Prevalence

200,000-500,000 TIAs occur in the U.S. each year and are the cause of 1.1 ED visits per 1,000 total visits yearly. The most important short-term risk of a TIA is stroke. The *early* risk of stroke following TIA is about 4-5% at two days and as high as 11% at seven days. A slightly higher incidence of TIAs is noted in African-American men compared to Caucasians and men compared to women.

Risk Factors

Risk factors patients can't change

- Family history
- Advancing age (> 55 years old)

- Male sex
- African-American ethnicity

Risk factors patients can do something about

- High blood pressure
- Carotid artery disease (CAD) peripheral vascular disease (PVD)
- Cigarette smoking
- Physical inactivity
- Diabetes
- Diet high in animal fat and salt (in salt sensitive patients)
- Low HDL, high LDL, high TG, high homocysteine levels, high C-reactive protein (CRP)
- Obesity
- Too much alcohol intake
- Use of cocaine and other drugs
- Birth control pills should be avoided if obesity, diabetes, or high blood pressure exist.

Mechanism Producing the Red Flag

The mechanism of injury is generally small emboli that dislodge from carotid plaques or form in the heart and travel to cerebral vessel where they get stuck and block blood flow. TIAs and CVA are therefore caused by the same mechanism, but blockage in TIA is brief and leaves no permanent damage. Plaques can be large enough to decrease the blood flow through an artery or parts of the plaque can break off and/or blood clots can form around them and travel to distant sites.

Other Important Considerations

- Although the great majority of patients who take oral contraceptives do so safely, there is some risk in taking them, especially in older females and those with risk factors of obesity, hypertension, and others listed in risk factor section.
- Supplementary non-bioidentical estrogen and even bioidentical estrogen given orally increase risk of blood clots in postmenopausal women. Thus, the safest route for replacement is through the skin.
- Progesterone supplementation should be bio-identical only in post-menopausal women. Synthetic alternatives increase blood clot risk.

Specific red flags: *Slow onset of patchy numbness and weakness of >1 body areas*

Condition assumed present until proven otherwise:
Multiple sclerosis (MS) – MS is the most common of several autoimmune demyelinating diseases in the brain and spinal cord.

Possible consequences of missing the condition:
Disability or possible death

Stabilization, referral and management:

1. **Stabilization:** There are no immediate stabilizing steps to take.
2. **Consultation and Referral Options, Transportation:** The referral should generally be on a timely basis because MS is a slow moving disease. The only exception would be a patient with a drastic complication of fairly advanced MS, like urosepsis from bladder dysfunction which might necessitate referral to the ED.

Relevance to acupuncturists: Because MS is not uncommon, patients who have the condition will be encountered by acupuncturists, some undiagnosed. Although there is no cure for MS at the time of this writing, proper management of this condition can often delay the onset of serious disability and possible death from associated conditions and prepare the patient for a cure when it is found. For these reasons, it is important to detect this illness and consult regarding it early.

ACTUAL CASE

- **History:** A 30-year-old female accountant presented for acupuncture treatment for what she said had been diagnosed by her medical doctor as a "pinched skin nerve." Her complaint at that time was an area of numbness on the outside of her left thigh. She was told it would go away on its own if she wore a looser belt around her waist ("superficial femoral cutaneous neuropathy"). The numbness had indeed faded, only to be replaced by patchy areas of numbness on both legs, some of which also came and went. She also noticed some weakness in her left leg when getting up out of chairs and had an episode of blurry vision a week earlier that had lasted two days.

- **Physical findings:** The patient looked generally well. Her subjectively numb areas did seem to be slightly less sensitive to light touch using a cotton ball than other normal areas. Her eye movement (extraocular muscle) exam was normal and the pupils were bilaterally symmetrical and reacted to light normally. There was mildly decreased quadriceps strength in her left leg compared to her right. There were no pathological reflex changes.
- **Impression:** Possible multiple sclerosis
- **Plan:** The patient's PCP was contacted by phone and informed of the change in her patient's condition.
- **Follow up:** The patient was seen one week later by her PCP and an MRI confirmed the presence of scattered demyelinated areas in the brain. She was started on vitamins, minerals, and fish oils, but her symptoms began worsening dramatically. She was given a course of steroids and had dramatic remission of almost all of her symptoms. The steroids were eventually stopped. She was left with only a mild amount of weakness in her quadriceps and has not had another setback in the last several months.

DISCUSSION

History and Symptoms

The most common presenting symptoms of MS are paresthesias and/or areas of patchy numbness in one or more extremities, trunk, or face, and/or weakness or clumsiness of a leg or hand. When numbness occurs, it does so in a way that is somewhat distinct from other illnesses. It tends to be patchy, often skipping over dermatomes. The areas can come and go in as quickly as in a few days to a few weeks. This is a rather distinct feature of MS when it occurs. Double vision due to ocular palsy is also fairly common, though not as common initially as skin tingling and skeletal muscle weakness.

Other common early symptoms include a feeling of slight stiffness of a limb, minor gait disturbances, difficulty with bladder function, and vertigo. Warm weather or a hot bath may temporarily exacerbate symptoms. In some cases, mild cognitive impairment, apathy, poor judgment, emotional liability, or depression may also occur. However, these latter symptoms are so non-specific that they rarely help with diagnosis unless the weakness and numbness are present. Depression may be reactive or partly due to cerebral lesions of MS. Fatigue is also very common in MS patients. Problems with speech and swallowing are also possible.

Muscle spasticity, bladder dysfunction, and bowel dysfunction (inadequate emptying in both cases) are very common as MS progresses. This is because upper motor neurons (UMNs) in the brain and spinal cord exert an antispasmodic (inhibitory) effect on many muscles, including sphincter muscles. With the loss of UMNs, there is a loss of inhibition and spasticity develops. Lower motor neurons (LMNs) in the spinal cord can also be affected, leading to flaccidity of muscle, so the advanced MS patient can have problems with both spasticity in some areas of the body and flaccidity in others.

Since white matter in the cerebellum is often damaged, MS patients can develop ataxia, imbalance, and difficulty with coordination. When added to the difficulty with sensation, loss of position sense (in the spinal column) and generalized weakness in muscles, balance problems can eventually make ambulation impossible, leaving such patients wheelchair bound and in need of significant assistance in activities of daily living (ADLs). The inability to ambulate can add to stasis of urine in the already dysfunctional bladder and urosepsis can occur, leading to death if bladder infections are not aggressively controlled.

Although this worst case scenario paints a rather grim picture of MS, some MS patients do remarkably well over a long period of time with minimal symptoms. The neurological problems associated with MS can go along in cycles of exacerbations and remission or pauses in their progression several times a year.

Physical Exam Findings

The physical exam for MS can be quite lengthy and we need only review some of the most important signs and tests that can be performed by interested acupuncturists. As in all other areas of neurology, you are referred to a standard text on physical exam for greater detail. In general, however, you should always start with the most general signs you can glean from inspection, like gross ataxia, lack of balance, weakness, or balance problems in ambulation and a brief assessment of mental status as described under the previous red flag. You will obviously want to test areas the patient claims are numb with a soft object, like the tuft of a cotton ball. Major muscles should be tested for strength. The limb reflexes should be elicited. In all of these tests, both sides should be tested and compared with one another. There are many special neurological tests that can be done, but only a few will be listed for the sake of interest here. Some of these are the same as those described under the red flag regarding spinal cord injuries because the spinal cord can also be affected in MS.

- Romberg's sign – a test for incoordination or clumsiness of movement (ataxia) in which the patient stands with feet together and eyes closed
- Gait and coordination tests can be done by observing the patient walk heel-to-toe and by having the patient rapidly perform finger-to-nose touching repeatedly.
- A standard vision test should be done due to the high incidence of optic neuritis in MS.
- Vibration and position sense of toes (see neck pain and spinal cord injury section)
- The Babinski reflex test (see neck pain and spinal cord injury section)

Incidence and/or Prevalence

MS is usually a young person's disease that often strikes people in their prime. Disease onset usually occurs between 20-40 years of age and is more common in women. The prevalence in the U.S. is 0.14% or 388,571 people.

Risk Factors

- People with a family history of MS
- MS is more likely to occur in the cooler climates. Highest incidence occurs in northern Europe, northern U.S., southern Australia and New Zealand.

Mechanism Producing the Red Flag

MS is a progressive neurodegenerative disease. It is caused by damage to the myelin sheath, the protective covering that surrounds nerve cells and allows for faster conduction of impulses along neurons. This causes nerve impulses to slow down or stop. The damage is caused by inflammation due to an autoantibody reaction. Repeated episodes of inflammation can occur in any area of the brain and/or spinal cord. The most common theories of etiology point to an antibody reaction against a virus or genetic predisposition, or more likely, a combination of the two.

Some nerve cell damage is also possible, but less likely. Fibrous plaques become disseminated throughout the CNS, primarily in white matter in the lateral and posterior columns of the spinal cord (especially in the cervical cord), optic nerves, and periventricular areas of the brain. Tracts in the midbrain, pons, and cerebellum are also affected.

Other Important Considerations

- According to a recent study by Munger et. al. in *Neurology* 2004; 62:60-65, Vitamin D intake can significantly protect against the development of MS
- The author of this book considers the above suspicions for why people in the northern latitudes get MS more often. Vitamin D_3 is produced in the skin from sun exposure. People in the northern latitudes get less sun exposure, and hence, make less vitamin D_3.

Review What You Have Learned
Chapter 19 Sensory and Motor Problems

1. A patient with a clear history of a transient ischemic attack such as unilateral arm and leg tingling, numbness and/or loss of function lasting 5-15 minutes

a. Should be advised to take one baby aspirin daily until their consult is achieved unless they have a prior history of peptic ulcer or esophageal irritation or bleeding
b. Has an 80% chance for a stroke within 10 days of the original attack
c. Should be advised to quit taking an oral contraceptive if they are taking one
d. A and C

2. Some differences between multiple sclerosis (MS) and recurrent TIAs would be

a. The onset of MS is slow whereas the onset of a TIA is rapid
b. MS effects motor nerve fibers first whereas TIAs effect sensory nerve fibers first
c. TIAs are more common in females whereas MS is more common in males
d. All of the above

Chapter 20: SKIN PROBLEMS, LUMPS & BUMPS

Most adults know that anything growing on or under the skin that is not supposed to be there is abnormal. This chapter tells you which skin abnormalities are red flags for which conditions and how they should be screened.

The task of detecting skin and subcutaneous cancer is too big and important to be in the hands of any one type of physician alone. It requires vigilance and a "high index of suspicion" by all providers, including acupuncturists who arguably look at the skin as much as any other type of practitioner. It requires awareness on the part of patients as well. All patients should be taught about the warning signs by health care providers who are familiar with these lesions. The rule for any provider who notices a potentially dangerous lesion should be "when in doubt, refer."

Skin cancers are the most common of cancers, accounting for approximately half of all cancers. The worst type is melanoma because melanoma is metastatic (spreads through the blood stream to distant sites). It is explored under its own specific red flag in this chapter. The next two lesions we'll consider are not metastatic, but can grow extensively in local tissue: basal cell and squamous cell carcinomas. They are not examined under specific red flags, but deserve special comment here because, while not often deadly, they can be quite disfiguring.

Basal cell carcinomas are generally nodular and develop pearly surfaces. They may start to grow suddenly (over weeks to months) and can grow large enough to necessitate removing big areas of skin that can result in significant scarring. Squamous cell carcinomas are often less nodular. They may be more ragged and spread out in appearance. Basal and squamous cell carcinomas are very similar, but squamous cell carcinoma tends to be more invasive than basal cell carcinoma and can grow into bone and other tissues beside skin. Both should be removed early.

The best way to strengthen your understanding about these lesions is to study these lesions visually by consulting a standard dermatology text or online site with pictures of them. The other nodules we consider as specific red flags in the chapter cannot be easily seen because they are under the dermis, but can be easily felt on palpation.

Specific red flags:
Growth or change in dark skin lesion

Condition assumed present until proven otherwise:
Malignant melanoma

Possible consequences of missing the condition:
Metastasis and death

Stabilization, referral and management:

1. **Stabilization:** There are no immediately stabilizing steps to take
2. **Consultation and Referral Options, Transportation:** Finding what appears to be a malignant melanoma is a semi-urgent situation warranting consultation with the patient's PCP if one is available or a dermatologist if there is no PCP. This is one of those fairly unique situations wherein referral to a free-standing urgent care center is not an equivalent option because it may be staffed by physicians with little dermatology training or those not trained to do biopsies (general internists, for example). They could refer that patient onward, however, if no arrangement can be made with an FP or a dermatologist.

Relevance to acupuncturists: Acupuncturists will see malignant lesions, including malignant melanomas due to their high incidence (see incidence below). Due to the high probability of widespread metastasis, spotting these lesions and teaching patients about how to spot them early can be lifesaving. Again, we are not asking acupuncturists to diagnose malignant melanoma but to know which dark skin lesions to refer.

ACTUAL CASE

- **History:** A 28-year-old Caucasian female yoga teacher came to the acupuncture clinic for treatment of menstrual irregularities. While on the table, the acupuncture student noticed a small, irregular, dark lesion on her abdomen. The patient claimed she had many such "moles" on her body, but they had been checked by her family doctor a year earlier and she was told "not to worry about them." She was instructed to return to have them checked again in one year, but she had not returned for a recheck due to her busy schedule.
- **Physical findings:** The patient had many scattered tan to dark moles on her torso, almost all of which were elevated and many of which had some hair growth on them (signs that they were probably benign). The lesion in question was periumbilical in location and was approximately 2cm in diameter, entirely flat, asymmetrical, irregular bordered and multicolored, but mostly dark brown to black. It did not look like the other moles and the patient finally realized on questioning that it had grown in the preceding three months.
- **Impression:** Possible malignant melanoma
- **Plan:** The patient was sent to her PCP at the direction of the attending acupuncture teacher.
- **Follow up:** The patient's PCP checked her for regional lymph nodes and checked the patient's liver enzymes (to check for local metastasis and widespread metastasis respectively) and found the nodes to be nonpalpable and the liver enzymes negative. He thought the lesion was highly suspicious for melanoma despite its small size and excised it with wide margins. The pathology report was positive for melanoma. The report also stated that the tumor was completely excised and the margins of the excised skin were negative for tumor cells. The patient's surgical site was watched closely for recurrence, as was the remainder of her skin for other suspicious areas. She had an additional small melanoma removed the following year and several benign melanocytic nevi as well.

Discussion

History and Symptoms

There are no symptoms of malignant melanoma unless there is metastasis, in which case there are the usual symptoms of cancer as discussed in other sections of this book.

Physical Exam Findings

Melanomas are usually dark, like melanocytic moles, but can be identified as suspicious when they grow in an unregulated way, unlike a mole. They can exhibit one or usually more of the A, B, C, D, E's of melanoma: Asymmetry because if folded, the two sides would not look alike. Borders are irregular or blurred. Color is often dark and contains mixed shades. Diameter is *usually* greater than six mm. Evolving skin lesion that looks different from others in shape, size or color.

Incidence and/or Prevalence

Even though melanomas account for less than 5% of all skin cancers, they cause the great majority of skin cancer deaths. The statistics are alarming. The incidence of melanoma is approximated 3% of the U.S. population yearly making for over nine million people who get this potentially deadly malignancy. Approximately 8,600 die from it. One in 50 Caucasian Americans will get melanoma sometime in their lives.

Risk Factors

- Ultraviolet A (UVA) and ultraviolet B (UVB) exposure: There is a dose response relationship between melanoma and exposure. The higher the total exposure (intensity x total time exposed), the higher the risk for melanoma. Sunlight and tanning beds are the main sources of both UVA and UVB.
- Dysplastic nevi: Dysplastic nevi look half way between normal moles and melanoma. A small number of them develop into melanomas, but most never do. Lifetime melanoma risk may be > 10% for those with many dysplastic nevi, however (*dysplastic nevus syndrome runs in families*). Patients with many dysplastic nevi and close relatives with melanoma have a 50% or greater lifetime risk of developing melanoma.
- Congenital melanocytic nevi: Moles present at birth also present some increased risk of melanoma (0–10%, depending on the size of the nevus, with higher risk for larger nevi.
- Fair skin, freckling, and light hair: The risk of melanoma is >10 times higher for white skinned people than for African-Americans. Red-haired people have the highest risk.
- Family history of melanoma: Approximately 10% of all people with melanoma have a family history of the disease. The increased risk might be due to family lifestyle (frequent sun exposure), a tendency for fair skin, inherited gene mutations, or combinations of these factors.
- Personal history of melanoma: Patients who have had

melanoma are at increased risk of getting melanoma again (5%–10% will develop a second one).
- Suppressed immune systems.
- Increasing age: Although melanoma is less related to aging than most other cancers, all other factors being equal, melanomas are more common as people age. This association is not as great a factor as most other cancers however, and melanoma is one of the most common cancers in people < 30 years old, especially if heredity is a factor.
- Males have higher incidence rates than females.
- Xeroderma pigmentosum (XP): Melanomas, basal cell, and squamous cell carcinomas are more common in people with XP, a rare, inherited condition causing a defect in an enzyme that repairs damage to DNA.

Mechanism Producing the Red Flag

The mechanism of melanoma formation, like other cancers, is the result of damage to the DNA within cells, which gives melanoma the same aggressive tendencies of other cancer cells discussed elsewhere in this book

Specific red flags:
Unilateral, painless lymph node swelling in the neck, arm or groin

Condition assumed present until proven otherwise

Lymphoma – a cancer involving lymphocytes in lymph nodes

Possible consequences of missing the condition

Death from metastasis and blood disease

Stabilization, referral and management

1. **Stabilization:** There are no specific stabilizing steps to take.
2. **Consultation and Referral Options, Transportation:** Patients with solitary lymph nodes should be referred on a timely basis to the patient's PCP within a week. Most will turn out to be benign on biopsy. It may be reassuring to let patients know this. Nonetheless, the referral for biopsy must be made to catch the malignant lesions. The PCP will most likely refer to a surgeon for the biopsy. A free-standing medical clinic will be appropriate if no PCP is available or referral can be made directly to a surgeon.

Relevance to acupuncturists: Lymph node swellings are common in patients. They may be discovered on acupuncture points. Knowing which of these represent the possibility of cancer is extremely important because patients with lymphomas that are treated early, especially Hodgkin's lymphomas, can almost always be cured.

ACTUAL CASE

- **History:** The patient was a 23-year-old college student who was being treated with acupuncture for neck pain.
- **Physical findings:** In palpating the muscles of his neck we noticed a solitary, nonpainful nodule in the patient's left anterior neck with no similar lesion on the other side or lymphadenopathy in any other area.
- **Impression:** Lymphadenopathy; rule out lymphoma
- **Plan:** The patient was referred to the college health care center. He saw a PCP there and was referred to a local surgeon.
- **Follow up:** The patient had a biopsy that turned out positive for Hodgkin's lymphoma (HL). Fortunately, the lymphoma was rated as a stage one lymphoma (lymphoma is rated as stage one if cancer is found in only one lymph node or in one area or organ outside the lymph node). He was treated with radiation therapy and has not had a recurrence of his lymphoma in the five years from its appearance and this writing.

DISCUSSION

History and Symptoms

The first symptom of lymphoma is often the patient's discovery of a painless swelling in the neck, underarm or groin. Experienced primary care physicians know the great majority of such discoveries are found to be normal bony protuberances, benign cysts, or bilaterally palpable lymph nodes in which the patient doesn't notice the contralateral nodule. Nevertheless, patients will occasionally discover a genuine solitary swollen lymph node.

Most people with early lymphoma have no other symptoms. An enlarged lymph node, however, may occasionally compress a vein or lymphatic vessel and cause swelling in an arm or leg or press against a nerve and cause pain, numbness, or tingling. Since the spleen contains a great deal of lymphatic tissue, patients with lymphoma, usually advanced, may have abdominal pain or discomfort from a swollen spleen or occasionally from pressure against the stomach.

Other symptoms of lymphoma may include fevers, chills, unexplained weight loss, night sweats, fatigue, or itching. These symptoms are notoriously non-specific and could be caused by any number of other conditions unrelated to cancer. In these cases, however, we would expect that they would come and go. In lymphoma, as in other cancers, symptoms like these are persistent or even progressive over time and cannot be explained by infection or other diseases.

Physical Exam Findings

The clinician should carefully check to see if lymphadenopathy is really unilateral, like the patient thinks. If a similar node can be found on the contralateral side, this discovery makes it much less likely that lymphoma is present. Also, tenderness of a node makes it much more likely to be a "reactive" lymph node from a nearby infection that is draining through the node region than a lymphoma. Tonsillar inflammation, for example, commonly causes bilateral anterior submandibular lymphadenopathy. *Solitary reactive lymphadenopathy* can be caused by local skin infections and can masquerade as a cancerous lymph node, but the source of infection, often a scratch or abrasion of nearby skin, can usually be found. The signs of advanced lymphoma are basically the same as for other types of cancer because advanced lymphomas will not stay confined to predominantly lymphatic tissue only but will eventually metastasize and invade other tissues throughout the body.

Incidence and/or Prevalence

Lymphoma is the most common type of blood cancer in the United States. It is the seventh most common cancer in adults and the third most common in children. Lymphomas fall into two major categories: Hodgkin's lymphoma (HL, previously called Hodgkin's disease) and all other lymphomas (non-Hodgkin's lymphomas or NHLs). Non-Hodgkin's lymphomas are far more common than Hodgkin's lymphoma. The incidence of both is increasing. HL has the greatest survival rate of all types of lymphoma and is most common in young adults between 16-34 years of age. Non-Hodgkin's lymphomas are more likely in older people. About 66,000 new cases of NHL and 8,500 new cases of HL were diagnosed in 2009. There were approximately 19,500 deaths due to NHLs and 1,290 due to HL.

Risk Factors

- Age: The incidence of NHLs increases with advancing age. HL in the elderly is associated with a poorer prognosis than in younger patients.
- Infections: HIV, Epstein-Barr virus (EBV) *Helicobacter pylori*, hepatitis B or C virus
- Autoimmune disease
- Immune suppressive therapy, as used following organ transplant
- Inherited immunodeficiency diseases
- Exposure to toxic chemicals: pesticides, herbicides, benzene and other solvents
- Black hair dye has been linked to higher rates of NHL for at least 20 years

Mechanism Producing the Red Flag

The lymphomas can derive from either abnormal B or T cells. There are five subtypes of Hodgkin's disease and about 30 subtypes of non-Hodgkin's lymphomas that can be distinguished only by unique genetic markers. Hodgkin's disease, for example, develops from a specific B lymphocyte lineage. The two types produce the same symptoms and signs regardless of cell type. The cancerous lymph cells grow so much that they cause swelling of tissues in which lymphocytes are prevalent such as lymph nodes, the spleen, tonsils, bone marrow, and the thymus gland.

Another Important Consideration

- Lymphomas are staged from stage I through stage IV with worsening prognosis the higher the staging. Many stage I and II lymphomas are completely cured by modern methods.

Specific red flags:
Painless and hard area within the testicle of a young adult male

Condition assumed present until proven otherwise

Testicular cancer

Possible consequences of missing the condition

Potentially rapidly fatal

Stabilization, referral and management

1. **Stabilization:** There are no specific stabilizing steps to take
2. **Consultation and Referral Options, Transportation:** It is preferable to refer patients with this red flag on a semi-urgent basis, although a delay of a week can often occur if the patient will see the urologist. As always, an attempt to refer the patient to their PCP, if they have one, is probably the best way to expedite this process.

Relevance to acupuncturists: The presence of a testicular lump or mass may come to your attention via a question from your patient, as it did in our actual case study below. This is another one of those situations, like postmenopausal vaginal bleeding or gross hematuria in older men, wherein recognition of an early sign of cancer and appropriately referring the patient may mean the difference between a complete cure versus an agonizing death for your patient.

Actual Case

- **History:** A 25-year-old male came in for acupuncture treatment of a "stiff neck." While we were taking his history, he mentioned that he found a hard area on his left testicle that was not painful. He wondered what we thought about it.
- **Physical findings:** Since the genital exam is not within the acupuncture scope of practice, the patient was referred for his question.
- **Impression:** Possible testicular carcinoma
- **Plan:** The patient did not have a PCP and the two urologists we contacted were only taking referrals from a PCP. The patient was therefore referred to a free-standing medical clinic.
- **Follow up:** The patient was seen by a physician at a free standing medical clinic who could not make the determination about what the testicular swelling was. A urologist was consulted who performed a scrotal ultrasound. Fortunately, the lump was benign and not a testicular cancer. The patient, who returned for acupuncture treatments, was quite grateful for his care and relieved by the consult.

DISCUSSION

History and Symptoms

Most patients with testicular cancer have no symptoms. Some are fortunate enough to have found a non-tender, pea sized lump on a testicle in its early stage. Rarely, there can be a dull ache in the lower abdomen or groin or a sensation of scrotal heaviness. In late stages, of course, patients will have all of the full-blown symptoms of metastatic cancer.

Physical Exam Findings

The sign of testicular cancer is a smooth, non-tender lump or area of induration (hardness) within the body of the testicle (not on top of the testicle).

Incidence and/or Prevalence

Testicular cancer accounts for only 1% of all cancers in males, but 11-13% of all cancer deaths in men between the ages of 15-35. It peaks before the age of 40 years old (90% of cases) and again after 50 years old (a small second peak). It is most common in Caucasians, especially of Scandinavian descent. The incidence rate has more than doubled among Caucasians in the past 40 years, but has only recently begun to increase in African-Americans.

Risk Factors

- Undescended testicle (cryptorchidism): Normally, the testicles descend from inside the abdomen into the scrotal sac before birth. The risk of testicular cancer is greatly increased in testicles that do not descend. The risk does not decrease after surgery to move the testicle into the scrotum.
- Congenital abnormalities: Men born with abnormalities of the testicles, penis, or kidneys or with inguinal hernias may be at increased risk.
- History of testicular cancer: Men who have had testicular cancer in one testicle are at increased risk of developing cancer in the opposite testicle.
- Family history of testicular cancer: The risk for testicular cancer is greater in men whose brother or father has had the disease.

Mechanism Producing the Red Flag

There are two major types of testicular cancer, seminomas and nonseminomas. Like all other cancer, the problem starts with changes in the DNA of the seminal vesicle cells in seminomas and nonseminal cells in nonseminomas. After metastasis of the cancer, the typical changes of metastatic cancer are seen.

Another Important Consideration

- Men should be instructed to perform a testicular cancer self-exam each month while standing up, preferably after a hot shower or bath to relax the muscles because testicular cancer has a cure rate of almost 100% if found in early stages.

Review What You Have Learned

Chapter 20 Skin Problems, Lumps and Bumps

1. Which list of skin lesions is arranged correctly from least to most dangerous?

a. Basal cell carcinoma, squamous cell carcinoma, melanoma
b. Basal cell carcinoma, melanoma, squamous cell carcinoma
c. Squamous cell carcinoma, basal cell carcinoma, melanoma
d. Melanoma, basal cell carcinoma, squamous cell carcinoma

2. The ABCDE of melanoma refers to

a. Asymmetry, Black color, Cauliflower-like shape, Diameter, Evasive
b. Asymmetry, Burgeoning, Color, Dirty looking, Evolving
c. Asymmetry, Bold, Cold, Diameter, Everywhere
d. Asymmetry, Borders, Color, Diameter, Evolving

3. What characteristics of enlarged lymph nodes would cause most concern for malignancy?

a. Very tender and warm bilateral lymph nodes in the cervical region
b. A solitary, hard, fixed, unilateral lymph node in the neck
c. Bilateral large lymph nodes in the groin area
d. All of the above

4. The internationally famous athlete Lance Armstrong fought and won a public battle with testicular cancer. What is true about testicular cancer?

a. The peak incidence is in men older than 50 years old
b. Risk factors include history of an undescended testicle
c. Men with history of testicular cancer in one testicle are at higher risk for it in the other testicle
d. All of the above
e. B and C

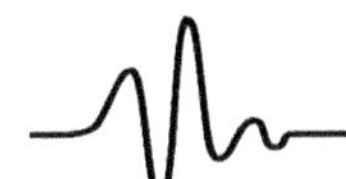

Chapter 21: SWELLING

Swelling that is not self-limiting can be a very serious symptom. In this chapter, we learn about three types of swelling that can be symptomatic of very serious disease and which require further screening and possible emergency medical intervention.

Specific red flags:
One-sided ankle/distal calf swelling or asymmetric bilateral swelling (> 3 cm difference)

Condition assumed present until proven otherwise:

Blood clot in a deep vein of the calf (deep venous thrombosis – DVT)

Possible consequences of missing the condition:

Dislodged clot can travel through veins to the lungs causing pulmonary embolus (PE). PE can cause death within minutes. (Red flags for PE are discussed separately under chest pain.)

Stabilization, referral and management:

1. **Stabilization:** There are no specific stabilizing actions to take except to tell the patient to avoid walking as much as possible to prevent dislodgment of a clot. The patient should also avoid coagulant ("stop bleeding") herbs and physical techniques applied to the legs like massage, *gua sha, tui na*, or cupping to avoid the possibility of dislodging a clot.
2. **Consultation and Referral Options, Transportation:** DVT *without* the additional red flag for pulmonary embolism (chest pain and shortness of breath) should be referred for same-day care at an ED in a nearby hospital with private transport, preferably with a friend or family member driving. DVT *with* the additional red flag of pulmonary embolism (chest pain and shortness of breath) warrants immediate activation of emergency medical services with a call to 911 (see red flag for PE under chest pain).

Relevance to acupuncturists: Ankle swelling is frequently encountered in primary care practices. Acupuncturists will note ankle edema in routine palpation or needling of acupoints. "Pitting" ankle edema (an indentation remains in the skin after pressure from the examining finger is removed) is sometimes a sign of serious and sometimes even life-threatening conditions. If present, further history and physical exam is warranted to assess for the presence of such conditions. Having "big" ankles from genetics or obesity is not the same as pitting edema, although patients often won't know the difference between the two. Patients with big ankles may develop pitting edema, however, adding to the overall size of the ankle.

Actual Case

- **History:** A 38-year-old Chinese American female came to the office with complaints of ankle swelling that had begun after a plane ride when returning from a visit to China. She had a prior history of ankle swelling after long flights, but this time the swelling seemed to last longer than usual. She denied overt pain, but said the back of her left calf felt "full" and looked "a little red." Oral contraceptives were her only medication.
- **Physical findings:** The patient looked fit and trim. Vital signs, including respirations, were normal. She had a trace of pitting edema of the right ankle and 2+ pitting edema of the left ankle and distal calf midway up the calf. The difference was 3.5 cm between the right and left ankles with the left being larger. There was some tenderness of the left calf to pressure and slight red duskiness of the skin of the posterior calf. Homan's test (forceful dorsiflexion of the ankle) was negative, *i.e.*, there was no significant pain. Her lungs were clear.
- **Impression:** Despite negative Homan's sign, probable DVT of left calf

- **Plan:** The patient was sent to the ED of a nearby hospital. A call was made to the triage nurse that we were sending in a patient with a possible DVT of her left calf.
- **Follow up:** A venous Doppler study of the left leg was performed in the ED and was positive for a distal calf DVT. The patient was admitted and placed on anticoagulant therapy until the clot became stable (adherent within the vein so it could not dislodge and travel to the lung). The patient was discharged on ongoing anticoagulation with Coumadin® to prevent further clots.

Discussion

History and Symptoms

The presentation of DVTs ranges from mild pitting edema without other signs to significant swelling, pain and redness in the area over the clot. Usually DVTs present with unilateral symptoms, bilateral asymmetric edema is also fairly common, especially in the elderly.

Physical Exam Findings

Swelling may be limited to the ankle, but usually extends up to the mid calf. Dark redness and palpable deep tenderness of the posterior calf muscle is often present, but may not be present in early cases. A positive Homan's sign is usually found on exam. The edema is "pitting." Your thumb or finger will leave an indentation after pressure, whereas the indentation will not remain in non-pitting edema.

Incidence and/or Prevalence

Calf vein DVTs are common. The incidence is 7/1,000 in females and 5/1,000 in males.

Risk Factors

- Recent surgery or trauma involving the affected leg
- Smoking
- Leg immobilization or lack of physical activity (including post-fracture casting, recent airplane travel, prolonged bedrest, and/or generally sedentary occupation and lifestyle)
- Obesity
- Recent or current chemotherapy
- History of prior blood clots, coagulopathy (thick blood)
- Estrogen or progestin containing birth control pills or hormone replacement
- General vascular pathology risk factors

Mechanism Producing the Red Flag

Clotting in the deep veins of the calves, thighs, or pelvis causes back pressure in the veins resulting in fluid egress from the veins into the loose subcutaneous tissue of the ankle and calf causing the pitting edema.

Another Important Consideration

- There may be simultaneous non-urgent edema from superficial thrombophlebitis (clots and inflammation in superficial veins) or skin infection (cellulitis), which may throw the practitioner off the track of a concurrent DVT. Regardless of the presence of edema from other causes, we must respond as if a DVT is present when confronted with the presence of this red flag.

Specific red flags:
Bilateral, pitting ankle swelling with shortness of breath

Condition assumed present until proven otherwise:

Congestive heart failure (CHF) – Heart failure (HF) is the inability of the heart to provide enough cardiac output to supply the metabolic needs of the body. When cardiac output decreases to a critical amount, blood begins to back up through the into the blood vessels of the lungs, causing CHF. As the pressure rises even more, it pushes backward into the vena cava and blood vessels of the legs, causing ankle edema. Thus, ankle edema should be recognized as signifying a late stage of CHF.

Possible consequences of missing the condition:

Disability and death

Stabilization, referral and management:

1. **Stabilization:** Patients can sometime be stabilized by resuming their heart and blood pressure medications if they have skipped doses or stopped them. Cutting back on sodium in their diet can also help tremendously until the consult is obtained.
2. **Consultation and Referral Options, Transportation:** Who and/or where to refer to depends on the level of decompensation as indicated by the degree of SOB of other

signs of inadequate cardiac output like cerebral insufficiency, symptoms of fainting, fatigue, etc., as well as ankle edema. Mildly decompensated patients (a little pitting edema and perhaps mild SOB) should be referred to their family physician on a semi-urgent basis. Moderately decompensated patients with moderate SOB and moderate to severe edema should be sent to the nearest ED by quick transport, perhaps with a relative driving. Added symptoms of chest pain, severe dyspnea, and/or cyanosis require a 911 call for emergency transportation.

Relevance to acupuncturists: All clinicians will see so many patients with some degree of ankle swelling that we can well underestimate its significance. A key finding is to see if the edema is pitting. Even though there are non-serious causes for pitting edema like poor venous competence or inflammatory swelling of the skin, pitting edema may also have a serious cause, like CHF or renal disease, and recognition of this as a red flag is very important.

ACTUAL CASE

- **History:** A 35-year-old Hispanic female presented for acupuncture treatment for anxiety, fatigue and shortness of breath. She saw her "regular doctor" for the problems who did some lab tests that were "within normal limits." She was sent to a pulmonary specialist, who had treated her with inhalers for presumed asthma, which did not help. He sent her back to her doctor, who did not seem to know what to do and told her that her shortness of breath was from anxiety. The only other complaint was a five pound weight gain over the previous months and a feeling that she would smother when she laid flat in bed at night. She wondered if acupuncture could help her.
- **Physical findings:** The patient was 5'3" and 155 pounds. She appeared mildly dyspneic at rest. Her blood pressure was 140/90. Her lungs were clear. She had 1 + pitting ankle edema bilaterally. When asked about this, she said she had always had "fat ankles," but that they had "gotten bigger lately."
- **Impression:** Possible CHF
- **Plan:** The patient refused to go back to her former PCP. She was able to locate a new physician, but the wait was three weeks. We called the new physician. He agreed to see her in a few days.
- **Follow up:** The new physician saw the patient and diagnosed her as "cardiac asthma," one way that early CHF can show up. This was based on her weight gain, mild ankle edema, shortness of breath, cough, fatigue, inability to lie flat at night, nonresponsiveness to bronchodilator inhalers, and a positive Pro-BNP on her lab test (Pro-BNP is positive in CHF). The major confusing factors that had delayed diagnosis were her SOB, young age, and minimal ankle swelling. The high blood pressure was thought to be the major problem and it was lowered over several days to 120/80mmhg. The patient felt much better and is currently stable under treatment.

DISCUSSION

History and Symptoms

Many people with CHF present with florid signs and symptoms. 50% of people with CHF, however, are difficult to diagnose. One of the reasons is because symptoms like fatigue, nausea, and edema can be indicative of other diseases (are non-specific) and also because dyspnea and sometimes cough can be from lung problems, throwing us off the track to making the diagnosis of CHF.

Other possible early symptoms of CHF will often vary among individuals according to the particular organ systems involved and can be quite general. An early symptom is often fatigue. While fatigue, for example, is a sensitive indicator of possible underlying CHF, it is obviously a nonspecific symptom that may be caused by many other conditions. A person's ability to exercise may diminish. Patients may not even sense this decrease and may automatically reduce their activities to accommodate this limitation. Accumulation of fluid in the liver and intestines may also cause nausea, abdominal pain, and decreased appetite.

As the lung and body become overloaded with fluid from CHF, however, swelling of ankles and legs or abdomen will be noticed. Regardless of early manifestations, patients with florid CHF will invariably have moderate to severe shortness of breath and sometimes massive ankle edema. In addition to shortness of breath with exercise or even at rest, the symptom of paroxysmal nocturnal dyspnea (PND), will often occur. Such patients are awakened at night, gasping for air and are often unable to sleep unless sitting upright.

Physical Exam Findings

Many patients with CHF will appear anxious because the body senses CHF as an urgent threat and catecholamines (epinephrine and norepinephrine) are released from neurological tissues and the adrenal medulla. Some will be sweating. Some will appear short of breath at rest if the case is advanced. If there is enough pulmonary congestion, allopathic physicians will hear moist lung sounds and sometimes abnormal heart sounds. All will see ankle edema, a little in early cases, and a massive amount later. The patient's weight will reflect fluid gain or losses and is often charted by allopaths to measure response to medication and/or a low-salt diet.

Incidence and/or Prevalence

The prevalence of heart failure (HF) in the U.S. is five million people, 6-10% of people over 65 have HF. The incidence is 500,000 new cases annually. *CHF results in one million admissions to hospitals/year, making it the most common reason for hospital admission in patients over 65.*

Risk Factors

The typical history and risk factors for CHF are the same as those previously listed for PND. It's useful to think of them in five general categories of causation of CHF: (1) coronary artery disease, (2) hypertension, (3) valvular heart disease, (4) cardiomyopathy, and (5) conduction and rhythm problems. These are listed below, followed by their risk factors.

1. Risk factors for heart failure from coronary artery disease (CAD)

- Positive family history
- Male sex
- Smoking
- Abnormal lipids
- High C-reactive protein (CRP)
- Sedentary lifestyle
- Diabetes mellitus
- Also see risk factors in the chest pain section for angina.

2. Risk factors for hypertension

- Renal arterial disease
- Advancing age
- African-Americans have higher incidence rates than Caucasians
- Family history of high blood pressure
- Obesity
- Sedentary lifestyle
- Cigarette smoking (nicotine use)
- Too much salt (sodium) in the diet (for sodium-sensitive people)
- Potassium deficiency
- Vitamin D deficiency (probable)
- Too much alcohol
- Stress
- Idiopathic

3. Risk factors for heart failure from valvular disease and dysfunction

- Congenital valvular disorders
- History of a severe sore throat when young (causing rheumatic heart disease as autoantibodies to streptococcus attacking the valves)

4. Heart failure from cardiomyopathy (primary disease of the heart muscle itself)

- Alcoholism
- Diabetes mellitus
- Viruses

5. Heart failure from conduction and rhythm problems

- Same as for the above four categories

Mechanism Producing the Red Flag

Again, these mechanisms of red flags are listed according to the five categories of etiology for CHF

1. Heart failure from coronary artery disease (CAD)

Blockage by plaque and/or emboli within coronary arteries (atherosclerosis) reduces the flow of oxygen carrying RBCs to heart muscle cells (myocytes), weakening the heart and decreasing cardiac output.

2. Heart failure from hypertension

High blood pressure causes backward pressure into the heart. The pressure is exerted during each systole, decreasing the cardiac output as the heart muscle pumps against a pressure gradient, and also during diastole when the heart is at rest.

3. Heart failure from valvular heart disease

Aortic and/or mitral valves that are either too loose or too tight can cause decreased cardiac output by respectively allowing either too much regurgitation backwards into the heart or not allowing enough blood flow outward.

4. Heart failure from cardiomyopathy

Damaged heart muscle from risk factors listed above decreases cardiac output and leads to the signs of HF and then CHF as the weakness progresses.

5. Heart failure from arrhythmias and conduction problems

Many arrhythmias can lead to acute heart failure, but some can lead to slower onset CHF. "Sick sinus syndrome," for example, is caused by a sick pacing node in the atrium causing a slow heartbeat (bradycardia) that will not respond to increasing exercise demand. (Its red flag is listed in this book under dizziness.) At other times, heart failure can be the result of abnormal (aberrant) conduction or blocked conduction across the AV node of the heart.

Another Important Consideration

- While the symptoms of cardiac asthma may be similar to asthma, it is not asthma in its typical form. Spasm of the bronchial tube in cardiac asthma is not the result of reactions to allergens (as in extrinsic asthma), but is due to spasm of bronchial tubes because the pulmonary vessels are so full (pulmonary vascular congestion).

Specific red flags:
Swelling of one arm with shoulder and/or armpit (axillary) pain

Condition assumed present until proven otherwise:

Subclavian vein deep venous thrombosis (SVDVT)

Possible consequences of missing the condition

Severe pain and dysfunction

Stabilization, referral and management:

1. **Stabilization:** Rest and arm elevation may relieve symptoms until referral can be accomplished.
2. **Consultation and Referral Options, Transportation:** The consult is a semi-urgent matter rather than an urgent matter because, unlike DVT of the calf, there is no danger of pulmonary embolus and sudden death. The referral should be to the patient's PCP or urgent care center if no PCP is available.

Relevance to acupuncturists: This red flag can be easily missed because the onset is often quite subtle and because this condition is seldom discussed. For these reasons, and even though it is far less frequent than DVT of the lower extremities, we include this red flag to help raise the acupuncturist's "index of suspicion" so it can be recognized when it appears.

ACTUAL CASE

- **History:** The star player on a college volleyball team, a 19-year-old Caucasian female, presented to the office with complaints of shoulder pain that her coach told her was probably a rotator cuff problem. The patient did the usual exercises recommended by her trainer for rotator cuff dysfunction, but the aching in her shoulder was getting worse instead of better. She had also recently noticed mild swelling in her hand and arm. Her only meds were oral contraceptives.
- **Physical findings:** The patient was a healthy and muscular looking young woman, 5'10, 140 pounds, with mild swelling of the right hand and arm. Her right shoulder and arm exam were otherwise normal. Right radial pulse was normal.
- **Impression:** Probable subclavian vein thrombosis of right arm
- **Plan:** Referral to cardiologist was made due to the fact that she had no PCP.
- **Follow up:** Patient's studies indicated subclavian vein thrombosis. She was started on anticoagulant medications and was told to discontinue her oral contraceptive. Her swelling receded and she was doing well at last check. She is again playing volleyball on the collegiate level.

DISCUSSION

History and Symptoms

Some patients who get this condition are rare exceptions to the general rule that unhealthy people get illnesses more often than healthy people. This problem can occur in young and healthy people who use their arms excessively. Many patients with early stages are asymptomatic or have only mild shoulder or axillary pain. Later, there can be moderate arm swelling with aching shoulder and/or axilla pain worse with activity and better with rest. The other group who get this problem can be on the opposite end of the health spectrum, however. These are patients with subclavian vein catheterization who get meds and IV fluids, often for cancer. Trauma patients with SVDVT present with the history of neck and/or shoulder trauma. SVDVT may occasionally occur in patients without obvious associated history or risk factors due to anatomical anomalies (see risk factors below).

Physical Exam Findings

The examiner will usually see mild to severe swelling in the arm and axillary region. Edema is generally nonpitting. There are no changes in pulses because this is a venous rather than an arterial problem.

Incidence and/or Prevalence

Subclavian vein thrombosis accounts for approximately 2% of all DVT, and is rising (see incidence of calf DVT for comparative figures).

Risk Factors

- Trauma to affected upper extremity, in particular, clavicular fractures.
- Strenuous use of arm (> 50% of cases): particularly repeated shoulder hyperabduction, external rotation, downward rotation. greater than 80% of cases occur in dominant arm.
- Factors that cause hypercoagulability: oral contraceptives, unopposed estrogen hormone replacement, thrombotic hematologic abnormalities.
- Factors causing external compression on the subclavian vein: anomalous subclavius or anterior scalene muscle, long transverse process of cervical spine, cervical rib, abnormal insertion of the first rib, etc.
- Central vein access procedures to give IV fluids in extreme situations.

Mechanism Producing the Red Flag

Clot formation causes backpressure on the veins of the distal arm and causes the swelling. Causes for clot formation are probably multifactorial: compressive and injurious changes to the vessel wall and intima (inner lining of blood vessels), stasis of blood and hypercoagulability, and direct trauma. Strenuous use of the arm and shoulder may cause microscopic tears of the intima and temporarily block venous flow and increase coagulability.

Another Important Consideration

- In a few cases where the diagnosis remains unknown, subclavian DVTs are later identified as stemming from lung cancer, the most common being the Pancoast tumor.

Specific red flags:
Swelling and itching of lips following insect sting or food, herb, supplement, or drug ingestion

Condition assumed present until proven otherwise:
Impending anaphylactic reaction

Possible consequences of missing the condition
Sudden death

Stabilization, referral and management:

1. **Stabilization:** If the patient has been prescribed medicines for allergy or asthma or an epinephrine injector for anaphylaxis, he or she should immediately self-administer the medications as directed by their medical doctor.
2. **Consultation and Referral Options, Transportation:** All stages of anaphylaxis are urgent and require that the patient be seen right away. The transportation used is determined by the severity and stage of the anaphylactic reaction (see symptom progression under history and symptoms section below). Emergency transport should be called via 911 for any patient in acute respiratory distress. Patients with anaphylactic symptoms but without acute respiratory distress may be transported by private vehicle to urgent care. A patient with only the mildest symptoms of itching and warmth may self-transport to their primary care physician's office or to an urgent care facility.

Relevance to acupuncturists: This is an important red flag because the condition is common, can occur rapidly in the acupuncturist's office, and can be fatal. Prior to prescribing herbs, supplements, and foods, it is advisable to inquire about known allergens and also to educate the patient about the warning signs and symptoms of anaphylaxis. When prescribing herbs and supplements, education about anaphylaxis should be repeated along with advice to contact the acupuncturist immediately in the event of a suspected allergic reaction and to seek urgent care or call 911 in the event of acute respiratory distress. If a patient contacts the acupuncturist's office regarding a suspected allergic reaction to herbs or supplements, immediate and careful questioning is necessary to determine the severity and stage of the reaction so that the patient may be advised appropriately according to the guidance given in this section.

ACTUAL CASE

- **History:** A 30-year-old Caucasian male patient came to the office for treatment of back pain. Just before coming to the office he stopped at a local street vendor stand and had a hot dog, potato chips, and a soda. During the patient interview, he began to complain of itching and warm skin and began to develop red welts. He remembered that he'd had a prior episode similar to this after eating lobster about a year earlier that landed him in the hospital ED. The patient's wife, who was in the waiting room, was summoned. By the time she came into the room, the patient's throat was itching and his lips were beginning to swell, but he was not short of breath. He did not have any medications to self-administer and was sent to the ED.
- **Physical findings:** Physical findings confirmed the above anaphylaxis features. The patient was not wheezing.
- **Impression:** Anaphylactic reaction
- **Plan:** Patient was transported to the emergency room and the emergency room physician was informed over the phone that a patient was being sent in for a possible anaphylactic reaction.
- **Follow-up:** The patient developed severe SOB in the ED. He was successfully treated with epinephrine, steroids, and antihistamines. Upon release from the hospital, he was seen by his family physician and prescribed an epinephrine injector in case this ever happened again. He and his PCP tried to determine what may have caused the anaphylactic reaction. The remainder of the followup will be highly condensed.

  The patient's PCP thought there might have been an additive in the hotdog that caused the allergic reaction. The patient wrote the company to inquire about the ingredients so he could avoid the possible allergen in the future. They released a short list of ingredients. The PCP thought the list must be incomplete because no preservatives or artificial ingredients were listed. After a year-long legal challenge by the patient, the company finally released the complete and lengthy list of ingredients. The patient has avoided substances most likely to be offending allergens from the list. Five years later, the patient is doing well and has not had another anaphylactic episode. He carries an epinephrine injector.

DISCUSSION

History and Symptoms

Patients with anaphylactic reactions may complain of problems with rashes, itching, and swelling of the skin (urticaria and eczema) and eyes (conjunctivitis), nasal discharge and congestion (rhinorrhea, rhinitis), wheezing and difficulty breathing (asthma), and digestive upset. The severity ranges from minor discomfort to death. The reaction usually takes several minutes from the time of exposure to the antigen to about an hour but at times can be delayed several hours. They generally evolve as below:

1. Symptoms of flushing, warmth, itching, hives
2. Feelings of anxiety and/or doom
3. Throat and tongue swelling and hoarseness
4. Difficulty breathing (asthmatic wheezing) and nasal discharge
5. 25% will proceed to full anaphylactic reaction with vasodilatation, acute respiratory distress, and falling blood pressure, dizziness, and loss of consciousness.

Physical Exam Findings

Physical findings match the symptoms progression listed. The rash will be red at first. Welts will follow. The swelling of lips can be extreme in the end, but starts gradually and may be accompanied by other facial swelling, especially around the eyes. Wheezing can eventually be audible even without a stethoscope and is an ominous finding. Acute respiratory distress is marked by labored breathing, use of the accessory respiratory muscles of the anterior neck, and panic. In the extreme, patients can faint and become cyanotic.

Incidence and/or Prevalence

The first recorded death from anaphylaxis was the Egyptian Pharaoh Menses in 2641 BCE from an insect sting. 1-15% of the US population are estimated to be "at risk" for anaphylactic reactions. The overall incidence of full-blown anaphylactic reactions is 0.05% in the U.S. Among these there is a 1% incidence of fatality from food induced anaphylaxis and a 3.3% fatality from insect sting induced anaphylaxis. Other causes of anaphylaxis are less likely to be fatal.

Risk Factors

- Asthma
- Family history of multiple allergens or asthma

Common allergens capable of triggering anaphylaxis include:

- Foods (in roughly descending order of prevalence): peanuts, walnut, hazel nut/filbert, cashew, pistachio nut, Brazil nut, pine nut, almond, shellfish, cow's milk, eggs, cotton seed, sesame, psyllium, mustard, some fruits and vegetables
- Medications
- Venomous insect stings and bites
- Latex
- Contrast dyes used in medical imaging

Mechanism Producing the Red Flag

Anaphylaxis is an example of a Type I hypersensitivity reaction, also known as an immediate hypersensitivity reaction. Immediate hypersensitivity is mediated by the immunoglobulin IgE. The primary cells involved are the mast cells or basophils, which carry granules of vasoactive and other immune-active substances within their cytoplasm. The hypersensitivity reaction is amplified and/or modified by other cells—platelets, neutrophils, and eosinophils. A biopsy of the reaction site will demonstrate mainly mast cells and eosinophils.

IgE is produced in response to certain antigens. IgE has a high affinity for its receptor on mast cells and basophils. A subsequent exposure to the same allergen triggers the release of IgE molecules that bind to the mast cells' receptors and cause degranulation of the inflammatory substances. The most important are histamine (causes bronchoconstriction, mucous production, vasodilatation, and vascular permeability) and leukotriene C-4 and D-4 (same effects as histamine, but more potent) as well as prostaglandin D-2 (edema and pain).

Mast cells may also be triggered by other stimuli such as exercise, emotional stress, and various chemicals. These non-IgE anaphylactic-like reactions are called "anaphylactoid" reactions. Both are considered together as anaphylactic reactions in this red flag because they produce the same clinical syndrome as anaphylaxis.

Other Important Considerations

- In general, the more rapid an anaphylactic reaction, the more severe its course will be and the more urgent the medical response needs to be.
- Food-associated, exercise-induced anaphylaxis may occur when individuals exercise within 2-4 hours after ingesting a food they are allergic to. The combination may cause anaphylaxis, whereas neither will individually.
- The venom in the stings of bee, wasp, yellowjacket, hornet, and fire ant (Hymenoptera species) contain enzymes capable of causing anaphylaxis.

Review What You Have Learned
Chapter 21 Skin Problems, Lumps and Bumps

Chapter 21—Swelling, One-Sided Ankle

1. Unilateral ankle swelling is a red flag for deep venous thrombosis of the calf which can lead to
a. A pulmonary embolus
b. Sudden death
c. Dislodgment and travel to the lung
d. All of the above

Chapter 21—Swelling, Both Ankles

1. Bilateral ankle swelling is a red flag if
a. There is accompanying severe shortness of breath
b. There is accompanying angina-type chest pain
c. There is accompanying cyanosis of nail bed and lips
d. All of the above

2. Causes of congestive heart failure (CHF) include
a. CAD
b. Uncontrolled hypertension
c. Cardiomyopathy
d. Valvular heart disease
e. All of the above

Chapter 21—Swelling, Arm

1. Factors associated with subclavian vein DVT include
a. History of upper extremity overuse
b. Substances that cause hypercoagulability like oral contraceptives
c. Clavicular fractures
d. All of the above

Chapter 21—Swelling, Facial

1. What statement(s) is (are) false about anaphylactic reactions?

a. Self-administration of prescribed epinephrine is advised for patients having reactions

b. Respiratory distress is a rare occurrence with anaphylactic reactions

c. Anaphylactic reactions can occur as the result of insect stings and food allergies

d. Anaphylactic reactions are more common in patients with allergies

Chapter 22: VISION PROBLEMS

All humans value vision over almost every other form of perceiving the world. While vision problems are not the most common complaints in acupuncture clinics, they do occur as both primary and more often as secondary symptoms. In this chapter, we learn about a few serious eye symptoms and how to spot them in our patients.

Specific red flags:
Sudden, painless loss of vision in one eye

Condition assumed present until proven otherwise:
Detached retina – separation of the light sensitive inner layer of the eye from underlying layers with blood vessels and nerves that support it.

Possible consequences of missing the condition:
Permanent blindness

Stabilization, referral and management:

1. **Stabilization:** There are no stabilizing steps to take.
2. **Consultation and Referral Options, Transportation:** The consult is semi-urgent and should ideally be done through the patient's PCP. This should not delay referral to an ophthalmologist who will perform a sight-saving procedure as soon as possible to prevent further retinal detachment and permanent blindness.

Relevance to acupuncturists: This is an important red flag for all clinicians to recognize because the patient may only get one warning before total blindness. It is also a sign that many patients minimize. Prompt referral will often save the patient's vision.

ACTUAL CASE

- **History:** A 60-year-old Caucasian female came to the acupuncture office with complaints of visual disturbances. She had a long history of migraine when younger. She always had flashes of light in her visual fields prior to her headache. Recently, she had some flashes of light, but they had been replaced by a dark area in her central vision in her left eye only and she never got the headache afterwards.
- **Physical findings:** The patient's physical exam was normal except for slightly decreased vision in one eye by her report.
- **Impression:** : Possible retinal detachment
- **Plan:** A call was placed to the patient's PCP who called back the next day with recommendations that the patient go directly to a retinal specialist that she had called to prepare for the patient's arrival.
- **Follow up:** The patient was seen by the retinal specialist and did indeed have a retinal detachment. The hole in the retinal was repaired with laser surgery and the loose piece of retina was reattached to the choroid.

DISCUSSION

History and Symptoms

Retinal detachment produces a sudden and painless loss of vision in one eye. Because the problem is painless and the vision may improve a little temporarily, many patients underestimate the problem and may not present for it until it is too late. The patient will report the sudden appearance of one or more of the following *in one eye.*

- **Floaters** – spots or string-like objects that float across the visual field (debris in the eye). These should not be confused with a normal amount of floaters that most people have as they age. The floaters in retinal attachment are more abundant.
- **Sudden flashes of light in one eye.** These should not be confused with ophthalmic migraine, in which case the bright lights go away.
- **A sudden shadow** over a portion of the visual field
- Sudden, persistent **blurring of vision**

Physical Exam Findings

The patient may have decreased visual acuity on the affected side. Visual fields can help isolate the location of the retinal detachment if done carefully. Pupillary reaction should be checked to exclude a neurological problem. The eye doctor will do ophthalmoscopy to see the exact location of the retinal detachment.

Incidence and/or Prevalence

Six percent of the general population has retinal breaks, but most of these will not lead to retinal detachment. The prevalence of retinal detachment is 0.3% in the U.S. and the annual incidence is approximately one in 10,000 or about one in 300 over a lifetime.

Risk Factors

- Aging – more common in people older than age 40
- Previous retinal detachment in one eye (15% risk for other eye)
- A family history of retinal detachment
- Extreme nearsightedness (myopia > 6 diopters)
- Previous eye surgery, such as cataract removal
- Previous severe eye injury or trauma
- Weak areas on the sides (periphery) of the retina
- Patients with prior cataract removal surgery

Mechanism Producing the Red Flag

Retinal detachment is caused by separation of the inner layers of the light sensitive retina from the underlying, nutritive retinal pigment epithelium (choroid). Over time these detached areas may expand, like wallpaper that slowly peels off a wall. Parts of the retina that detach lose their blood supply and stop functioning. Separation of the sensory retina from the underlying choroid occurs by one of the following three basic mechanisms.

1. Vitreous humor can leak through a retinal tear or tiny holes in the retina that have thinned due to aging and accumulate under the retina.
2. Adhesions on the surface of the retina caused by inflammation can tether to the vitreous humor in the eyeball. As the vitreous gel shrinks with age, these adhesions can pull areas of the retina away from the underlying choroid.
3. Exudation of material under the retina from retinal vessels as the result of inflammation, hypertension, central retinal venous occlusion, vasculitis, tumor, or papilledema can cause detachment of the retina without a break in it.

Another Important Consideration

- Retinal detachments were uniformly blinding until Jules Gonin, MD pioneered the first repair of retinal detachments in Lausanne, Switzerland in the 1920s, thus ushering in the age of sight-saving modern surgical techniques.

Specific red flags: *Transient, painless "curtain" coming down over vision of one eye then lifting*

Condition assumed present until proven otherwise

Amaurosis Fugax (AF) – Brief and fleeting attacks of monocular partial or total blindness lasting seconds to minutes. "Amaurosis fugax" is derived from Greek roots for "darkening" and "fleeting" or "fugitive."

Possible consequences of missing the condition

Amaurosis Fugax also serves as a warning for possible stroke or MI because of atherosclerosis in the circulation to the eye or elsewhere in the body.

Stabilization, referral and management

1. **Stabilization:** There are no particular stabilizing steps. The patient should be on one baby aspirin a day, just like patients with TIA, until consult is accomplished.
2. **Consultation and Referral Options, Transportation:** The patient should be seen by their PCP on a semi-urgent basis or a free standing medical clinic if they have no PCP. They will need to be referred for a carotid doppler study to determine the extent of disease in the internal carotid arteries.

Relevance to acupuncturists: Acupuncturists and other clinicians need to understand the importance of this red flag as a warning for future ischemia or infarction in eye, brain, or heart.

ACTUAL CASE

- **History:** The patient was a hypertensive 55-year-old man who came to the acupuncture clinic for treatment of shoulder pain. During the interview, he mentioned that he had two episodes of "a curtain coming down over my eye" that lasted for 10 seconds or so in the prior week. He thought he had something in his eye and flushed it with water and the episode resolved. He had a past medical history of cholesterol problems and his mother had died of MI at age 63.

- **Physical findings:** The patient appeared healthy and had a normal physical exam.
- **Impression:** Probable amaurosis fugax
- **Plan:** A consultation request was sent to the patient's PCP regarding the situation.
- **Follow up:** The patient was seen three days later by his PCP. Carotid studies were ordered and the patient had a significant blockage of his right ICA. He opted for carotid surgery to clear the blockage. In preparation for the surgery, an exercise stress test was done to assess for possible CAD. The test was halted early due to ischemic changes on the ECG tracing. An angiogram of the coronary arteries revealed a 98% blockage of the patient's left anterior descending artery (LAD), the main artery serving the heart muscle. A stent was placed in the LAD to open the LAD and stabilize the patient. After the patient was stable the plaque was removed from his right ICA. He is currently doing well.

DISCUSSION

History and Symptoms

The symptoms in the red flag are typical, but patients may also present with longer attacks that last minutes rather than seconds. Since ischemia (as opposed to infarction) is temporary and reversible, there will always be recovery in this condition, but it should be obvious that the same region threatened by ischemia could eventually experience infarction, resulting in permanent blindness. For this reason, risk factors like hypertension, hypercholesterolemia, and diabetes should be sought out, as well as family history of such conditions.

Physical Exam Findings

Vision testing should be done to exclude a permanent defect in the visual field. The examination also should include complete cardiac and neurologic evaluation, including murmurs and carotid bruits.

Incidence and/or Prevalence

Estimates of the incidence of AF are difficult to come by in the literature, perhaps because the symptoms are fleeting and under-reported. It has been estimated by some experts at approximately 14 per 100,000 per year. This is approximately 25-30% of the reported incidence of TIA. Caucasian men have the highest incidence of ICA origin atherosclerosis. The AF and the male/female ratio is 2/1.

Risk Factors

The risk factors for AF are the same as the risk factors for TIA and coronary artery disease. They are the risk factors for atherosclerosis since this is the vasculopathology that underlies all of these conditions.

Demographic

- Advancing age
- Male gender

Lifestyle

- Tobacco smoking
- Sedentary lifestyle
- High-stress
- Diet high in animal fats, trans-fats, and refined carbohydrates, and low in anti-inflammatory essential free fatty acids

Disease Risk Factors

- Coronary-prone (Type A) behavior or personality
- Post-menopausal status
- Diabetes mellitus
- Hypertension
- Obesity
- Personal history of atherosclerotic disease
- Low and/or pro-inflammatory type HDL cholesterol
- C-reactive protein elevation
- Homocysteine elevation
- Lipoprotein (a) elevation
- Apolipoprotein B elevation
- Low Apolipoprotein A-1 level
- Lp-PLA2 elevation (an enzyme that causes deposition of LDL into arterial walls)
- Small, dense LDL particle size elevation
- High fibrinogen levels

Family/Inherited

- Positive family history of coronary artery disease, peripheral artery disease or stroke
- Family history of lipid disorder

Mechanism Producing the Red Flag

AF is due to transient ischemia due to blocking emboli that originate in the internal carotid artery (ICA) breaking off and getting temporarily trapped in the retinal artery of one of the eyes, causing transient ischemia of the retina and fleeting vision loss.

Another Important Consideration

- Sudden vision loss is a common complaint among patients of different ages with variable presentations and is a red flag regardless of the fact that it has benign causes like transient vision loss from migraine or vasospasm in people under 45 years of age.

Specific red flags:
Double vision following blunt trauma to one eye that subsequently appears lower than the other eye

Condition assumed present until proven otherwise:

"Blowout fracture" of the eye orbit with entrapment of inferior rectus muscle in the fracture

Possible consequences of missing the condition:

Permanent loss of vision and removal (enucleation) of the eyeball

Stabilization, referral and management:

1. **Stabilization:** Patients should protect themselves from further eye trauma.
2. **Consultation and Referral Options, Transportation:** The situation is urgent, but does not require a 911 call. The best option would be a call to the patient's PCP, if one is available explaining the situation. The PCP will refer immediately to an ophthalmologist for surgery to repair the fracture before permanent damage is done. If a PCP is not available, the call to an ophthalmologist should be attempted. If neither of these is successful, the patient should be directed to the nearest ED, because surgery will be necessary and an ophthalmologist will be assigned in the ED.

Relevance to acupuncturists: This type of injury and its sequelae will be seen rather rarely by acupuncturists, but the outcome can be so disastrous if the red flag is not recognized that it is well worth knowing.

ACTUAL CASE

- **History:** A 20-year-old Caucasian male presented to the office for acupuncture with the complaint of eye pain. He was drinking with friends the night before and was struck in the eye while trying to break up a fight. He did not lose consciousness and didn't think much more of it until he woke the next morning with pain. His sister told him that acupuncture worked well for pain, so he came in for treatment. His only other complaint was some double vision.
- **Physical findings:** The patient seemed like an intelligent young man with moderate bruising around the right eye. When we held up two fingers for a check of gross vision, he said that he was seeing a "double shadow" around the fingers. Looking directly at the patient's face, it appeared that his right eye was slightly lower than the left eye.
- **Impression:** Possible blowout fracture of the inferior floor of the right eye orbit
- **Plan:** The patient did not have a PCP. We called the college health service where he went to school and the patient was directed to an ophthalmologist who saw him the same day.
- **Follow up:** The ophthalmologist confirmed the patient's fracture of the orbital floor bones with an MRI scan and took the patient to surgery. The surgeon rescued the inferior rectus muscle from where it had slipped into a jagged fracture fragment in the orbital floor and repaired the orbital floor with "microplating." The patient recovered well and now has normal vision.

DISCUSSION

History and Symptoms

The history is always associated with some kind of high velocity trauma secondary to impact with a hardball or similar-sized object, usually in a young male. It can occur in fights, sports, motor vehicle accidents, etc. There is usually quite a bit of pain, contusion, and ecchymosis around the eye, but sometimes there is a little bruising. The symptom of double vision is present only if the fracture in the inferior floor of the orbit is sufficient to allow the inferior rectus muscle to drop into it and become trapped.

Physical Exam Findings

The clinician may notice that one eye is lower than the other when the patient is observed face on. The injured eye may not track with the other eye while following a moving finger if the patient complains of double vision (diplopia).

Incidence and/or Prevalence

Orbital floor fractures alone or with other facial skeletal

fractures are the most commonly encountered midfacial fractures, second only to nasal fractures. Trauma centers, especially in urban settings, see a higher incidence of this injury type.

Risk Factors

- Anything that puts a patient at risk for more frequent trauma
- More common in males, especially young males

Mechanism Producing the Red Flag

Orbital floor fractures are secondary to a sudden increase in intraorbital hydraulic pressure from objects small enough to put sudden pressure on the eyeball, but too large to penetrate the eye. The infraorbital floor is the part of the bony socket that usually sustains a fracture because this is where the bones are thinnest. When the inferior rectus is trapped in the fracture crack the contribution to movement of the inferior rectus is impossible. Blood vessels within the muscle can also be occluding, causing ischemic necrosis in the muscle. Since the floor of the orbit is lower due to the fracture, the affected eyeball can appear lower to an examiner who looks straight at the face compared to the normal eye. The fracture must be fixed and the eye muscle entrapment released fairly soon to keep from having permanent damage to the eye.

Another Important Consideration

- Smith and Regan coined the term "blow-out fracture of the orbit" in 1956 to indicate entrapment of the inferior rectus muscle and decreased ocular mobility, but the problem had been described as early as 1844 in France.

Specific red flags:
Blurry vision, frequent urination, increased hunger and fatigue in an adult

Condition assumed present until proven otherwise

Adult Onset Diabetes Mellitus (Type 1)

Type I: Usually diagnosed in childhood. The body makes little or no insulin in this type and daily injections of insulin are needed.

Type II: This is far more common than type I. It usually occurs in adulthood, but young people are increasingly being diagnosed with it (see mechanisms of red flag).

Gestational diabetes: This is high serum glucose that develops during pregnancy in a woman who usually does not have diabetes after pregnancy.

Possible consequences of missing the condition

Disability, blindness, neuropathy, loss of lower limbs, renal failure, heart disease, death

Stabilization, referral and management

1. **Stabilization:**

Stabilizing the noncritical diabetic patient

In patients with relatively stable diabetes, as in the red flag, the patient should be encouraged to engage in a mild walking program if there are no cardiopulmonary concerns until their blood sugar can be brought down by the consultant. This simple step can be amazingly helpful initially. Also, the patient should be advised to avoid high glycemic index foods and to balance carbohydrate intake with at least 30% protein intake at every meal.

Stabilizing a diabetic patient who lapses into coma

It is unlikely, but not impossible that the acupuncturist will see a diabetic patient lapse into coma, either a *hypoglycemic* or a *hyperglycemic* coma. If this happens before you see the patient, it will be difficult, if not impossible to tell which type of coma it is and your only option will be to send the patient to the ED. If, however, you are present when a diabetic patient starts on their way into a coma, you will have an excellent opportunity to know which type it is and to stabilize the patient in a way that might be lifesaving.

This would happen specifically with a patient on their way to a *hypoglycemic* coma due to erroneously giving themselves too much insulin. They could have done so on their way to your office and it could kick in when they arrive. In this case, the patient would pass through a 10-30 minute stage of plunging blood sugar with sympathetic nervous system activation resulting in anxiety, tremors, racing pulse, sweating, etc.

Such patients can and should be stabilized well before a coma ensues and it is well within the ability of acupuncturists to do so. In fact, it is necessary. This brings us to another specific red flag. **Known insulin-taking diabetic patients who present with anxiety, tremor, sweating and racing pulse** should be assumed to be having a ***hypoglycemic reaction*** until proven otherwise.

The patient should immediately be given any source of glucose available, to be followed by protein containing foods like peanut butter to keep the glucose from crashing again. This is not a time to worry about too much blood sugar. The blood sugar must be immediately raised to stabilize the patient.

2. **Consultation and Referral Options, Transportation:**

   Hyperglycemic coma

   One type of coma is reviewed above, the hypoglycemic coma. The other type of diabetic coma is a *hyperglycemic* coma, which is a very high blood sugar rather than a blood sugar that is too low. In this case, there is no preceding fight or flight reaction and the only way to stabilize it is with insulin, which is generally done in a hospital and thus requires the patient to be transported to the ED, usually by a 911 call.

   This coma would occur generally in people who have advanced diabetes and are unaware of it or those who have been on insulin who decide not to take it. This also requires a 911 call.

   If the patient presents with the red flag described in the beginning, they will be stable enough for a semi-urgent consultation with their PCP on a same day or perhaps a next day basis, but should be instructed to go to the ED if they suddenly become worse before they obtain their consult.

Relevance to acupuncturists: The acupuncturist will see many patients with adult onset diabetes in their practices at all stages of overt diabetes. They will see even more insulin-resistant and glucose-intolerant patients who are months to years away from overt diabetes who make up the much larger "iceberg under the sea" portion of the glucose dysregulation population than those with overt diabetes (see mechanisms of red flag). Overt diabetes can often be prevented in these at-risk patients through adequate lifestyle modifications. Many of these patients can be identified by risk factor analysis.

Acupuncturists will also see patients with chronic complications of previously diagnosed diabetes, like vascular and neurological deficiencies in the feet, partial or total blindness from diabetic retinopathy, heart disease, and renal insufficiency. They may particularly see referred patients with peripheral neuropathy in the feet because modern scientific medicine solutions for this condition are relatively ineffective.

ACTUAL CASE

- **History:** A 45-year-old Hispanic man presented to the clinic for a tingling sensation in both feet which he thought was from standing on them all day at work. In passing, he mentioned that he needed to get some new glasses because he was having blurry vision. He also noticed more frequent urination and greater appetite for the last two months.
- **Physical findings:** The man was mildly obese, but otherwise had a normal physical exam including neurological exam.
- **Impression:** Possible diabetes mellitus, type II, with possible early peripheral neuropathy.
- **Plan:** The patient was sent back to his PCP, who he had not seen for two years.
- **Follow up:** The patient had a fasting blood sugar of 220mg/dl (< 105mg/dl normal) and a hemoglobin A1C of 8.8mg/dl (<6.0mg/dl normal)

DISCUSSION

History and Symptoms

Adult onset type II diabetes mellitus develops quite slowly. Most people have no symptoms until blood sugar levels rise to >200 mg/dl for some time. Diabetes is quite advanced (although not immediately dangerous) by the time these red flag symptoms develop. In addition, since many of the early symptoms of diabetes are non-specific (like fatigue), or can be caused by other problems (frequent urination from bladder infection or blurry vision from refractive error), early symptoms can easily be minimized by patients and clinicians alike.

It is the *clustering* of these mild, early symptoms that is so revealing to the alert clinician. For example, even though a 45-year-old female patient may well need eyeglasses, have a bladder infection and feel tired, will she also have some tingling in her feet? The clustering of blurry vision, frequent urination and tingling feet, like the red flag cluster, makes the clinician suspicious of the presence of diabetes. Similarly, the classical presentation of the "3 P's" of diabetes—polyphagia (increased hunger), polydipsia (increased thirst), and polyuria (increased urination) may not present initially, but when it does, diabetes is likely.

Patients with sufficiently advanced diabetes will also paradoxically report weight loss in spite of an increased appetite and increased food intake. This reflects what is happening at the cellular level. The patient's cells are "starving in a sea of plenty." Though the serum glucose is high and the cell is surrounded by lots of glucose, the insulin receptor is unresponsive so that the gate mechanism to let glucose into the cells is faulty and a patient's cells are literally starving.

Patients with later complications of diabetes have symptoms (and signs) compatible with large vessel atherosclerotic disease like coronary artery disease, peripheral vascular disease, erectile dysfunction, transient ischemic attacks, stroke, etc. They will also have disorders associated with small blood vessel problems like diabetic nephropathy (kidney insufficiency), diabetic retinopathy leading to vision loss, diabetic neuropathy leading to numbness (from small vessel disease feeding neurons), and hyperlipidemia from shunting of excess glucose into lipids. Infections of the skin and urinary tract will be prevalent due to microorganisms that feed on glucose.

Physical Exam Findings

The patient is almost always overweight in the insulin resistance and glucose dysregulation stages (see mechanisms below) and usually in the early overt diabetes stage. Later, there can be some measurable weight loss in late diabetes, not well controlled with insulin. Many diabetics remain obese. An exam should be performed consistent with the problems that may occur with overt diabetes if it is present. In other words, the feet should be examined for signs of ulceration and foot pulses should be palpated for adequacy. A cardiovascular exam commensurate with acupuncturist's ability should also be done.

Incidence and/or Prevalence

Overt type II diabetes mellitus affects more than 20 million Americans. Over 40 million North Americans have prediabetes glucose dysregulation with minimally abnormal blood sugars. If we also include those with insulin resistance, the figure is even higher, perhaps even as high as 30-40% of North Americans (see red flag mechanisms for these stages).

Risk Factors

- Having a first degree relative with diabetes
- Being > 45 years old
- Gestational diabetes or delivering a baby weighing more than nine pounds
- Sedentary lifestyle
- High glycemic index diet (simple, refined carbohydrates)
- Unfavorable serum lipid levels
- Obesity
- Polycystic ovarian syndrome (PCOS)
- Insulin insensitivity and glucose in tolerance
- African-Americans, Native Americans, Asians, Pacific Islanders, and Hispanic Americans have a higher incidence of diabetes than other ethnic groups.

Mechanism Producing the Red Flag

Overt diabetes is the end stage of a long process that occurs over years. We can basically chart the process in the following three stages.

1. **Insulin resistance stage.** In this stage, the patient's blood sugar is normal, but the blood insulin level spikes in an effort to stimulate as many dull insulin receptors as possible to open the cellular gate to allow glucose to enter cells. The only symptom a patient may have at this stage is weight gain (because some of the oversupply of insulin causes deposition of glucose into fat cells) and possibly "reactive hypoglycemia" from crashing blood sugars. In crashing blood sugar, the glucose is suddenly allowed to enter cells when the insulin gets high enough, which leaves a patient with temporarily low blood sugar 1-3 hours after a meal. Eating protein with each meal lowers this insulin spike and relieves reactive hypoglycemia.

2. **Glucose dysregulation.** In this stage, there is still insulin resistance and the insulin level is still high, but the body cannot produce enough insulin to lower the blood sugar into the normal range so that there is periodic hyperglycemia as well as hyperinsulinemia. Some physicians call this stage "prediabetes."

3. **Overt diabetes.** In this stage, the production of insulin begins to fall due to exhaustion of the pancreatic beta cells that produce insulin. At this point, the blood sugar is high most or all of the time and the insulin is low.

There are stages of overt diabetes beyond this last stage, but they are continuations of the same insulin depletion state. Eventually, the rate of atherosclerosis and damage to large and small blood vessels is heightened. Neurological changes, numbness and tingling in the feet and also in the arms and hands to a lesser extent, are due to small vessel damage that affects the nerves.

The symptom of blurry vision has an interesting underlying pathophysiological mechanism. The lens of the eye normally absorbs some of the serum glucose. If the glucose level remains elevated, the lens absorbs more and swells. When it swells, it changes the diameter of the lens and causes a decrease in visual acuity. In a way, the lens acts in a similar way to the most accurate exam for determining the average amount of blood sugar elevation, the hemoglobin A1C test. Both hemoglobin A1C (HA1C) elevation and the swelling of the lens phenomenon give us ways to tell that the average blood sugar has been high over a long period of time.

Other Important Considerations

- Although the dietary and lifestyle education of a patient with diabetes can be quite involved, the most important measures are simple.
  1. Protein with every meal: a palm full of protein for every fist full of carbohydrate, preferably low glycemic index carbohydrate that the body has to work to break down, for example, whole grain like brown rice rather than white rice, etc.
  2. Regular aerobic exercise at least 30 minutes a day to burn off excessive blood sugar. The author has never seen a marathon runner with type 2 diabetes, although he or she might exist.

Review What You Have Learned
Chapter 22 Vision Problems

Chapter 22—Vision Problems, Loss of Vision

1. What is true about acute vision loss?
a. Acute vision loss is a red flag only if accompanied by pain in the eye
b. Retinal detachments repair themselves if the eye is rested for two weeks
c. Retinal detachments are painless
d. Retinal detachments are unrelated to age

Chapter 22—Vision Problems, Curtain over Vision

1. Amaurosis Fugax (from Greek "darkening fugitive") is the result of
a. Retinal detachment
b. A direct blow to the eye
c. Embolic occlusion of the retinal artery
d. Embolic occlusion of the retinal vein

Chapter 22—Vision Problems, Double Vision

1. A powerful, direct blow to the eye can cause permanent eye damage that can ultimately result in loss of the eye. What is the likely mechanism for this kind of severe damage to the eyeball?
a. Damage to the bones of the eye socket and entrapment of intraocular muscles
b. Damage to the retina from the blow
c. Damage to the optic nerve similar to that seen in diabetes
d. Damage to the cornea

Chapter 22—Vision Problems, Blurry Vision

1. The mechanism for blurry vision in the early phases of diabetes mellitus is
a. Damage to the retina
b. Swelling of the lens from absorbed glucose
c. A direct effect of high insulin levels
d. None of the above

Chapter 23: WEIGHT FLUCTUATIONS

Weight fluctuations in all age groups are important to note, especially if they manifest over a short period of time. While most of us are more worried about weight gain, unexplained weight loss is usually more serious. It can be a symptom of many types of major chronic illnesses, the most fearsome being cancer.

Weight fluctuations are so common in all age groups that its significance can easily be overlooked. Fluctuations from "normal" and "usual" body weight in those who have attained maturation can signal the possible presence of dangerous conditions, however. This chapter will examine weight fluctuations in general, especially weight loss, which is of more concern from a red flag point of view than weight gain (putting aside morbid obesity, which is dangerous in its own right).

Unexplained and/or unintended weight loss < 5% of body weight in an adult or child should be regarded as a red flag for ***cancer, metabolic diseases like hyperthyroidism or diabetes, major chronic disease, malnutrition, serious psychiatric illness including eating disorders like anorexia and bulimia, or some combination of these problems.*** With such a broad list of potential causes, unexplained weight loss is the general flag without equal and is valuable due to its broad implications.

The significance of unexplained weight loss is especially apparent when we consider that, in the absence of a concerted effort to lose weight, the natural tendency through the lifespan (excluding the very elderly) is to gain weight. We must therefore assume that a patient who loses weight "for no reason" actually has a serious cause that remains to be discovered. Even weight loss in the very elderly (>75, for example), *though commonly accepted*, is still a red flag, as insurance companies acknowledge by charging higher premiums for underweight seniors.

Specific red flags that we have already covered in which weight loss is one sign include:

1. Cancers of all kinds
2. Hyperthyroidism
3. We now add all kinds of ***undiagnosed major chronic illnesses*** that have a general debilitating effect on the body like liver disease, kidney disease, and lung disease. Heart disease is already covered under the heart failure section.

Specific red flags:
Mild weight gain (5-10 pounds) with lethargy, dry hair and cold extremities

Condition assumed present until proven otherwise:

Hypothyroidism, overt (clinical)—Clinical hypothyroidism is caused by failure of the thyroid gland to produce enough thyroid hormones, the thyronines—L-thyroxine (T4) and/or triiodothyroxine (T3)—to meet the minimal metabolic rate for the body. The problem can be with the thyroid gland itself (primary hypothyroidism – the most common type), the pituitary (secondary hypothyroidism), or the hypothalamus (tertiary hypothyroidism).

Possible consequences of missing the condition:

Debilitation and increased risk for cardiovascular and other problems leading to untimely death

Stabilization, referral and management:

1. **Stabilization:** There are no specific stabilizing steps to take.
2. **Consultation and Referral Options, Transportation:** The consult can generally be secured in a timely manner since thyroid disorders (with the exception of thyroid storm) usually evolve slowly.

Relevance to acupuncturists: This is an important red flag for acupuncturists to know about for several important reasons. Firstly, hypothyroidism is common and debilitating if not treated. Secondly, it is associated with significantly increased risk for cardiovascular and psychiatric problems. Thirdly, it passes through a stage of unnoticeable or barely noticeable symptoms (subclinical hypothyroidism) on its way to overt illness making it difficult to detect. Finally, it can be easily treated once it is definitively diagnosed.

ACTUAL CASE

- **History:** The patient was a 65-year-old male widower who had been receiving acupuncture for many years for a variety of minor complaints, most recently knee pain. He said he was getting more aches and pains lately and found it difficult to keep warm in his house even when it was just a little cool.
- **Physical findings:** The patient had always been rather stoic, careful with his words, and slow to respond to questions. Over the prior six months, however, the reception staff and his treating acupuncturist both noticed that his speech rhythm and his verbal responses to questions had become particularly slow. He seemed more forgetful and his hair appeared drier. He had developed some mild bilateral ankle edema which was new for him.
- **Impression:** Possible hypothyroidism
- **Plan:** The patient was referred to his PCP.
- **Follow up:** The PCP obtained a thyroid profile. The TSH was 120mg/dl (< 4.0 mg/dl is normal) and the free T4 and free T3 were both very low. The patient was placed on thyroid supplementation and improved gradually.

DISCUSSION

History and Symptoms

Patients with clinical hypothyroidism usually have no complaints in early (subclinical) stages of the illness. Later, they can complain of slow thinking, memory problems, depressed feelings, mild weight gain, sometimes constipation, and dry skin and hair. They need not have all of these symptoms, however. In fact, they seldom do. Cold intolerance is also a common complaint as is muscle aching and stiffness. Some patients will notice that their body temperature is lower than usual.

Women will sometimes complain of irregular menstruation and, if they are in the reproductive years, an inability to get pregnant. When hypothyroidism occurs in the elderly, which it often does, it is easy to blame their symptoms on "old age." Even in middle-aged and younger patients, however, the onset of symptoms can be so slow that patients aren't sure they have a problem for months, years, or even decades!

Physical Exam Findings

Many of the symptoms noted above can be verified in the physical examination by corresponding signs. The general observation of the patient can be the most rewarding window into the problem. In the actual case presented, the patient's responses to questions were considerably slower than usual, he was slower to understand questions, and his voice had become thick and gravelly. Even if this is a new patient to you and there is no premorbid state to compare a patient to, these signs can be quite noticeable.

The weight gain can be measured objectively, but weight gain can be the result of other factors. Therefore, it is not that reliable to make the diagnosis, except as supporting data. The skin and hair can appear dry, but the more pathognomonic sign, when it is present, is a quite characteristic thickening of the skin (myxedema) and sometimes a trace of edema at the ankles. The patient can also become so mentally slow in severe cases that it may appear they are becoming demented.

If a patient brings you his or her labs, they are confirmatory in that the patient's thyroid stimulating hormone (TSH) will be high (in primary hypothyroidism) in an attempt to stimulate the thyroid gland. However, the thyroid hormones themselves will be low because the thyroid gland cannot respond. If the TSH is low and the thyroid hormones are low, the fault is in the pituitary not putting out enough TSH to stimulate the thyroid gland (secondary hypothyroidism).

Incidence and/or Prevalence

The incidence of clinical (overt) hypothyroidism is 40/10,000 women and 6/10,000 men yearly (6:1 ratio). The prevalence is 9.3% in women and 1.3% in men. The incidence of subclinical hypothyroidism is much higher. Although unknown for the entire population, we do know that up to 10% of women over age 60 have subclinical hypothyroidism. The incidence of both subclinical and clinical hypothyroidism increases with age.

Risk Factors

- Lack of iodine in the diet – The incidence of hypothyroidism is higher in areas where the iodine content of food is low because iodine is an essential part of all thyroid hormones.
- Autoimmune diseases
- Pernicious anemia (especially in middle-aged women)
- Chronic autoimmune thyroiditis

- Prior radioactive iodine treatment or surgical removal of the thyroid
- Prior hyperthyroidism—In autoimmune thyroiditis hypothyroidism is often preceded by hyperthyroidism
- Adverse drug effects (e.g., amiodarone and lithium)
- Pregnancy, due to silent or postpartum thyroiditis

Mechanism Producing the Red Flag

There are other thyronines besides T4 and T3, but only these two are metabolically active enough to be considered here. The thyroid gland produces twenty times more T4 than T3, but T3 is three to four times more metabolically active than T4. It is actually only the unbound "free" fraction of both hormones that can pass into cells, so it is ideal to measure free T4 and free T3, rather than total T4 and T3 (along with TSH), when assessing thyroid function. Both free hormones can easily pass through cell membranes to enter the cytoplasm.

They do so in almost every cell in the body whereupon they are also able to penetrate into the nucleus of the cells. In the nucleus, they bind to their receptors on DNA and cause myriad effect, including, but not limited to: increasing basal metabolic rate, increasing the rate of protein synthesis, regulating growth of bone and neurons in synergy with growth hormone, and increasing sensitivity to catecholamines such as epinephrine. They also regulate protein, fat, and carbohydrate metabolism.

The thyroid hormones are also essential to proper development and differentiation of all cells of the human body. Since the thyroxines increase the basal metabolic rate and do so many critical things like make possible the proper development and differentiation of all cells in the human body, reductions in the concentrations of these hormones below certain critical levels have the numerous effects noted throughout this chapter and below.

Most subclinical and overt hypothyroidism is caused by autoimmune thyroid disease (anti-thyroid antibodies attack the thyroid gland). Subclinical hypothyroidism also occurs in patients with infectious, silent, or postpartum thyroiditis, those on excessive doses of anti-thyroid medications, patients on lithium and other medications, those with hypothyroidism on inadequate replacement, and patients with diminished thyroid function related to permanent treatment for hyperthyroidism like radioactive ablation or thyroidectomy.

Other Important Considerations

- The major debate about thyroid disorders in the U.S. has to do not with what constitutes subclinical hypothyroidism (SH) but what the effects of SH are. Until fairly recently, SH was considered a benign condition. However, that is no longer the case.
- Western medicine first realized that the earlier "normal" reference value for TSH serum levels (up to 20) was far too high. The range was gradually lowered to the most recent range for normal as 3.0. It is readily apparent, therefore, that many patients considered to have had "borderline" hypothyroid problems in the recent past actually had overt hypothyroidism by today's TSH criteria.
- A general agreement has arisen that patients have subclinical hypothyroidism if they have minor or no symptoms of hypothyroidism and their TSH is between 5-10 even if serum T4 is "within normal limits."
- I, among others, do not believe this is an adequate definition of subclinical hypothyroidism, however, because it doesn't take into account the important role of T3 which is even more metabolically active than T4. If T3 is low, and the patient has symptoms, regardless of the TSH or T4, we believe the thyroid function is inadequate.
- Problems with the reference range for TSH was only the first wake-up call for medical scientists regarding subclinical hypothyroidism. The next occurred when studies were completed that see if SH had adverse health effects even if the TSH was only minimally elevated, such as in the 5-10 range. Today SH is well-known to be associated with the following list of problems.

1. Unfavorable lipid levels
2. Increased cardiac abnormalities (including MI, CHF, congestive heart failure, atrial fibrillation)
3. Latency of motor nerve conduction
4. Increased intraocular pressure
5. Arthralgia
6. Depression refractory to both antidepressant drugs and thyroid hormone alone, sometimes needing both.
7. Neuropsychological impairments in cognitive function tests, memory tests, reaction time, and self-rating mood scales
8. More clinical memory impairment, anxiety, and somatic complaints
9. Earlier frailty, dementia, and death

Specific red flags:
Weight loss and/or failure to maintain adequate body weight due to body image concerns

Condition assumed present until proven otherwise:

Anorexia nervosa—Obsession about weight and food with subsequent starving and possibly over-athleticism

Related eating disorders, bulimia nervosa (binging on food then purging by vomiting, laxatives, or excessive exercise), or binge eating disorder (frequently consuming overly large amounts of food with loss of control) are not directly part of this red flag but are also considered to some extent.

Possible consequences of missing the condition:

Heart disease, depression, suicidal thoughts or behavior, amenorrhea and subsequent osteoporosis, stunted growth, seizures, renal damage, severe tooth decay, high or low blood pressure, type 2 diabetes, gallbladder disease, anemia, and death

Stabilization, referral and management:

1. **Stabilization:** The patient with an eating disorder must be managed carefully to ensure that they maintain enough trust to confide about their problem and seek help. A calm, positive, and non-judgmental demeanor on the part of the practitioner is critical.
2. **Consultation and Referral Options, Transportation:** An eating disorder is one of those difficult problems usually best handled by a team of clinicians including the acupuncturist, a PCP who can do necessary tests, and an eating disorder counselor, at the very least. The referrals can start with the PCP.

Relevance to acupuncturists: Every acupuncturist will see patients with eating disorders due to its high prevalence (see incidence and prevalence section). Although these patients will usually be reticent to discuss their disorder, rapport is necessary so that a patient can receive needed help. It starts with the recognition of this red flag.

ACTUAL CASE

- **History:** The patient was a 23-year-old female and former gymnastics athlete who was seeking acupuncture for abdominal pain. The patient was hesitant to discuss issues having to do with diet, but finally confided that her stomach pain was worse lately because she had been skipping meals and increased her jogging to "stay in shape and lose a couple of pounds."
- **Physical findings:** The patient was quite lean and muscular 5'3" and 100 pounds. She appeared hypervigilant at times, but also lapsed into sad spells during the interview.
- **Impression:** Possible anorexia nervosa
- **Plan:** The patient at first declined any help for her problem, but was eventually directed to see an eating disorder psychologist. She wanted to continue to use her gynecologist as a PCP "if necessary."
- **Follow up:** The patient has been seen periodically for other issues having to do with amenorrhea, but has declined to discuss her eating disorder further.

DISCUSSION

History and Symptoms

The typical anorexic is an achievement oriented female from an achievement oriented family structure. She is generally quiet, serious and discreet, and tends to be avoidant when issues about eating and food come up. There may be an extreme focus on small areas of normal adiposity like in the thighs or abdomen. Some anorexics are quite knowledgeable about nutrition. All are obsessed with food. The average anorexic is quite aware of her problem, but talking about it may be the last thing she wants to do.

An indirect and subtle approach is the best in this situation with a gentle probing into what her life has been like and an invitation to share how she handles the inevitable stresses in life. Discussing the relationship of stress to health is a good place to start. Rarely will the anorexic come seeking help. Rather, it can be gently offered when the time is right. A very important initial strategy is to focus on health, rather than weight or food.

Physical Exam Findings

Anorexics, unless in remission, will be thin, sometimes painfully so. Bulimics may be any weight. The examiner will notice a mental and emotional disconnect in the patient between how a patient thinks she looks and how she actually looks and may also intuit a sense of shame that the patient holds regarding their issues with food.

Incidence and/or Prevalence

A best estimate is that 8 million people in the U.S. have an eating disorder. The female to male ratio is 7:1. One in

200 women suffers from anorexia while six in 200 suffer from bulimia. Eating disorders have the highest mortality rate of any mental illness. The mortality rate associated with anorexia nervosa alone is twelve times higher than the death rate of all other combined causes of death for females between the ages of 15-24 years old. Five to ten percent of anorexics die within 10 years after disease onset and 18–20% die within 20 years. Only 30-40% will fully recover. Many will prematurely die from complications, including suicide and heart problems. All ethnic groups seem to have similar incidence statistics.

Risk Factors

- Teenage girls and young women are more likely to have eating disorders than males.
- Although eating disorders can occur at any age, they are much more common during the teens and early 20s.
- Eating disorders are significantly more likely to occur in families wherein parents or siblings have had an eating disorder.
- People who feel insecure about their appearance due to overly critical parents or siblings, being teased about appearance, or coming from families in which appearance is a strong focus, are at higher risk for eating disorders.
- People with depression, anxiety, and obsessive-compulsive disorder are more likely to also have an eating disorder.
- Eating disorders can start in susceptible people by repeated positive comments from others while dieting that their appearance is improved.
- People are at higher risk of developing an eating disorder if there is stress from life transitions.
- Social, play, and work influences: actors and actresses, people on television, dancers (especially ballerinas), models, and some athletes (especially gymnasts, runners, wrestlers) are at higher risk of eating disorders than the general population. Coaches and parents may contribute to the development of eating disorders by encouraging young athletes to unwisely lose weight.

Mechanism Producing the Red Flag

The mechanism for anorexic weight loss is obviously an inadequate intake of calories from macronutrients to keep up with caloric needs driven by an unrealistic "body image" that an anorexic has. There is also inadequate ingestions of micronutrients like vitamins and minerals. The low levels of certain minerals, like potassium, for example, can be exacerbated by purging – diarrhea and/or vomiting. A patient who is anorexic and bulimic is especially at risk for heart rhythm disturbances from inadequate minerals and purging, leading to fatal arrhythmias in some cases.

Review What You Have Learned
Chapter 23 Weight Fluctuations

Chapter 23—Weight Fluctuations, Weight Gain

1. Which statement(s) is(are) false about the thyroid hormones (the thyroxines)?

a. All thyroid hormones are made from the amino acid tyrosine and iodine atoms
b. T4 is more abundant that T3, but T3 is more metabolically active than T4
c. When T4 and T3 are high, TSH is usually high as well
d. Thyroid hormone set the overall metabolic rate of the body

2. What statement(s) is (are) true about hypothyroidism?

a. Overt hypothyroidism is serious, but subclinical hypothyroidism has no significant negative health consequences
b. The onset of hypothyroidism can be so slow, it can be easily missed by patients and clinicians
c. Hypothyroidism can follow hyperthyroidism
d. B and C

Chapter 23—Weight Fluctuations, Weight Loss

1. Anorexia nervosa

a. Is seven times more common in females than males
b. Has a fatality rate of 5-10% in ten years and 20% in twenty years
c. Patients who have it often don't bring up the problem unless encouraged to do so
d. All of the above

Appendix A: SAMPLE REFERRAL FORM, SAMPLE REFERRAL LETTER

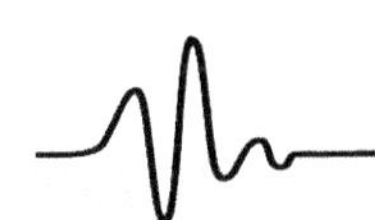

John Needles, L.Ac
Any Street
Any City, State ZIP
Phone 000-111-2222, Fax 000-111-2223

Consultation request for: ____________________________ DOB ________________
Pt. phone # ________________________
Today's date ___________________________

Dear ____

I hope this consultation request finds you in good health and spirits.

I'm sending my patient, ___________________________, to you in consultation for

symptoms/signs of ____.

I'm specifically concerned about the possibility of ______________________________.

I am sending this patient specifically to you for purposes of:

1. __ Evaluation and suggestions for treatment options that I'll discuss with patient
2. __ Evaluation and co-treatment of referred problem with me
3. __ Evaluation and your treatment of this problem until it is resolved

Thank you in advance for your consultation and consultation report.

Sincerely,

John Needles, L.Ac

(SAMPLE FORMAT OF LETTER TO CONSULTANT)

Your letterhead including contact information

Name of consultant
Address
Date:
RE: Patient's name and phone number

Dear (   )

I hope this consultation request letter finds you in good health. I'm sending my patient (   ) to see you because of complaints and finding of (   ). I recognize these symptoms and signs as red flags for possible (   ) and am sending this patient to determine whether or not (   ) is present.

Other *relevant or significant* PMH for this patient include (insert here)

I am sending this patient specifically for:

() Your evaluation and suggestions for treatment of this problem, which I will discuss with the patient to help with their decision making process

() Your evaluation and co-treatment with me for the referred condition

() Your evaluation and treatment for the referred condition

I await your thoughtful opinion regarding (   ) and thank you ahead of time for your correspondence, e-mail, or phone call regarding this patient.

Respectfully yours,

Mini-Mental State Examination (MMSE)

Patient's Name: ______________________________ Date: ____________

Instructions: ***Ask the questions in the order listed. Score one point for each correct response within each question or activity.***

Maximum Score	Patient's Score	Questions
5		"What is the year? Season? Date? Day of the week? Month?"
5		"Where are we now: State? County? Town/city? Hospital? Floor?"
3		The examiner names three unrelated objects clearly and slowly, then asks the patient to name all three of them. The patient's response is used for scoring. The examiner repeats them until patient learns all of them, if possible. Number of trials: ___________
5		"I would like you to count backward from 100 by sevens." (93, 86, 79, 72, 65, …) Stop after five answers. Alternative: "Spell WORLD backwards." (D-L-R-O-W)
3		"Earlier I told you the names of three things. Can you tell me what those were?"
2		Show the patient two simple objects, such as a wristwatch and a pencil, and ask the patient to name them.
1		"Repeat the phrase: 'No ifs, ands, or buts.'"
3		"Take the paper in your right hand, fold it in half, and put it on the floor." (The examiner gives the patient a piece of blank paper.)
1		"Please read this and do what it says." (Written instruction is "Close your eyes.")
1		"Make up and write a sentence about anything." (This sentence must contain a noun and a verb.)
1		"Please copy this picture." (The examiner gives the patient a blank piece of paper and asks him/her to draw the symbol below. All 10 angles must be present and two must intersect.)
30		TOTAL

(Adapted from Rovner & Folstein, 1987)

Source: www.medicine.uiowa.edu/igec/tools/cognitive/MMSE.pdf

Provided by NHCQF, 0106-410

Instructions for administration and scoring of the MMSE

Orientation (10 points):

- Ask for the date. Then specifically ask for parts omitted (e.g., "Can you also tell me what season it is?"). One point for each correct answer.
- Ask in turn, "Can you tell me the name of this hospital (town, county, etc.)?" One point for each correct answer.

Registration (3 points):

- Say the names of three unrelated objects clearly and slowly, allowing approximately one second for each. After you have said all three, ask the patient to repeat them. The number of objects the patient names correctly upon the first repetition determines the score (0-3). If the patient does not repeat all three objects the first time, continue saying the names until the patient is able to repeat all three items, up to six trials. Record the number of trials it takes for the patient to learn the words. If the patient does not eventually learn all three, recall cannot be meaningfully tested.
- After completing this task, tell the patient, "Try to remember the words, as I will ask for them in a little while."

Attention and Calculation (5 points):

- Ask the patient to begin with 100 and count backward by sevens. Stop after five subtractions (93, 86, 79, 72, 65). Score the total number of correct answers.
- If the patient cannot or will not perform the subtraction task, ask the patient to spell the word "world" backwards. The score is the number of letters in correct order (e.g., dlrow=5, dlorw=3).

Recall (3 points):

- Ask the patient if he or she can recall the three words you previously asked him or her to remember. Score the total number of correct answers (0-3).

Language and Praxis (9 points):

- Naming: Show the patient a wrist watch and ask the patient what it is. Repeat with a pencil. Score one point for each correct naming (0-2).
- Repetition: Ask the patient to repeat the sentence after you ("No ifs, ands, or buts."). Allow only one trial. Score 0 or 1.
- 3-Stage Command: Give the patient a piece of blank paper and say, "Take this paper in your right hand, fold it in half, and put it on the floor." Score one point for each part of the command correctly executed.
- Reading: On a blank piece of paper print the sentence, "Close your eyes," in letters large enough for the patient to see clearly. Ask the patient to read the sentence and do what it says. Score one point only if the patient actually closes his or her eyes. This is not a test of memory, so you may prompt the patient to "do what it says" after the patient reads the sentence.
- Writing: Give the patient a blank piece of paper and ask him or her to write a sentence for you. Do not dictate a sentence; it should be written spontaneously. The sentence must contain a subject and a verb and make sense. Correct grammar and punctuation are not necessary.
- Copying: Show the patient the picture of two intersecting pentagons and ask the patient to copy the figure exactly as it is. All ten angles must be present and two must intersect to score one point. Ignore tremor and rotation.

(Folstein, Folstein & McHugh, 1975)

Source: www.medicine.uiowa.edu/igec/tools/cognitive/MMSE.pdf

Interpretation of the MMSE

Method	Score	Interpretation
Single Cutoff	<24	Abnormal
Range	<21	Increased odds of dementia
	>25	Decreased odds of dementia
Education	21	Abnormal for 8th grade education
	<23	Abnormal for high school education
	<24	Abnormal for college education
Severity	24-30	No cognitive impairment
	18-23	Mild cognitive impairment
	0-17	Severe cognitive impairment

Sources:

- Crum RM, Anthony JC, Bassett SS, Folstein MF. Population-based norms for the mini-mental state examination by age and educational level. *JAMA*. 1993;269(18):2386-2391.
- Folstein MF, Folstein SE, McHugh PR. "Mini-mental state": a practical method for grading the cognitive state of patients for the clinician. *J Psychiatr Res*. 1975;12:189-198.
- Rovner BW, Folstein MF. Mini-mental state exam in clinical practice. *Hosp Pract*. 1987;22(1A):99, 103, 106, 110.
- Tombaugh TN, McIntyre NJ. The mini-mental state examination: a comprehensive review. *J Am Geriatr Soc*. 1992;40(9):922-935.

Adult ADHD Interview Form

DSM-IV-TR Criteria

The symptom must be frequent, impairing, and present across multiple settings. Mark S for self report, C for collateral report or information. Mark separately whether it was present in childhood and as an adult.

Inattention symptoms (need 6)

Child   Adult

___   ___ Poor attention to details

___   ___ Difficulty sustaining attention

___   ___ Does not seem to listen when spoken to directly

___   ___ Does not follow through on instructions and fails to finish tasks

___   ___ Disorganized

___   ___ Avoids tasks that require sustained mental effort

___   ___ Loses things

___   ___ Easily distracted

___   ___ Forgetful

Hyperactive/impulsive symptoms (need 6)

___   ___ Fidgety

___   ___ Difficulty remaining seated

___   ___ Feels restless

___   ___ Difficulty engaging in leisure activities quietly

___   ___ Is often "on the go"

___   ___ Talks excessively

___   ___ Blurts out answers

___   ___ Difficulty waiting turn

___   ___ Interrupts or intrudes on others

Tone of the Interview

___ Long-standing pain and frustration
___ Sense of lost opportunities or regret
___ Under-achievement or failure to work to potential
___ Interrupts you and himself
___ Wanders off topic
___ Forgets the question or answers a different question
___ Physically restless
___ Distracted by items in the office or extraneous noises

Collateral Information Sources

___ Previously diagnosed with ADHD
___ Family member or significant other, if present, mostly confirms self-report
___ Report cards or teacher comments are consistent with ADHD
___ Results of assessment instruments are consistent with ADHD
___ Family history of ADHD, especially in parents, siblings, or children

Comorbid Conditions

___ Depression
___ Bipolar disorder
___ Anxiety
___ Post-traumatic stress disorder
___ Learning disabilities
___ Antisocial personality disorder
___ Substance abuse or other addictions
___ Borderline personality disorder
___ Sleep deprivation
___ Head injury and medical conditions

Reprinted with permission from *Integrative Treatment for Adult ADHD: A Practical, Easy-to-Use Guide for Clinicians*. Ari Tuckman (2007). New Harbinger Publications. This handout and others are available free of charge at www.TuckmanPsych.com.

APPENDIX D

SAMPLE NO SELF-HARM CONTRACT

DATE:

I, ______________________ do hereby promise of my own free will that I will not seek to harm myself by any direct act of commission or any indirect act of omission while I am waiting to receive social and/or psychological support services for my depression.

Patient's name ________________________

Clinician's name __________________________

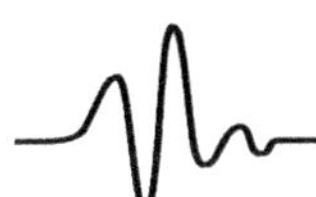

Chapter 3
1. C
2. B
3. D
4. D
5. D
6. D
7. D
8. E
9. E
10. A
11. D
12. B
13. C
14. D
15. B
Chapter 4
1. A
2. A
3. D
Chapter 5
1. B
2. A
3. B
4. A
5. C
6. C
7. D
8. B
Chapter 6
1. B
Chapter 7
1. B
2. D
3. E
4. B
Chapter 8
1. E
2. B
3. A
4. D
5. A
Chapter 9
1. D
2. E
Chapter 10
1. C
2. C
3. B
4. D
Chapter 11
1. C
2. B
Chapter 12
1. C
Chapter 13
1. D
Chapter 14
1. D
Chapter 15
1. E
2. E
Chapter 16, PAIN,General
1. D
2. E
3. B
4. D
5. E
6. D
Chapter 16, Abdominal
1. B
2. D
3. B
4. B
5. C
6. C
Chapter 16, Back
1. C
2. D
3. B
4. A
5. B
6. D
7. C
8. D
9. B
10. Λ
11. C
Chapter 16, Chest
1. D
2. D
3. B
4. B
5. B
6. A
7. E
Chapter 16, Ear
1. C
Chapter 16, Elbow
1. D
2. B
3. A
Chapter 16, Facial
1. D
Chapter 16, Foot & Toe
1. C
Chapter 16, Headache
1. D
2. E
Chapter 16, Hip
1. C
2. A
Chapter 16, Knee
1. C
Chapter 16, Calf
1. E
Chapter 16, Shin
1. D
Chapter 16, Neck
1. A
2. A
Chapter 16, Shoulder
1. E
Chapter 16, Throat
1. B
Chapter 16, Urination
1. D
Chapter 16, Wrist
1. E
2. D
Chapter 17, Anxiety
1. A
Chapter 17, Delusions
1. B
2. D
Chapter 17, Depression
1. D
Chapter 17, Mood Swings
1. B
Chapter 17, Drug Abuse
1. D
2. D
Chapter 18
1. D
2. B
3. C
4. E
5. B
6. C
Chapter 19
1. D
2. A
Chapter 20
1. A
2. D
3. A
4. E
Chapter 21, swelling, one ankle
1. D
Chapter 21, swelling both ankles
1. D
2. E
Chapter 21, arm swelling
1. D
Chapter 21, Facial swelling
1. B
Chapter 22, Loss of Vision
1. C
Chapter 22, Curtain over Vision
1. C
Chapter 22, Double Vision
1. A
Chapter 22, Blurry Vision
1. B
Chapter 23, Weight Gain
1. C
2. D
Chapter 23 Weight Fluctuations, Weight Loss
1. D

General Index

V

W

OTHER BOOKS ON CHINESE MEDICINE AVAILABLE FROM:

BLUE POPPY ENTERPRISES, INC.

Colorado: 1990 North 57th Court, Unit A, Boulder, CO 80301
For ordering 1-800-487-9296 PH. 303-447-8372 FAX 303-245-8362
California: 1725 Monrovia Ave. Unit A4, Costa Mesa, CA 92627
For ordering 1-800-293-6697 PH. 949-270-6511 FAX 949-335-7110
Email: info@bluepoppy.com Website: www.bluepoppy.com

ACUPOINT POCKET REFERENCE
by Bob Flaws
ISBN 0-936185-93-7
ISBN 978-0-936185-93-4

ACUPUNCTURE, CHINESE MEDICINE & HEALTHY WEIGHT LOSS Revised Edition
by Juliette Aiyana, L. Ac.
ISBN 1-891845-61-6
ISBN 978-1-891845-61-1

ACUPUNCTURE & IVF
by Lifang Liang
ISBN 0-891845-24-1
ISBN 978-0-891845-24-6

ACUPUNCTURE FOR STROKE REHABILITATION
Three Decades of Information from China
by Hoy Ping Yee Chan, et al.
ISBN 1-891845-35-7
ISBN 978-1-891845-35-2

ACUPUNCTURE PHYSICAL MEDICINE: An Acupuncture Touchpoint Approach to the Treatment of Chronic Pain, Fatigue, and Stress Disorders
by Mark Seem
ISBN 1-891845-13-6
ISBN 978-1-891845-13-0

AGING & BLOOD STASIS: A New Approach to TCM Geriatrics
by Yan De-xin
ISBN 0-936185-63-6
ISBN 978-0-936185-63-7

AN ACUPUNCTURISTS GUIDE TO MEDICAL RED FLAGS & REFERRALS
by Dr. David Anzaldua, MD
ISBN 1-891845-54-3
ISBN 978-1-891845-54-3

BETTER BREAST HEALTH NATURALLY with CHINESE MEDICINE
by Honora Lee Wolfe & Bob Flaws
ISBN 0-936185-90-2
ISBN 978-0-936185-90-3

BIOMEDICINE: A TEXTBOOK FOR PRACTITIONERS OF ACUPUNCTURE AND ORIENTAL MEDICINE
by Bruce H. Robinson, MD Second Edition
ISBN 1-891845-62-4
ISBN 978-1-891845-62-8

THE BOOK OF JOOK: Chinese Medicinal Porridges
by Bob Flaws
ISBN 0-936185-60-6
ISBN 978-0-936185-60-0

CHANNEL DIVERGENCES Deeper Pathways of the Web
by Miki Shima and Charles Chase
ISBN 1-891845-15-2
ISBN 978-1-891845-15-4

CHINESE MEDICAL OBSTETRICS
by Bob Flaws
ISBN 1-891845-30-6
ISBN 978-1-891845-30-7

CHINESE MEDICAL PALM IS TRY: Your Health in Your Hand
by Zong Xiao-fan & Gary Liscum
ISBN 0-936185-64-3
ISBN 978-0-936185-64-4

CHINESE MEDICAL PSYCHIATRY: A Textbook and Clinical Manual
by Bob Flaws and James Lake, MD
ISBN 1-845891-17-9
ISBN 978-1-845891-17-8

CHINESE MEDICINAL TEAS: Simple, Proven, Folk Formulas for Common Diseases & Promoting Health
by Zong Xiao-fan & Gary Lis cum
ISBN 0-936185-76-7
ISBN 978-0-936185-76-7

CHINESE MEDICINAL WINES & ELIXIRS
by Bob Flaws Revised Edition
ISBN 0-936185-58-9
ISBN 978-0-936185-58-3

CHINESE PEDIATRIC MASSAGE THERAPY: A Parent's & Practitioner's Guide to the Prevention & Treatment of Childhood Illness
by Fan Ya-li
ISBN 0-936185-54-6
ISBN 978-0-936185-54-5

CHINESE SCALP ACUPUNCTURE
by Jason Jishun Hao & Linda Lingzhi Hao
ISBN 1-891845-60-8
ISBN 978-1-891845-60-4

CHINESE SELF-MASSAGE THERAPY: The Easy Way to Health
by Fan Ya-li
ISBN 0-936185-74-0
ISBN 978-0-936185-74-3

THE CLASSIC OF DIFFICULTIES: A Translation of the Nan Jing
translation by Bob Flaws
ISBN 1-891845-07-1
ISBN 978-1-891845-07-9

A CLINICIAN'S GUIDE TO USING GRANULE EXTRACTS
by Eric Brand
ISBN 1-891845-51-9
ISBN 978-1-891845-51-2

A COMPENDIUM OF CHINESE MEDICAL MENSTRUAL DISEASES
by Bob Flaws
ISBN 1-891845-31-4
ISBN 978-1-891845-31-4

CONCISE CHINESE MATERIA MEDICA
by Eric Brand and Nigel Wiseman
ISBN 0-912111-82-8
ISBN 978-0-912111-82-7

CONTEMPORARY GYNECOLOGY: An Integrated Chinese-Western Approach
by Lifang Liang
ISBN 1-891845-50-0
ISBN 978-1-891845-50-5

CONTROLLING DIABETES NATURALLY WITH CHINESE MEDICINE
by Lynn Kuchinski
ISBN 0-936185-06-3
ISBN 978-0-936185-06-2

CURING ARTHRITIS NATURALLY WITH CHINESE MEDICINE
by Douglas Frank & Bob Flaws
ISBN 0-936185-87-2
ISBN 978-0-936185-87-3

CURING DEPRESSION NATURALLY WITH CHINESE MEDICINE
by Rosa Schnyer & Bob Flaws
ISBN 0-936185-94-5
ISBN 978-0-936185-94-1

CURING FIBROMYALGIA NATURALLY WITH CHINESE MEDICINE
by Bob Flaws
ISBN 1-891845-09-8
ISBN 978-1-891845-09-3

CURING HAY FEVER NATURALLY WITH CHINESE MEDICINE
by Bob Flaws
ISBN 0-936185-91-0
ISBN 978-0-936185-91-0

CURING HEADACHES NATURALLY WITH CHINESE MEDICINE
by Bob Flaws
ISBN 0-936185-95-3
ISBN 978-0-936185-95-8

CURING IBS NATURALLY WITH CHINESE MEDICINE
by Jane Bean Oberski
ISBN 1-891845-11-X
ISBN 978-1-891845-11-6

CURING INSOMNIA NATURALLY WITH CHINESE MEDICINE
by Bob Flaws
ISBN 0-936185-86-4
ISBN 978-0-936185-86-6

CURING PMS NATURALLY WITH CHINESE MEDICINE
by Bob Flaws
ISBN 0-936185-85-6
ISBN 978-0-936185-85-9

DISEASES OF THE KIDNEY & BLADDER
by Hoy Ping Yee Chan, et al.
ISBN 1-891845-37-3
ISBN 978-1-891845-35-6

THE DIVINE FARMER'S MATERIA MEDICA: A Translation of the Shen Nong Ben Cao
translation by Yang Shouz-zhong
ISBN 0-936185-96-1
ISBN 978-0-936185-96-5

DUI YAO: THE ART OF COMBINING CHINESE HERBAL MEDICINALS
by Philippe Sionneau
ISBN 0-936185-81-3
ISBN 978-0-936185-81-1

ENDOMETRIOSIS, INFERTILITY AND TRADITIONAL CHINESE MEDICINE: A Layperson's Guide
by Bob Flaws
ISBN 0-936185-14-7
ISBN 978-0-936185-14-9

THE ESSENCE OF LIU FENG-WU'S GYNECOLOGY
by Liu Feng-wu, translated by Yang Shou-zhong
ISBN 0-936185-88-0
ISBN 978-0-936185-88-0

EXTRA TREATISES BASED ON INVESTIGATION & INQUIRY: A Translation of Zhu Dan-xi's Ge Zhi Yu Lun
translation by Yang Shou-zhong
ISBN 0-936185-53-8
ISBN 978-0-936185-53-8

FIRE IN THE VALLEY: TCM Diagnosis & Treatment of Vaginal Diseases
by Bob Flaws
ISBN 0-936185-25-2
ISBN 978-0-936185-25-5

FULFILLING THE ESSENCE:
A Handbook of Traditional & Contemporary Treatments for Female Infertility
by Bob Flaws
ISBN 0-936185-48-1
ISBN 978-0-936185-48-4

FU QING-ZHU'S GYNECOLOGY
trans. by Yang Shou-zhong and Liu Da-wei
ISBN 0-936185-35-X
ISBN 978-0-936185-35-4

GOLDEN NEEDLE WANG LE-TING: A 20th Century Master's Approach to Acupuncture
by Yu Hui-chan and Han Fu-ru, trans. by Shuai Xue-zhong
ISBN 0-936185-78-3
ISBN 978-0-936185-78-1

A HANDBOOK OF CHINESE HEMATOLOGY
by Simon Becker
ISBN 1-891845-16-0
ISBN 978-1-891845-16-1

A HANDBOOK OF TCM PATTERNS & THEIR TREATMENTS
Second Edition
by Bob Flaws & Daniel Finney
ISBN 0-936185-70-8
ISBN 978-0-936185-70-5

A HANDBOOK OF TRADITIONAL CHINESE DERMATOLOGY
by Liang Jian-hui, trans. by Zhang Ting-liang & Bob Flaws
ISBN 0-936185-46-5
ISBN 978-0-936185-46-0

A HANDBOOK OF TRADITIONAL CHINESE GYNECOLOGY
by Zhejiang College of TCM, trans. by Zhang Ting-liang & Bob Flaws
ISBN 0-936185-06-6 (4th edit.)
ISBN 978-0-936185-06-4

A HANDBOOK of TCM PEDIATRICS
by Bob Flaws
ISBN 0-936185-72-4
ISBN 978-0-936185-72-9

THE HEART & ESSENCE OF DAN-XI'S METHODS OF TREATMENT
by Xu Dan-xi, trans. by Yang Shou-zhong
ISBN 0-926185-50-3
ISBN 978-0-936185-50-7

HERB TOXICITIES & DRUG INTERACTIONS: A Formula Approach
by Fred Jennes with Bob Flaws
ISBN 1-891845-26-8
ISBN 978-1-891845-26-0

IMPERIAL SECRETS OF HEALTH & LONGEVITY
by Bob Flaws
ISBN 0-936185-51-1
ISBN 978-0-936185-51-4

INSIGHTS OF A SENIOR ACUPUNCTURIST
by Miriam Lee
ISBN 0-936185-33-3
ISBN 978-0-936185-33-0

INTEGRATED PHARMACOLOGY: Combining Modern Pharmacology with Chinese Medicine
by Dr. Greg Sperber with Bob Flaws
ISBN 1-891845-41-1
ISBN 978-0-936185-41-3

INTRODUCTION TO THE USE OF PROCESSED CHINESE MEDICINALS
by Philippe Sionneau
ISBN 0-936185-62-7
ISBN 978-0-936185-62-0

KEEPING YOUR CHILD HEALTHY WITH CHINESE MEDICINE
by Bob Flaws
ISBN 0-936185-71-6
ISBN 978-0-936185-71-2

THE LAKESIDE MASTER'S STUDY OF THE PULSE
by Li Shi-zhen, trans. by Bob Flaws
ISBN 1-891845-01-2
ISBN 978-1-891845-01-7

MANAGING MENOPAUSE NATURALLY WITH CHINESE MEDICINE
by Honora Lee Wolfe
ISBN 0-936185-98-8
ISBN 978-0-936185-98-9

MASTER HUA'S CLASSIC OF THE CENTRAL VISCERA
by Hua Tuo, trans. by Yang Shou-zhong
ISBN 0-936185-43-0
ISBN 978-0-936185-43-9

THE MEDICAL I CHING: Oracle of the Healer Within
by Miki Shima
ISBN 0-936185-38-4
ISBN 978-0-936185-38-5

MENOPAIUSE & CHINESE MEDICINE
by Bob Flaws
ISBN 1-891845-40-3
ISBN 978-1-891845-40-6

MOXIBUSTION: A MODERN CLINICAL HANDBOOK
by Lorraine Wilcox
ISBN 1-891845-49-7
ISBN 978-1-891845-49-9

MOXIBUSTION: THE POWER OF MUGWORT FIRE
by Lorraine Wilcox
ISBN 1-891845-46-2
ISBN 978-1-891845-46-8

A NEW AMERICAN ACUPUNTURE By Mark Seem
ISBN 0-936185-44-9
ISBN 978-0-936185-44-6

PLAYING THE GAME: A Step-by-Step Approach to Accepting Insurance as an Acupuncturist
by Greg Sperber & Tiffany Anderson-Hefner
ISBN 3-131416-11-7
ISBN 978-3-131416-11-7

POCKET ATLAS OF CHINESE MEDICINE
Edited by Marne and Kevin Ergil
ISBN 1-891-845-59-4
ISBN 978-1-891845-59-8

POINTS FOR PROFIT: The Essential Guide to Practice Success for Acupuncturists 5th Fully Edited Edition
by Honora Wolfe with Marilyn Allen
ISBN 1-891845-25-X
ISBN 978-1-891845-25-3

PRINCIPLES OF CHINESE MEDICAL ANDROLOGY: An Integrated Approach to Male Reproductive and Urological Health by Bob Damone
ISBN 1-891845-45-4
ISBN 978-1-891845-45-1

PRINCE WEN HUI's COOK: Chinese Dietary Therapy
By Bob Flaws & Honora Wolfe
ISBN 0-912111-05-4
ISBN 978-0-912111-05-6

THE PULSE CLASSIC: A Translation of the Mai Jing
by Wang Shu-he, trans. by Yang Shou-zhong
ISBN 0-936185-75-9
ISBN 978-0-936185-75-0

THE SECRET OF CHINESE PULSE DIAGNOSIS
by Bob Flaws
ISBN 0-936185-67-8
ISBN 978-0-936185-67-5

SECRET SHAOLIN FORMULAS FOR THE TREATMENT OF EXTERNAL INJURY
by De Chan, trans. by Zhang Ting-liang & Bob Flaws
ISBN 0-936185-08-2
ISBN 978-0-936185-08-8

STATEMENTS OF FACT IN TRADITIONAL CHINESE MEDICINE
by Bob Flaws Revised & Expanded
ISBN 0-936185-52-X
ISBN 978-0-936185-52-1

STICKING TO THE POINT: A Step-by-Step Approach to TCM Acupuncture Therapy
by Bob Flaws & Honora Wolfe 2 Condensed Books
ISBN 1-891845-47-0
ISBN 978-1-891845-47-5

A STUDY OF DAOIST ACUPUNCTURE
by Liu Zheng-cai
ISBN 1-891845-08-X
ISBN 978-1-891845-08-6

THE SUCCESSFUL CHINESE HERBALIST
by Bob Flaws and Honora Lee Wolfe
ISBN 1-891845-29-2
ISBN 978-1-891845-29-1

THE SYSTEMATIC CLASSIC OF ACUPUNCTURE & MOXIBUSTION: A translation of the Jia Yi Jing
by Huang-fu Mi, trans. by Yang Shou-zhong & Charles Chace
ISBN 0-936185-29-5
ISBN 978-0-936185-29-3

THE TAO OF HEALTHY EATING: DIETARY WISDOM ACCORDING TO CHINESE MEDICINE
by Bob Flaws Second Edition
ISBN 0-936185-92-9
ISBN 978-0-936185-92-7

TEACH YOURSELF TO READ MODERN MEDICAL CHINESE
by Bob Flaws
ISBN 0-936185-99-6
ISBN 978-0-936185-99-6

TEST PREP WORKBOOK FOR BASIC TCM THEORY
by Zhong Bai-song
ISBN 1-891845-43-8
ISBN 978-1-891845-43-7

TEST PREP WORKBOOK FOR THE NCCAOM BIOMEDICINE MODULE: Exam Preparation & Study Guide
by Zhong Bai-song
ISBN 1-891845-34-9
ISBN 978-1-891845-34-5

TREATING PEDIATRIC BED-WETTING WITH ACUPUNCTURE & CHINESE MEDICINE
by Robert Helmer
ISBN 1-891845-33-0
ISBN 978-1-891845-33-8

TREATISE on the SPLEEN & STOMACH: A Translation and annotation of Li Dong-yuan's Pi Wei Lun
by Bob Flaws
ISBN 0-936185-41-4
ISBN 978-0-936185-41-5

THE TREATMENT OF CARDIOVASCULAR DISEASES WITH CHINESE MEDICINE
by Simon Becker, Bob Flaws & Robert Casañas, MD
ISBN 1-891845-27-6
ISBN 978-1-891845-27-7

THE TREATMENT OF DIABETES MELLITUS WITH CHINESE MEDICINE
by Bob Flaws, Lynn Kuchinski & Robert Casañas, M.D.
ISBN 1-891845-21-7
ISBN 978-1-891845-21-5

THE TREATMENT OF DISEASE IN TCM, Vol. 1: Diseases of the Head & Face, Including Mental & Emotional Disorders New Edition
by Philippe Sion neau & Lü Gang
ISBN 0-936185-69-4
ISBN 978-0-936185-69-9

THE TREATMENT OF DISEASE IN TCM, Vol. II: Diseases of the Eyes, Ears, Nose, & Throat
by Sionneau & Lü
ISBN 0-936185-73-2
ISBN 978-0-936185-73-6

THE TREATMENT OF DISEASE IN TCM, Vol. III: Diseases of the Mouth, Lips, Tongue, Teeth & Gums
by Sionneau & Lü
ISBN 0-936185-79-1
ISBN 978-0-936185-79-8

THE TREATMENT OF DISEASE IN TCM, Vol IV: Diseases of the Neck, Shoulders, Back, & Limbs
by Phi lippe Sion neau & Lü Gang
ISBN 0-936185-89-9
ISBN 978-0-936185-89-7

THE TREATMENT OF DISEASE IN TCM, Vol V: Diseases of the Chest & Abdomen
by Philippe Sionneau & Lü Gang
ISBN 1-891845-02-0
ISBN 978-1-891845-02-4

THE TREATMENT OF DISEASE IN TCM, Vol VI: Diseases of the Urogential System & Proctology
by Phi lippe Sion neau & Lü Gang
ISBN 1-891845-05-5
ISBN 978-1-891845-05-5

THE TREATMENT OF DISEASE IN TCM, Vol VII: General Symptoms
by Phi lippe Sion neau & Lü Gang
ISBN 1-891845-14-4
ISBN 978-1-891845-14-7

THE TREATMENT OF EXTER NAL DIS EASES WITH ACUPUNCTURE & MOXIBUSTION
by Yan Cui-lan and Zhu Yun-long, trans. by Yang Shou-zhong
ISBN 0-936185-80-5
ISBN 978-0-936185-80-4

THE TREATMENT OF MODERN WESTERN MEDICAL DISEASES WITH CHINESE MEDICINE
by Bob Flaws & Philippe Sionneau
ISBN 1-891845-20-9
ISBN 978-1-891845-20-8

UNDERSTANDING THE DIFFICULT PATIENT: A Guide for Practitioners of Oriental Medicine
by Nancy Bilello, RN, L.ac.
ISBN 1-891845-32-2
ISBN 978-1-891845-32-1

WESTERN PHYSICAL EXAM SKILLS FOR PRACTITIONERS OF ASIAN MEDICINE
by Bruce H. Robinson & Honora Lee Wolfe
ISBN 1-891845-48-9
ISBN 978-1-891845-48-2

YI LIN GAI CUO (Correcting the Errors in the Forest of Medicine)
by Wang Qing-ren
ISBN 1-891845-39-X
ISBN 978-1-891845-39-0

70 ESSENTIAL CHINESE HERBAL FORMULAS
by Bob Flaws
ISBN 0-936185-59-7
ISBN 978-0-936185-59-0

160 ESSENTIAL CHINESE READY-MADE MEDICINES
by Bob Flaws
ISBN 1-891945-12-8
ISBN 978-1-891945-12-3

630 QUESTIONS & ANSWERS ABOUT CHINESE HERBAL MEDICINE:
A Work book & Study Guide
by Bob Flaws
ISBN 1-891845-04-7
ISBN 978-1-891845-04-8

260 ESSENTIAL CHINESE MEDICINALS
by Bob Flaws
ISBN 1-891845-03-9
ISBN 978-1-891845-03-1

750 QUESTIONS & ANSWERS ABOUT ACUPUNCTURE
Exam Preparation & Study Guide
by Fred Jennes
ISBN 1-891845-22-5
ISBN 978-1-891845-22-2